Total Knee Arthroplasy

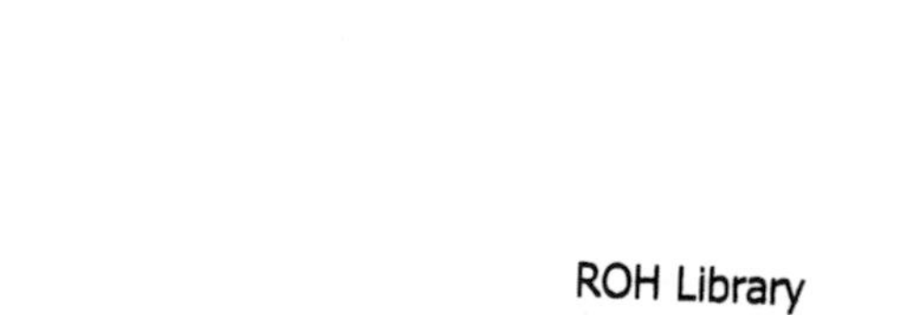

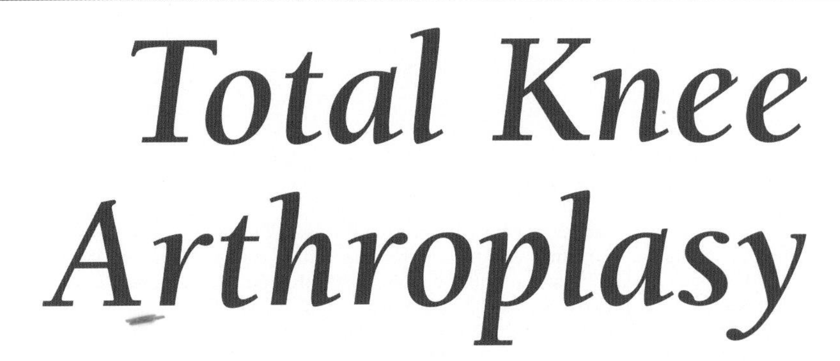

Total Knee Arthroplasy

Richard D. Scott, MD

Professor of Orthopaedic Surgery
Harvard Medical School
Boston, Massachusetts

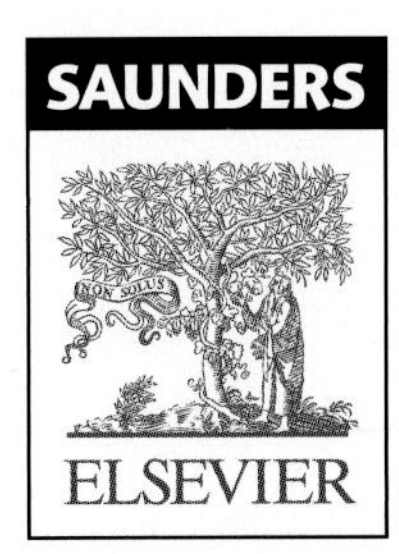

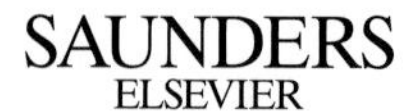

An Imprint of Elsevier

1600 John F. Kennedy Boulevard
Suite 1800
Philadelphia, Pennsylvania 19103

ISBN-13: 978-0-7216-3948-2
ISBN-10: 0-7216-3948-8

TOTAL KNEE ARTHROPLASTY

NOTICE

Neither the Publisher nor the Author assumes any responsibility for any loss or injury and/or damage to persons or property arising out of or related to any use of the material contained in this book. It is the responsibility of the treating practitioner, relying on independent expertise and knowledge of the patient, to determine the best treatment and method of application for the patient.

Library of Congress Cataloging-in-Publication Data
Total knee arthroplasty/Richard D. Scott.—1st ed.
p. cm.
ISBN 0-7216-3948-8
1. Total knee replacement. I. Scott, Richard D. (Richard David), 1943–

RD561.T6672 2005
617.5′820592–dc22

20050428

Publishing Director: Kim Murphy
Design Direction: Steven Stave
Publishing Services Manager: Joan Sinclair
Project Manager: Mary Stermel

Printed in China.

Last digit is the print number: 9 8 7 6 5 4 3 2 1

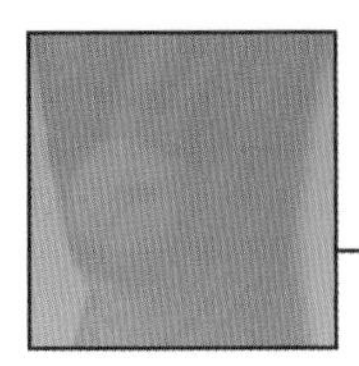

Preface

I began my orthopedic residency in Boston in 1971. The state of the art of knee arthroplasty consisted of McKeever metallic hemiarthroplasty and uniaxial metal hinge arthroplasty with the Walldius or Guepar prosthesis.

I was on the scene, therefore, in 1972, when the first metal-to-plastic knee replacements were performed. Over the next three decades, I witnessed and participated in the evolution of modern total knee arthroplasty and have personally performed between 3,000 and 4,000 primary replacements.

This book is a summary of these three decades of experience. I have made many mistakes and learned many lessons through the years. The concepts and techniques I describe in this book are certainly not the only way to approach various problems in knee arthroplasty (and may, in fact, not be the best way) but they have worked well for me.

I have had the privilege of training more than 500 orthopedic residents and joint arthroplasty fellows at the Brigham and Womens and New England Baptist Hospitals. I am indebted to them for what they have taught me in return. It is they who have stimulated me to undertake this project.

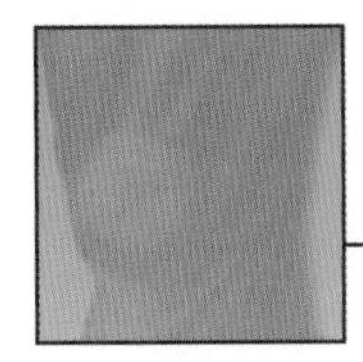

Dedication

To my inspiration at home: my wife, Mary, and sons, Jordan and Andrew.

To my inspiration at work: my own mentors and the hundreds of residents and fellows who allowed me to mentor them.

To my colleague and friend, Tom Thornhill, who traveled much of this road with me.

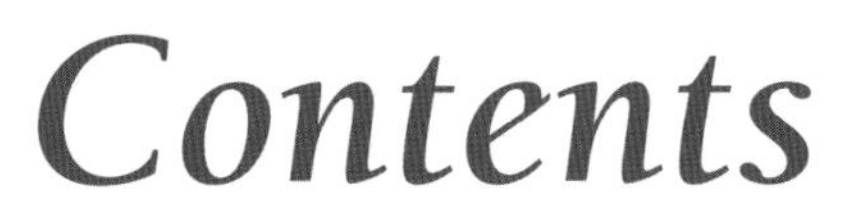
Contents

CHAPTER 1

A Brief History of Three Decades of Evolution of Total Knee Arthroplasty in Boston

BICOMPARTMENTAL ARTHROPLASTY

In the 1960s, the process of knee arthroplasty began its evolution in Boston with the MGH mold femoral hemiarthroplasty, pioneered at the Massachusetts General Hospital, and the McKeever metallic tibial hemiarthroplasty, pioneered at the Robert Breck Brigham Hospital (now Brigham and Women's Hospital).

In the late 1960s, patients with severe deformity not amenable to the McKeever technique began to receive metal hinged total knee arthroplasty (TKA) in the form of the Walldius or the Guepar prosthesis (Fig. 1–1). Early results were promising, but failures soon appeared as a result of component loosening, metastatic infection, metal synovitis, and degeneration of the unresurfaced patella on the flat metallic trochlear flange. McKeever prostheses continued to be implanted in less involved knees, but follow-up showed only 60% good midterm results in the rheumatoid patient.[1]

In 1972, based on the early success of metal-to-plastic hip arthroplasty, metal-to-plastic knee replacement began in Boston with the use of the Marmor prosthesis. Although this design is still a successful unicompartmental prosthesis, 10% of rheumatoid patients who received the early bicompartmental Marmor prostheses suffered from mediolateral subluxation of the tibiofemoral articulation (Fig. 1–2).

In 1973, the duocondylar prosthesis supplanted the Marmor for bicompartmental disease (Fig. 1–3). This design, however, had no provision for resurfacing either side of the patellofemoral compartment, and 2- to 4-year follow-up showed residual patellofemoral symptoms in 20% of both rheumatoid and osteoarthritic patients.[2]

In 1974, Drs. Peter Walker and Chit Ranawat journeyed from New York City to Boston to introduce the total condylar and duopatellar prostheses designed in conjunction with their colleague, Dr. J. Insall (Fig. 1–4). The total condylar called for sacrifice of both cruciate ligaments, whereas the duopatellar allowed their preservation. The total condylar had the advantage of higher conformity and contact area, but motion often was limited to 90 degrees. The less conforming posterior cruciate-retaining duopatellar allowed more rollback and motion, making it appealing for use in the rheumatoid patient with poor upper extremities (Fig. 1–5). Both designs had a trochlear flange and optional patellar polyethylene button for the patellar side of the patellofemoral joint. The cruciate-preserving technique was adopted in Boston mainly because of the needs of the rheumatoid patient. The trochlear flange was modified at the request of the Brigham surgeons into asymmetric right and left designs to diminish medial overhang in the rheumatoid knee of the small woman. The initial duocondylar design and the first duopatellar design had individual tibial components, separated by the patient's tibial spine (Fig.1–6). This allowed preservation of both cruciates, and the retained tibial spine isolated the two compartments from varus/valgus compression/distraction forces that could promote tibial component loosening of a one-piece design. Their relatively small surface contact with the tibial plateau, however, led to high focal forces in heavy patients with possible component subsidence, especially when limb alignment was abnormal (Fig.1–7).

By 1978, after some tibial component loosening was observed with the two-piece duopatellar design,[3] an all-plastic, one-piece tibial component was adopted similar in concept to the original total condylar plateau and stem (Fig. 1–8).

By 1979, metal backing was shown to be advantageous to the tibial component, and for the next 5 years, the Kinematic and Kinematic II designs were the prostheses most often utilized (Fig. 1–9). These knees had a nonmodular metal-backed tibial component, with the femur and tibia available in three sizes.

In the early 1980s, cementless fixation with porous coated components became popular along with the use of

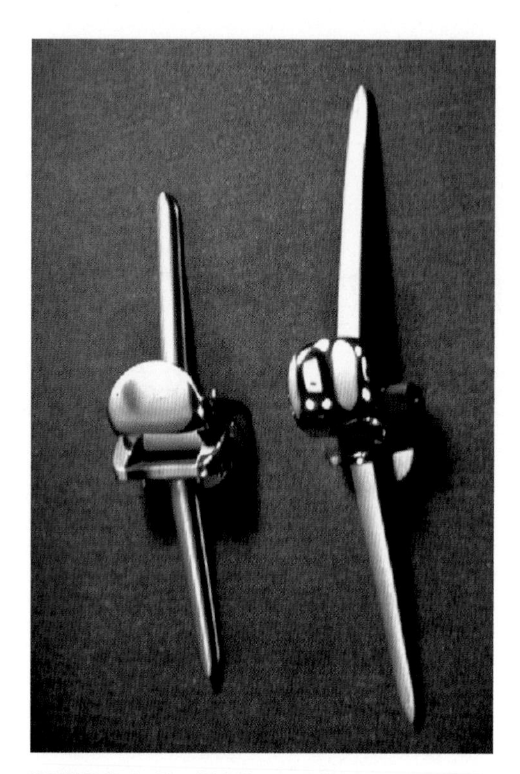

FIGURE 1–1. The Walldius and Guepar prostheses.

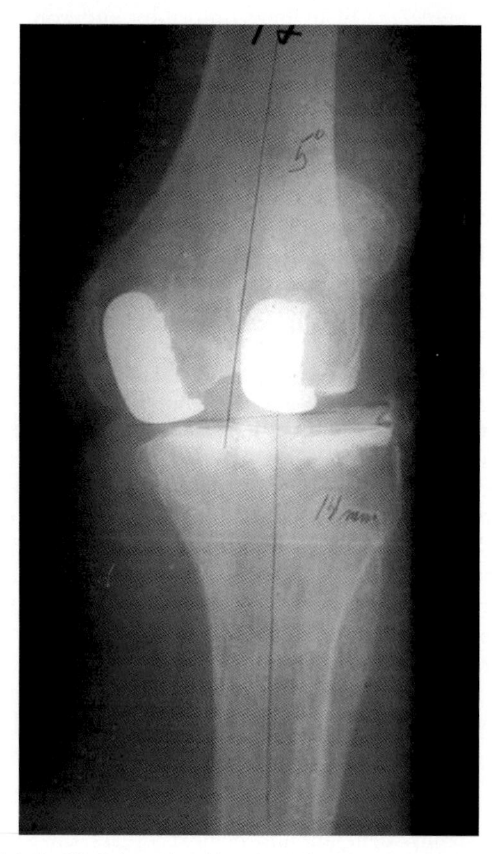

FIGURE 1–2. Mediolateral subluxation of a bicompartmental Marmor prosthesis.

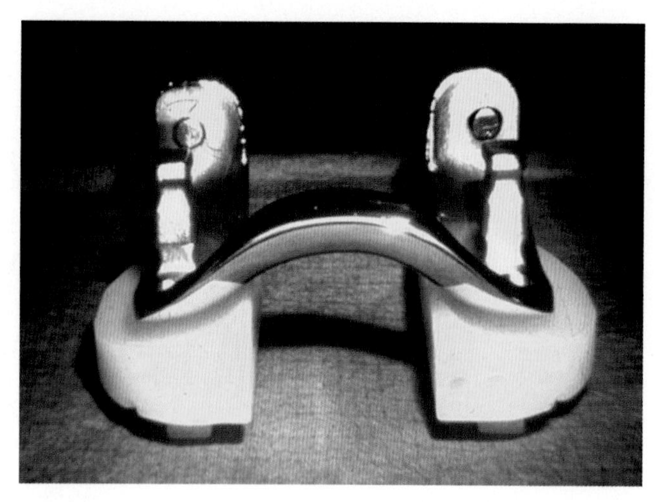

FIGURE 1–3. Duocondylar prosthesis with a two-piece tibial component.

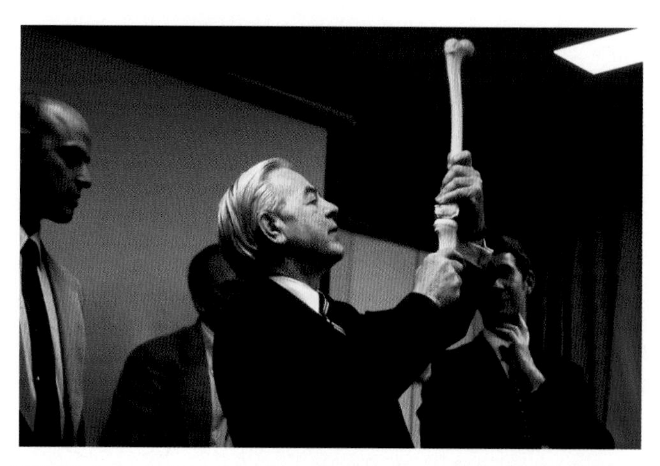

FIGURE 1–4. A visit to the Massachusetts General Hospital in 1974 by Chit Ranawat (*far left*) and Peter Walker (*far right*). William Jones is holding the knee, and William Harris stands behind him.

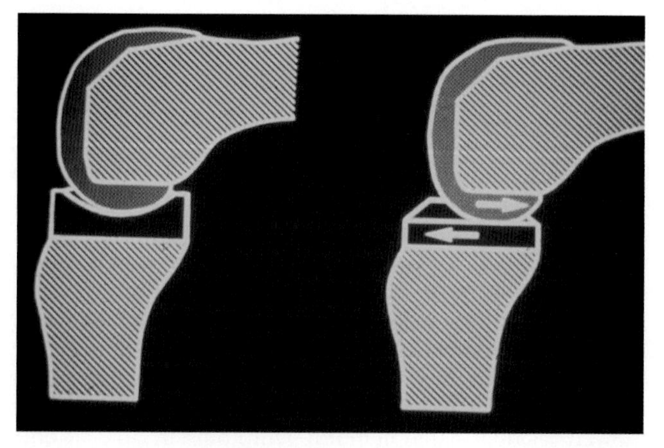

FIGURE 1–5. Diagram of the sagittal articulating topography of a total condylar and duopatellar prosthesis.

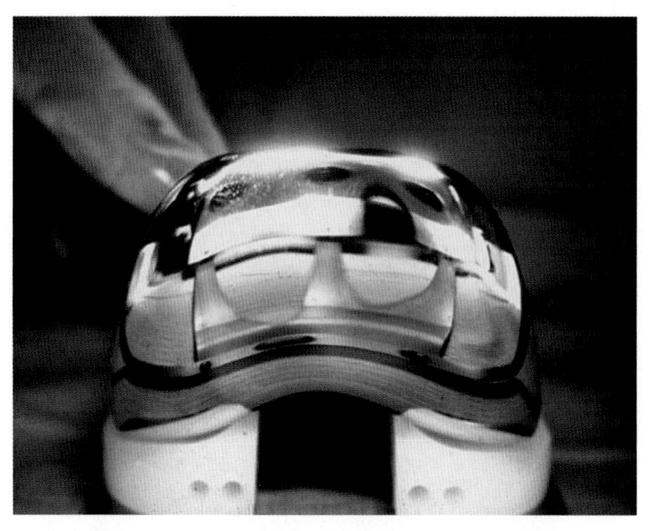

FIGURE 1–6. A first-generation duopatellar prosthesis with two separate tibial components.

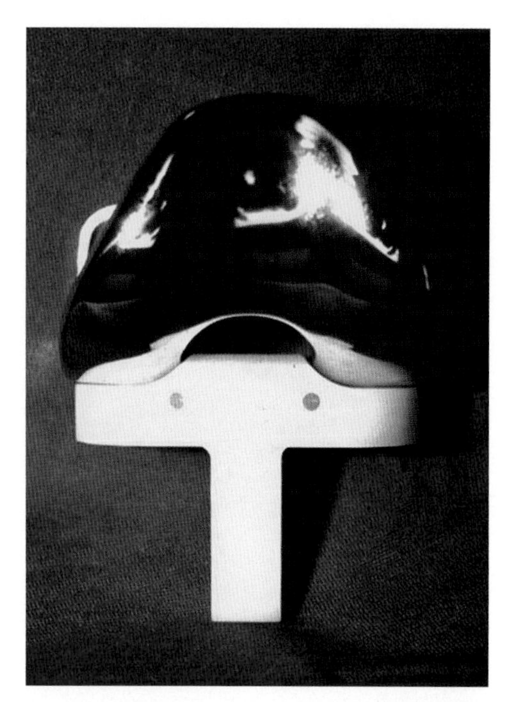

FIGURE 1–8. An all-polyethylene, one-piece tibial prosthesis with a central stem.

instrumentation for alignment and bone preparation. In response to this movement, Dr. Thomas Thornhill and I designed the press-fit condylar (PFC) total knee system; it was first implanted in November 1984 and was introduced nationally in 1986 (Fig. 1–10). Components were provided with and without porous coating for cementless or cemented fixation. Innovations included a broader spectrum of proportional sizes, tibial tray modularity, universal exchangeability among femoral and tibial sizes, and an oval sombrero-shaped patellar component for increased prosthetic-bone and metal-plastic contact (Fig. 1–11). Initially, the patellar component was available in a metal-backed design to allow cementless fixation, but this was abandoned by 1986 for an all-polyethylene design.[4]

Another innovation in the PFC design was the use of a cruciate keel in place of the traditional solid tibial stem. This concept enhanced tibial stem function while preserving

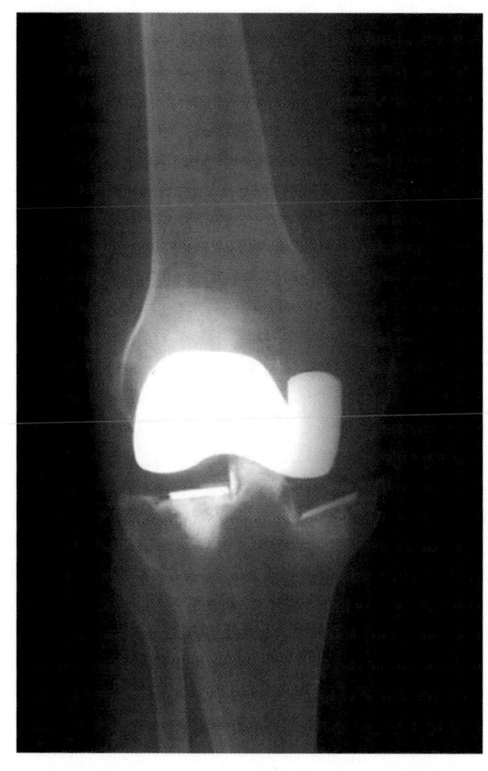

FIGURE 1–7. Loosening and subsidence of the medial tibial component of a duopatellar prosthesis.

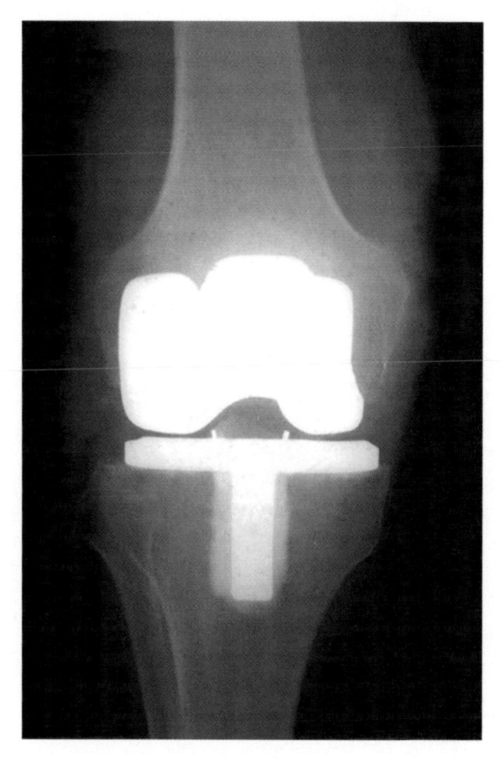

FIGURE 1–9. A nonmodular Kinematic metal-backed tibial component.

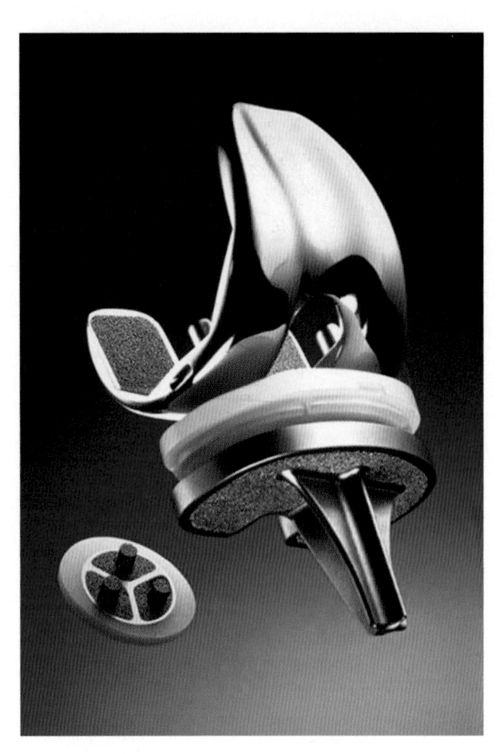

FIGURE 1–10. The first PFC prosthesis was implanted in 1984.

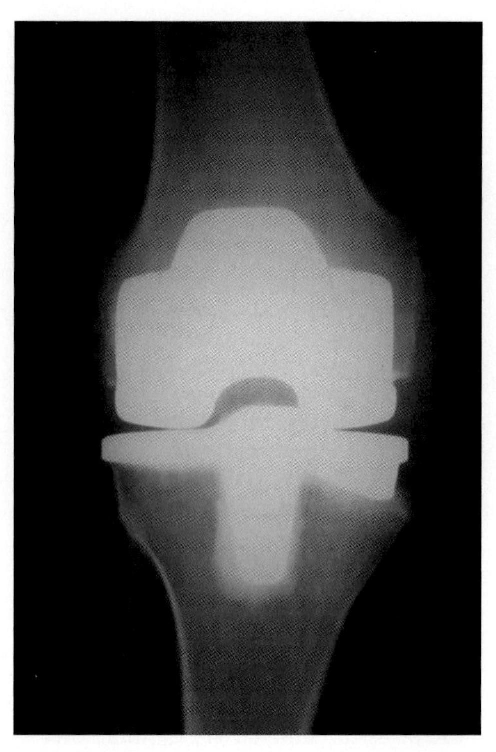

FIGURE 1–12. A medial tibial augmentation wedge implanted with the Kinematic system.

metaphyseal bone stock. At about the same time, a similar but longer keel design was incorporated in a press-fit non-ingrowth design for the Kinematic system. The keel concept grew from the McKeever cruciate keel experience, and a long-stem finned design had also been used previously in the Murray-Shaw variable axis knee.

Modular metallic tibial wedges were shown to be effective for restoration of tibial bone stock in a study performed in Boston by Peter Brooks, Peter Walker, and myself.[5] I implanted the first modular tibial wedge with the Kinematic II knee in September 1984 (Fig. 1–12), and subsequently good short-term success was reported with this technique.[6] This concept was incorporated into the PFC tibial tray by the mid-1980s.

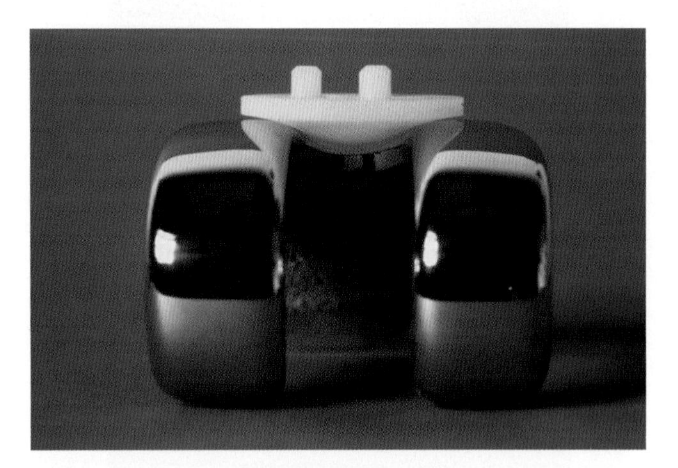

FIGURE 1–11. A sombrero-shaped patella for increased metal-to-plastic contact with the trochlea in flexion.

In 1986, the Omnifit knee (Osteonics Company) was designed by Thomas Thornhill and myself and first implanted a year later. Features included fixed extended stems for both femur and tibia for use in revision or complex primary surgery. Innovations included tibial insert modularity with various levels of prosthetic constraint from preserving and substituting the posterior cruciate to constraining the articulation for varus/valgus stability. Femoral components had identical coronal and sagittal topography with or without an intercondylar housing of two different depths for two levels of constraint. The Omnifit knee was also the first to provide modular femoral augmentation wedges for restoration of femoral bone stock.

A few years later, Dr. Thornhill and I joined with others to create the design of the PFC modular knee revision-system. The posterior stabilized femoral component had a deepened trochlear groove that was prolonged onto the femoral condyles to allow enhanced metal-plastic contact in flexion with a classic "dome" patella (Fig. 1–13). The closed intercondylar box of the femoral component allowed for use of modular femoral stems for press-fit or cemented use in variable diameters, lengths, and valgus angles. The finned tibial stem was of standard length but round and solid, and it could now accept modular tibial stems for press-fit or cemented use in variable diameters and lengths. A variety of augmentation wedges were available for both femoral condyles and tibial plateaus (Fig. 1–14). The locking mechanism for all trays was similar and remained unchanged for 20 years until slightly modified in 2004. The constrained designs have always had an additional reinforcing metal post as an endoskeleton within the conforming tibial polyethylene eminence that also extends into the hollow stem of the modular tray design.

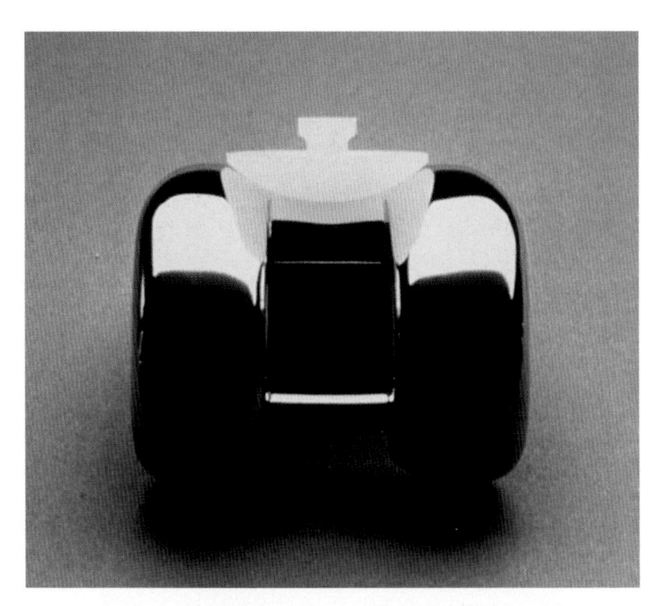

FIGURE 1–13. The trochlear groove is prolonged onto the femoral condyles for increased contact with a dome-shaped patellar prosthesis.

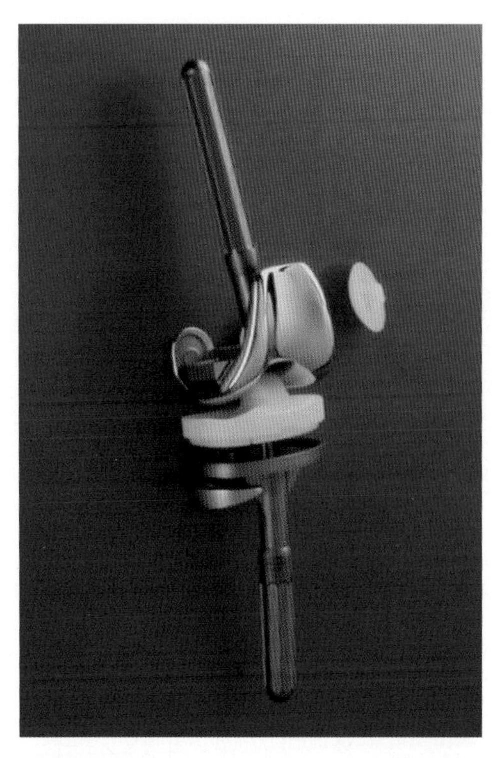

FIGURE 1–14. A variety of modular stems and augmentation wedges facilitate revision surgery.

While the PFC and Omnifit designs were evolving in the late 1980s and through the 1990s, the Kinematic system evolved in Boston into the Kinemax and Kinemax Plus designs. Like the PFC knee, the Kinemax system incorporated insert modularity, proportional sizing, variable prosthetic constraint, and modular femoral and tibial stems and wedges.

Although the PFC cruciate-preserving system and PFC modular cruciate-substituting system, designed by Dr. Chit Ranawat, shared the same tibial tray, femoral sagittal topography, and surgical instrumentation, they initially had different patellofemoral and coronal femoral geometry. In the mid-1990s, we elected to marry the two designs so that they were identical except for the presence or absence of a tibial eminence and a femoral intercondylar housing. The result was the PFC Sigma knee system introduced in April 1996. The tibial trays (keeled and modular) and the femoral sagittal geometry remained unchanged. Coronal condylar femoral geometry became rounded to minimize edge-loading for all components (Fig. 1–15). Both cruciate retaining and substituting femurs adopted the deepened trochlear groove, prolonged onto the femoral condyles to mate with a classic round or oval "domed" patella. For the revision system, more wedges and femoral stem positions were made available, as was an offset modular tibial stem option. The polyethylene, previously sterilized with gamma irradiation in air, was now gamma-radiation-sterilized and packaged in a vacuum.

The latest evolution of bicompartmental knees in Boston was the participation of Thomas Thornhill and myself in the addition of a mobile-bearing rotating platform to the PFC Sigma system (Fig. 1–16). In the mobile-bearing design, the femoral and patellar components are identical to the fixed-bearing design. A polished chrome-cobalt tray accepts highly conforming, PCL-preserving, -sacrificing, or -substituting tibial inserts that are free to rotate about a central post inside the tray. Potential advantages of mobile-bearing knees are enumerated in Chapter 3.

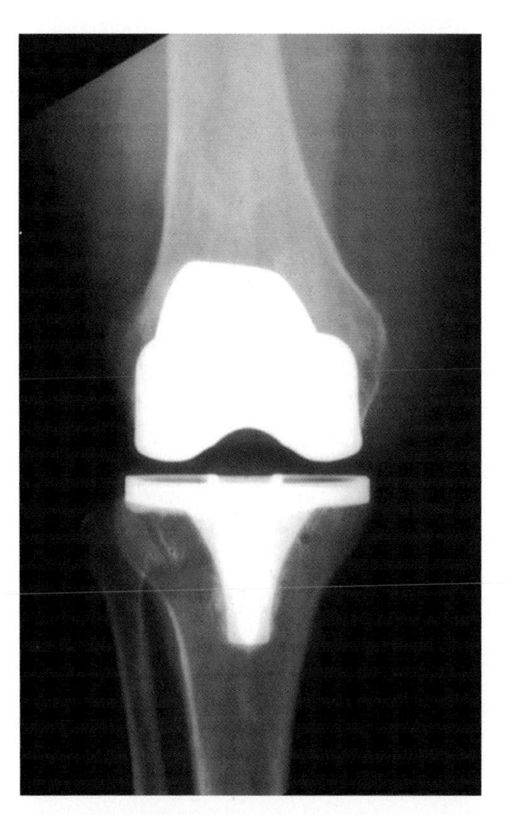

FIGURE 1–15. Rounded condylar coronal topography minimizes edge-loading.

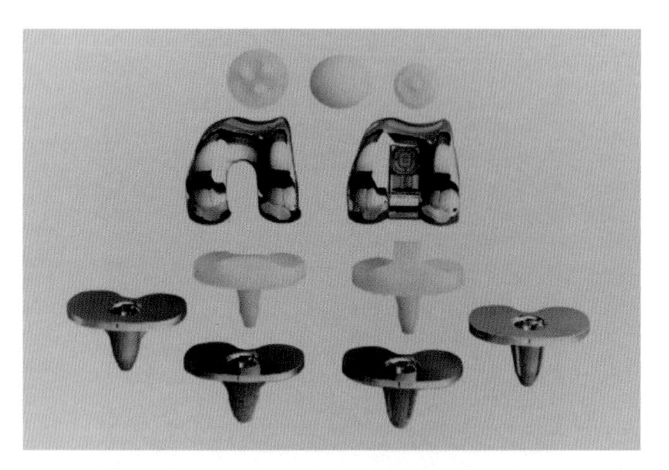

FIGURE 1–16. A mobile-bearing rotating platform prosthesis.

UNICOMPARTMENTAL ARTHROPLASTY

Unicompartmental replacement has been advocated in Boston since 1972. Initial experience began with the Marmor design and progressed to the unicondylar design in 1974, parallel with the duocondylar bicompartmental experience from that era (Fig. 1–17). Two- to six-year results with this design were published in 1981, with 92% good to excellent results.[7] When metal backing of bicompartmental tibial components came into vogue, Peter Walker and I designed the Robert Brigham unicompartmental knee, and it was first implanted in 1981 (see Chapter 18). This was a conservative resurfacing design that called for no distal femoral resection and removal of only 4 to 6 mm of posterior condylar bone.

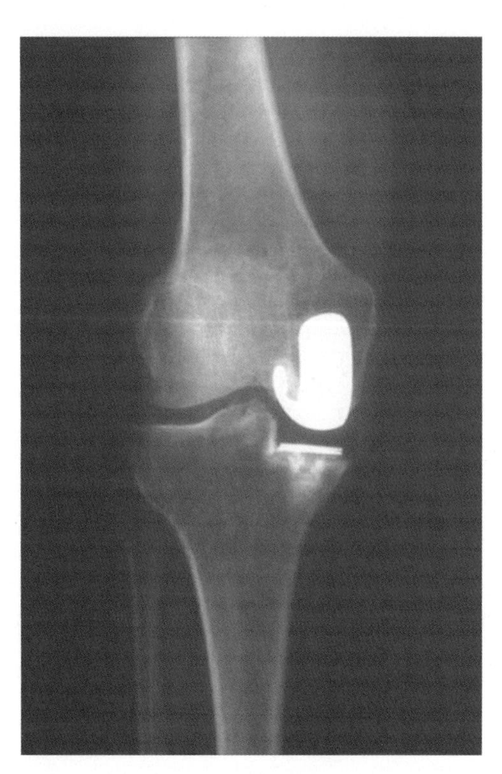

FIGURE 1–17. A unicondylar knee prosthesis from 1974.

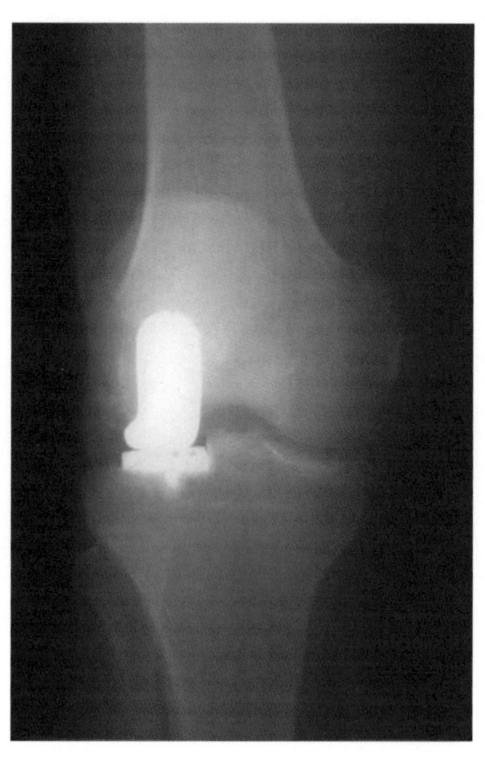

FIGURE 1–18. A composite 6-mm metal-backed unicompartmental knee prosthesis from 1981.

On the tibial side, a titanium-backed 6-mm composite thickness was similarly conservative (Fig. 1–18). Early excellent results were marred by a high incidence of polyethylene wear through to the metal backing in the 6-mm thickness when the femur articulated with the anterior or posterior quarter of the tibial component, where the polyethylene was only 2 mm thick.[8]

In 1990, Thomas Thornhill and I designed the PFC unicompartmental knee. Its tibial tray was anatomic in shape to maximally cap the resurfaced plateau. The metal-backed tibial component was modular, with a minimal thickness of 6 mm of polyethylene. An all-polyethylene tibial component also was available (Fig. 1–19). Femoral instrumentation could be intramedullary based. Distal femoral resection was 4 mm to allow for more conservative tibial resection. The articulating geometry was made more conforming to decrease wear stresses on the polyethylene surface, but the resulting constraint increased the incidence of component radiolucent lines and eventually led to an increased incidence of loosening of either component compared with nonconforming designs.[9] In 1996, we modified the PFC unicompartmental knee into the PFC Sigma design to decrease this conformity and also improve the fixation between the two femoral lugs and their surrounding cement mantle.

SUMMARY

Knee arthroplasty design has many of its roots in Boston. I am fortunate to have been present and to have participated along with many other surgeons in its evolution.

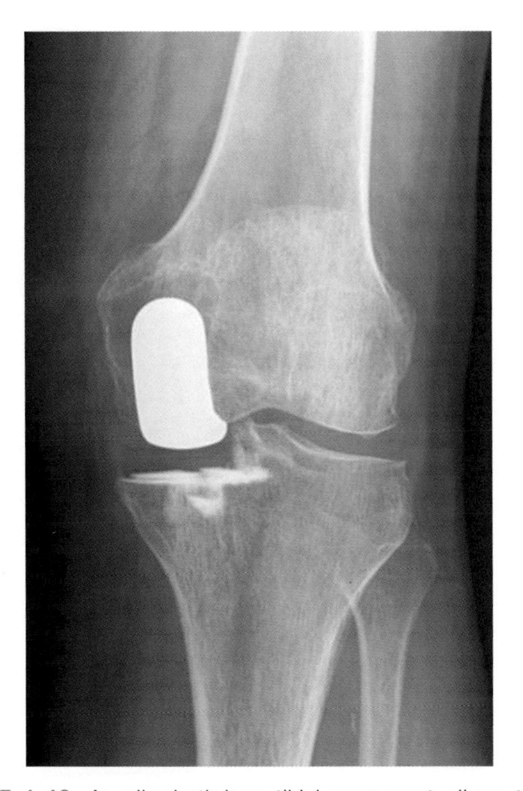

FIGURE 1–19. An all-polyethylene tibial component allows thinner sizes to have an adequate thickness of plastic.

References

1. Potter TA, Weinfeld MS, Thomas WH: Arthroplasty of the knee in rheumatoid arthritis and osteoarthritis: a follow-up study after implantation of the McKeever and MacIntosh prostheses. J Bone Joint Surg Am 1972;54:1–24.
2. Scott RD, Joyce MJ, Ewald FC, Thomas WH: McKeever metallic hemiarthroplasty of the knee in unicompartmental degenerative arthritis: long-term clinical follow-up and current indications. J Bone Joint Surg Am 1985;67:203–207.
3. Scott RD: Duopatellar total knee replacement: the Brigham experience. Orthop Clin North Am 1982;13:89–102.
4. Scott RD, Thornhill TS: Press-fit condylar total knee replacement. Tech Orthop 1986;1(4):41–58.
5. Brooks PJ, Walker PS, Scott RD: Tibial component fixation in deficient tibial bone stock. Clin Orthop 1984;183:302–308.
6. Brand MG, Daley RJ, Ewald FC, Scott RD: Tibial tray augmentation with modular metal wedges for tibial bone stock deficiency. Clin Orthop 1989;248:71–79.
7. Scott RD, Santore RF: Unicondylar unicompartmental knee replacement in osteoarthritis. J Bone Joint Surg Am 1981;63:536–544.
8. McCallum JD III, Scott RD: Duplication of medial erosion in unicompartmental knee arthroplasties. J Bone Joint Surg Br 1995;77:726–728.
9. Schai PA, Suh JT, Thornhill TS, Scott RD: Unicompartmental knee arthroplasty in middle-aged patients. J Arthroplasty 1998;13:365–372.

CHAPTER 2

Posterior Cruciate Ligament Retention versus Substitution

The controversy over whether to retain or substitute for the posterior cruciate ligament (PCL) has been ongoing since the advent of condylar total knee arthroplasty in the early 1970s. Three schools exist. One almost exclusively preserves the PCL, the second exclusively substitutes for it, and the third is selective. Boston is thought of as the school of PCL retention, whereas the New York school is one of substitution. In 1974, when I was chief resident in orthopedic surgery at the Massachusetts General Hospital, two New Yorkers, Drs. Chit Ranawat and Peter Walker, came to Boston to share their latest designs of condylar knee prostheses. Both were at the Hospital for Special Surgery at that time and collaborated with Dr. J. Insall on early knee prosthetic designs. A meeting was held in the Smith-Petersen room, and notable attendees included William Jones, Chief of the Knee Service, and William Harris, Chief of the Hip Service (see Fig. 1–4). We were shown two options. One was the total condylar prosthesis, which sacrificed the PCL, and the other was the duopatellar prosthesis, which preserved it. The total condylar had a dished sagittal topography, whereas the duopatellar was flat. With the PCL retained and functioning, this flat topography allowed the femur to roll back on the tibia and enhance potential flexion (Fig. 2–1). Users of the total condylar technique were reporting average flexion of approximately 85 degrees, while duopatellar users were often achieving more than 100 degrees of flexion. These findings were shared with surgeons at the Brigham Hospital, where 85% of patients undergoing total knee arthroplasty at that time had rheumatoid arthritis. Because the rheumatoid patient often had significant involvement of the upper extremities, the potential for enhanced flexion via retention of the posterior cruciate ligament was very attractive. Unless patients achieved well over 100 degrees of knee flexion, they would have difficulty arising from a chair and negotiating stairs and would depend on their upper extremities for these activities. The cruciate preserving technique, therefore, was adapted in Boston to better serve the rheumatoid population.[1] Nearly all Boston orthopedic residents and fellows were trained in this technique, whereas in New York the sacrificers predominated. This led to a friendly rivalry between the Boston and New York camps and spawned many formal and informal debates that have continued for decades.

PCL RETENTION

Advantages of PCL Retention

The potential advantages of preserving the PCL are many. Because stability is imparted by a biologic structure, the prosthesis can be less constrained, and therefore less force is imparted to the insert-tray interface and the prosthesis-

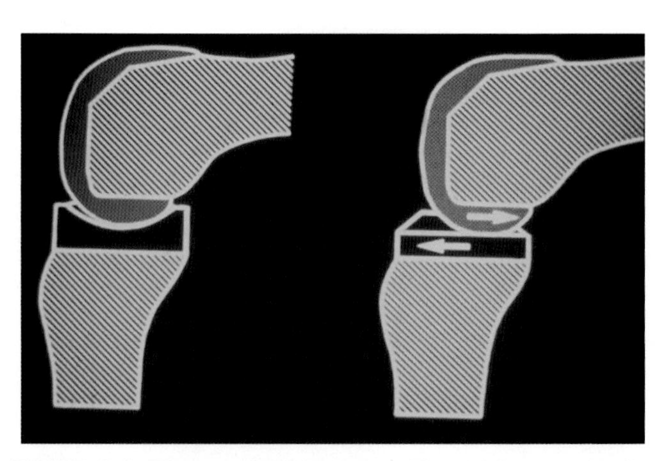

FIGURE 2–1. Diagram showing how a PCL-retaining round-on-flat articulation allows rollback and enhances potential flexion.

to-bone interface. Until cruciate substituting designs that mandated rollback by their sagittal topography became available, cruciate-retaining knees could achieve a greater potential range of motion than cruciate-sacrificing knees.

With posterior cruciate ligament retention, it is also possible to preserve the joint line at a near-normal location. When the posterior cruciate ligament is cut, the flexion gap increases and there is a requirement for thicker polyethylene for any given amount of bone resection. This thicker polyethylene in turn requires greater distal femoral resection to allow full extension of the knee. Thus, the joint line is elevated in both flexion and extension by several millimeters with cruciate-sacrificing designs. This means a mandatory distortion of the collateral ligament kinematics. Although it is possible to equalize the 90-degree flexion gap with the full extension gap, mid-flexion laxity is bound to occur to some extent when the joint line is elevated. Finally, cruciate-retaining knees allow for preservation of intercondylar bone stock for future revision, if it becomes necessary.

Candidates for PCL Retention

The belief that knees with severe deformity require posterior cruciate ligament sacrifice and substitution is a misconception in my personal experience. I believe that at least 98% of primary knees can be treated with PCL retention. This is because the PCL does not have to be "normal" to be retained. In knees with severe varus deformity, the PCL often is encased by intercondylar osteophytes, which must be débrided in order to define the ligament origin (Fig. 2–2). When medial structures are subsequently released (see Chapter 5) to balance lax lateral structures, the PCL indeed is usually too tight relative to these structures and must be released to some extent to balance the knee.

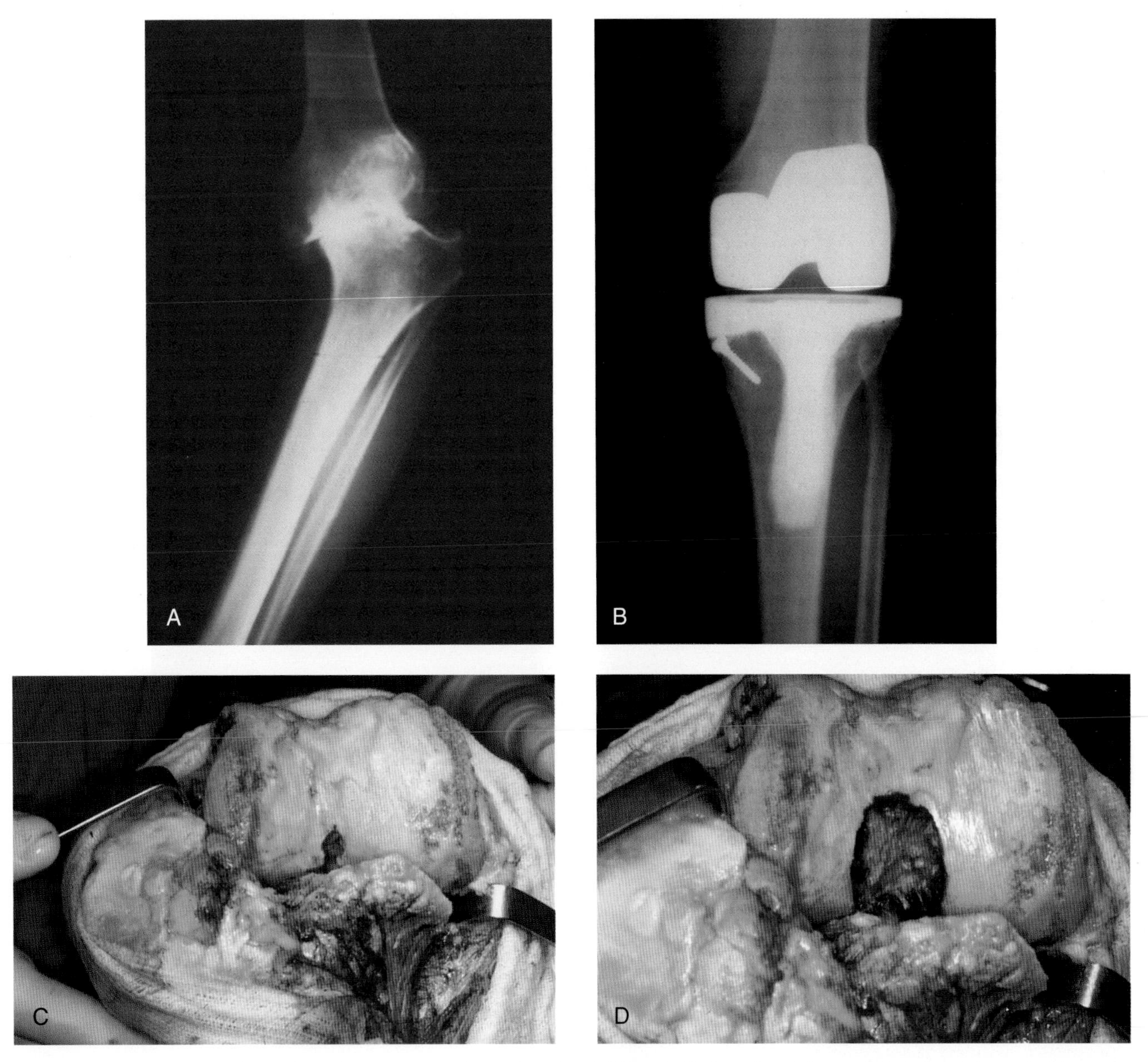

FIGURE 2–2 A–D. *A* and *B*, Correction of severe varus deformity without PCL substitution. *C* and *D*, The PCL is intact beneath intercondylar osteophytes but is not normal.

In severe valgus deformity, it is not only possible to preserve the PCL, but it may be preferred because of the medial stabilizing force of this ligament (see Chapter 6). Again, as in severe varus deformity, the ligament often has to be released after the tight lateral side is released to balance the lax medial side (Fig. 2–3).

Balancing the PCL

Another misconception is that balancing the PCL is a difficult and complicated maneuver. "Balancing" the PCL essentially means leaving the knee with a PCL that is neither too loose nor too tight.

I have developed a simple intraoperative test for PCL balancing that allows the surgeon to adequately assess these two possibilities and remedy either problem. The procedure is called the POLO (*p*ull-*o*ut *l*ift-*o*ff) test.[2] The pull-out test is to assess the knee for flexion laxity. With the trial components in place (the tibial component must always be placed before the femoral component), the knee is flexed 90 degrees. The surgeon then tries to pull out the tibial component from underneath the femur (Fig. 2–4). This test must be performed with an insert that has a curved sagittal topography. The one I use has a posterior lip that is approximately 3.5 mm higher than the midpoint of the articulation. In essence, the pull-out test is to determine whether at least 3.5 mm of laxity or distraction is possible in the flexion gap. Obviously, there are gradations between 1 mm and 3.5 mm of laxity or distraction capability in this test. I like the flexion gap to be on the tighter side of this spectrum. A corollary of the pull-out test is the push-in test. In this case, the surgeon pushes the tibial component into place underneath the femoral component, which has been previously inserted. If this is possible in a cruciate-retaining knee, my opinion is that the knee is too loose in flexion, unless the surgeon is using a flat sagittal topography. If the knee fails

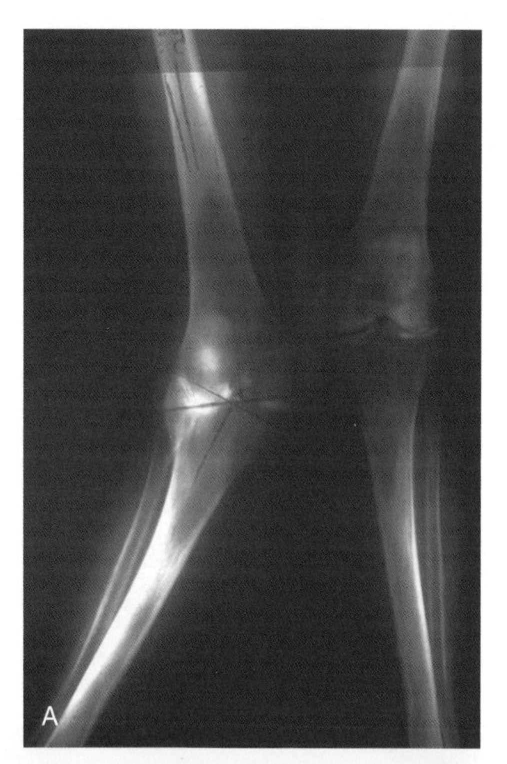

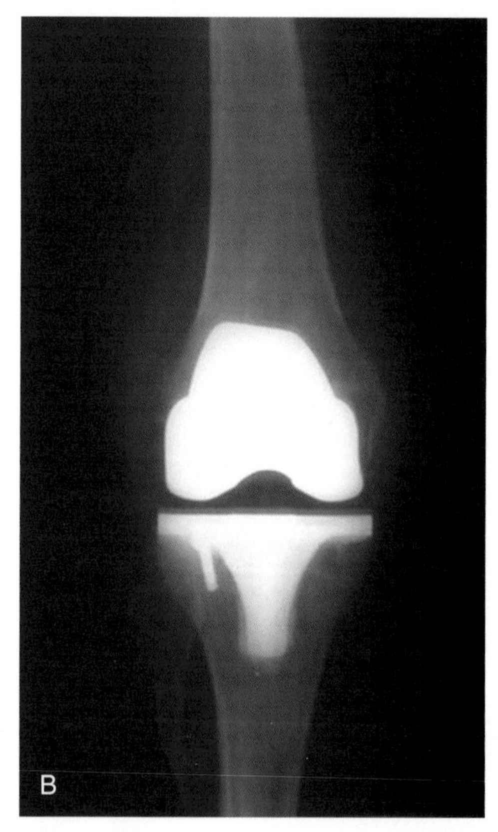

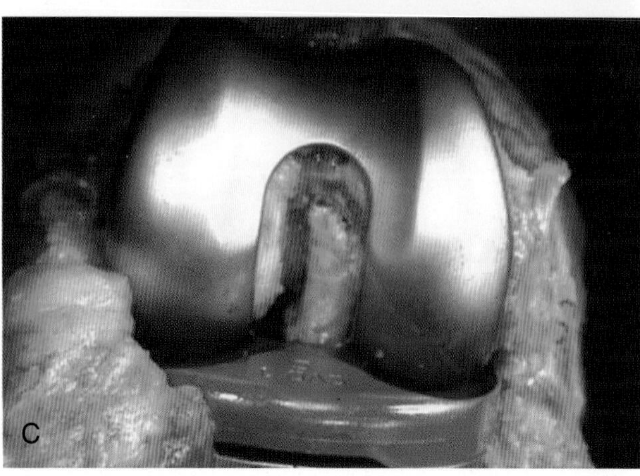

FIGURE 2–3. PCL retention in severe valgus deformity requiring a partial femoral release.

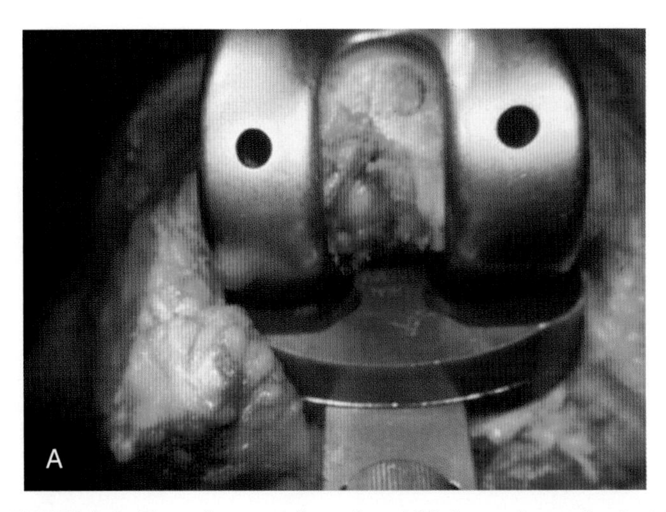

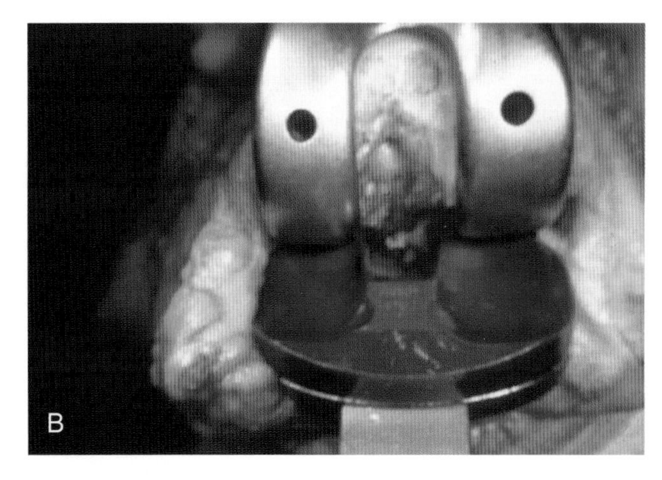

FIGURE 2–4. The pull-out test (knee flexed 90 degrees): negative test (*A*), positive test (*B*).

the pull-out test, thicker inserts are tried until pull-out no longer is possible.

Once the knee has proved to be not too loose, I make sure it is not too tight with the lift-off test. With the same trial components in place, the knee is flexed between 80 and 100 degrees. If the PCL is too tight, it will pull the femur posteriorly on the tibia, where the posterior condyles impinge on the posterior lip of the tibial insert, pushing it down in back with lift-off in front (Fig. 2–5). A tight PCL can usually be visualized as the source of the rollback, posterior impingement, and lift-off (Fig. 2–6). The tightest fibers are usually the more anterior and lateral fibers. My preference is to release the PCL under direct visualization with the trial components in place (Fig. 2–7). The release can be gradual and sequential until lift-off disappears. Some surgeons prefer to perform the release from the tibial attachment. This technique can be effective but does not allow a selective release with the trial components in place.

It is important to remember that lift-off can be caused by at least two factors other than a tight PCL. If the lift-off test is performed with the patella everted and the knee has a tight quadriceps mechanism (e.g., a preoperatively stiff knee), the everted quadriceps will artificially draw the tibia forward and into external rotation. In such cases, lift-off should be tested with the patella returned to the trochlear groove. If lift-off no longer takes place, a posterior cruciate release probably is not necessary. The second cause of lift-off, other than a tight PCL, is failure to clear the posterior

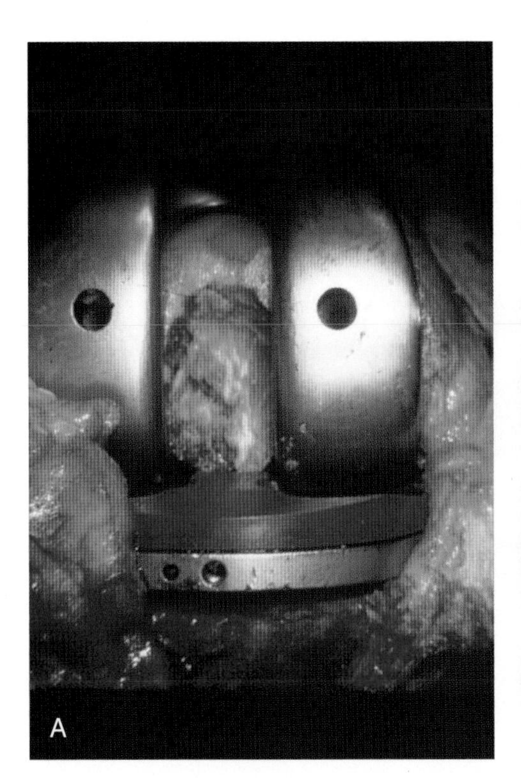

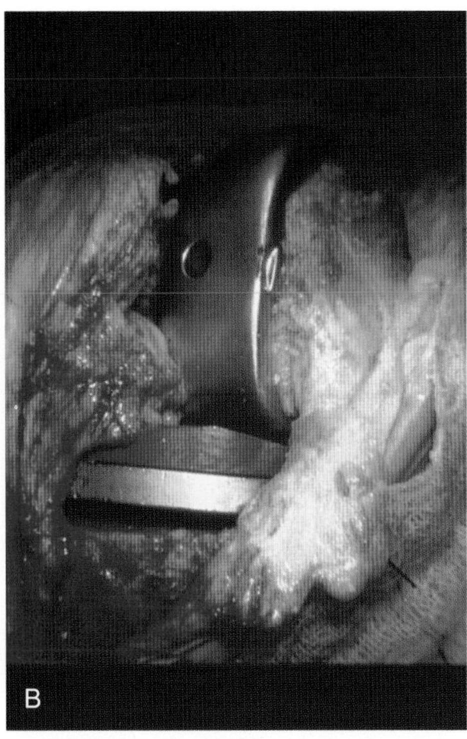

FIGURE 2–5. The lift-off test (knee flexed 80 to 100 degrees). The test is positive with both the patella everted (*A*) or returned to the trochlear groove (*B*).

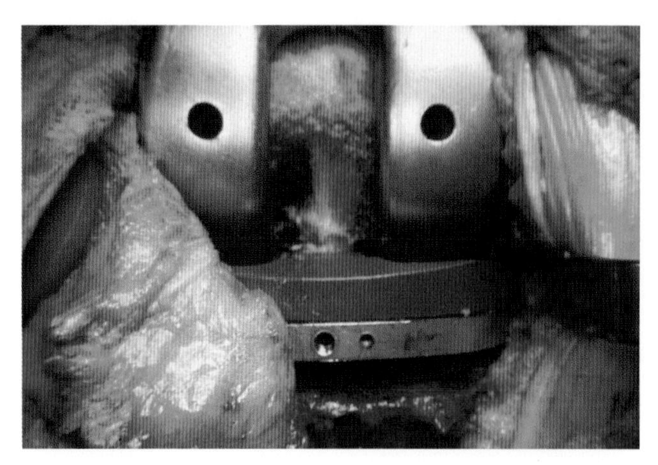

FIGURE 2–6. A tight PCL causing anterior tray lift-off.

femur of uncapped bone or retained osteophytes (Fig. 2–8). Impingement of the posterior lip of the tibial component on this bone will cause lift-off.

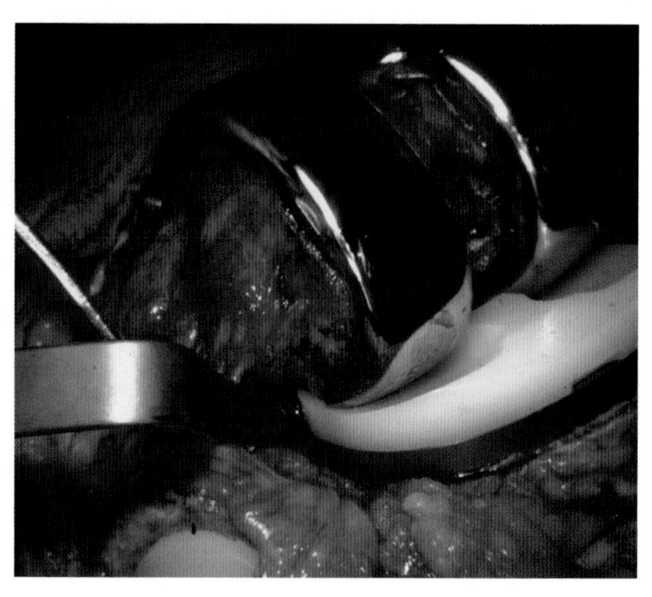

FIGURE 2–8. Posterior impingement also can cause lift-off.

Disadvantages of PCL Retention

Advocates of PCL sacrifice correctly point out some potential disadvantages of PCL retention. There is the possibility of late anterior-posterior instability if the PCL stretches over time. I have rarely seen this in my own practice and feel it is the result of a combination of a flexion gap left too loose initially and tibial topography that is flat in the sagittal plane. In addition, if the surgeon inadvertently applies an up-slope to the tibial resection, posterior subluxation of the tibia on the femur is more likely.

A second historical criticism of PCL retention was the apparent need for more frequent lateral release for patellar tracking. I believe this was true for early PCL experience when proper attention was not given to appropriate femoral and tibial component rotational alignment. With improvements in surgical technique and prosthetic designs that promote better patellar tracking, I believe there is no longer a difference in lateral release rate between cruciate-preserving and -substituting techniques.

A third historical criticism is a higher incidence of late polyethylene wear. Again, this was true in earlier experience for a number of reasons. The earliest PCL retention designs had high contact stresses from a round-on-flat articulation (Fig. 2–9). Stresses related to the conformity of the articulation and specifically to the difference between the radius of curvature of one articulation and of the other. The greater the difference, the higher are the stresses. For example, there is less stress with a round-on-round articulation such as a hip arthroplasty and a flat-on-flat articulation such as the undersurface of a rotating platform. A round-on-flat articulation, however, has a large difference between the radii of curvature and therefore high stresses. Since early designs of cruciate-retaining knees were mostly round-on-flat, the higher stresses led to a higher incidence of wear compared with cruciate-sacrificing designs with curved-on-curved articulations. Our retrievals of PCL retaining knees that failed owing to wear showed a common wear pattern. Most of these knees functioned well for a number of years with excellent range of motion but eventually showed late posterior wear due to excessive rollback of the femur on the tibia combined with the high stresses of a round-on-flat articulation (Fig. 2–10). In our early experience with posterior cruciate

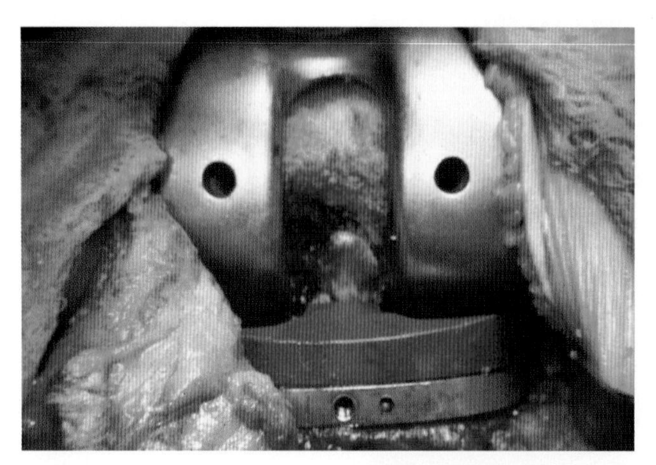

FIGURE 2–7. The lift-off resolves after femoral release of the PCL.

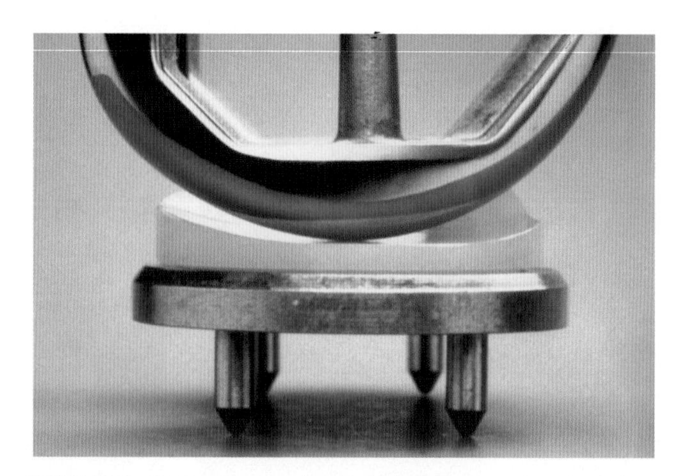

FIGURE 2–9. Point contact can lead to high stresses on the polyethylene.

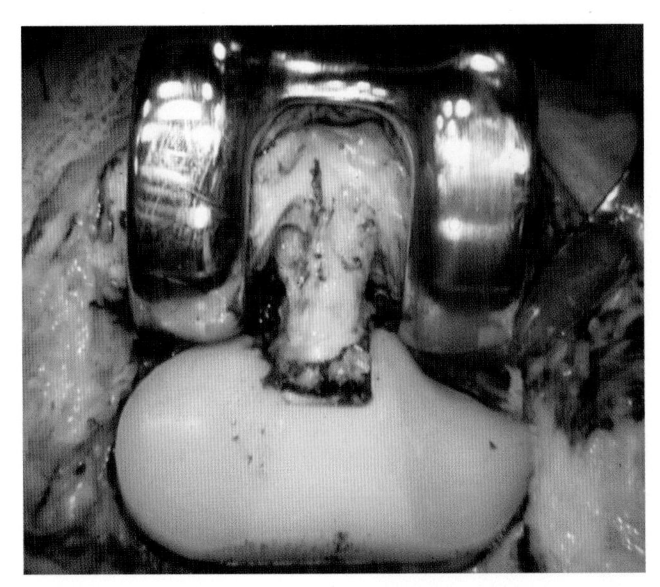

FIGURE 2–10. Late posterior wear can result from excessive rollback with a tight PCL.

ligament retention, we allowed the knee to adjust to the cruciate. If the cruciate was left too tight, the femur would have excessive rollback and possible late posterior wear. If the cruciate was left too loose, the tibia could undergo subluxation posteriorly and the wear pattern would move forward. This occurred in combination with the round-on-flat articulation. This experience led to the evolution of PCL-preserving designs with curved tibial topography in the sagittal plane.[3] The knee would no longer adjust to the cruciate, but the cruciate would have to be adjusted to each individual knee. This need to balance the PCL led me to the development of the POLO test described above. In the early 1990s, my experience progressed to virtually 100% use of curved inserts, with PCL release from the femur as needed.

PCL SUBSTITUTION

Indications for Posterior Stabilized Primary TKA

Since I "grew up" learning how to save and eventually balance the posterior cruciate ligament, it is unusual for me to perform a primary PCL-substituting TKA. I acknowledge, of course, that this procedure has definite advantages for selected patients. Currently, those patients make up 1% to 2% of my practice. Since I practice in a teaching environment, I feel that if I can teach residents and fellows to save and balance the PCL in almost all cases, they will understand ligament balance better and perform a better PCL substitution if they eventually choose that technique.

The advantages of PCL substitution are that it is easier and more forgiving to balance deformity. The knee is certainly more forgiving of slight flexion laxity. It is also easier to correct and stabilize a knee with a severe flexion contracture (see Chapter 9). Modern designs of cruciate substitution provide controlled rollback for better potential range of motion, especially in preoperatively ankylosed knees (see Chapter 8). Finally, the partial rotational constraint between the post and the femoral housing allows the surgeon more control in selecting the Q-angle of the knee to facilitate patellar tracking in cases having patellar instability. This rotational constraint, however, comes with the disadvantage of imparting rotational forces through the polyethylene to the insert-tray interface in modular tibial components (Fig. 2–11).

I propose that the following are ideal candidates for PCL substitution: the ankylosed knee, the knee with a severe flexion contracture, the knee with chronic patellar dislocation, and the postpatellectomy knee. Although the patellectomized knee possibly can be treated with PCL retention, it is vulnerable to late instability owing to a deficient quadriceps mechanism and an imbalanced, lax PCL is more likely to stretch, allowing instability to progress. Because PCL substitution is more forgiving, it should be used for borderline cases. Whether the PCL is retained or substituted in the patellectomy patient, I believe it is important to "tube" the quadriceps mechanism if it is thin and requires reinforcement (see Chapter 7).

Finally, most total knee revision arthroplasties are probably best handled with cruciate-substituting techniques. On the femoral side, this permits the use of modular stems for enhanced fixation, which often are combined with modular augments for the femoral condyles (Fig. 2–12).

Disadvantages of PCL Substitution

Several possible disadvantages can be enumerated for PCL substitution technique. As mentioned above, because of the higher constraint in the articulation, greater stress is imparted through the polyethylene to the modular insert-tray or bone-cement interface. In theory, these forces would lead to increased motion between the insert and tray and increase back-side wear. These same forces could also increase the potential for loosening of the prosthesis at the fixation interface in both modular and nonmodular designs.

A second problem that is unique to PCL-substituting designs is the patellar clunk syndrome. This occurs when there

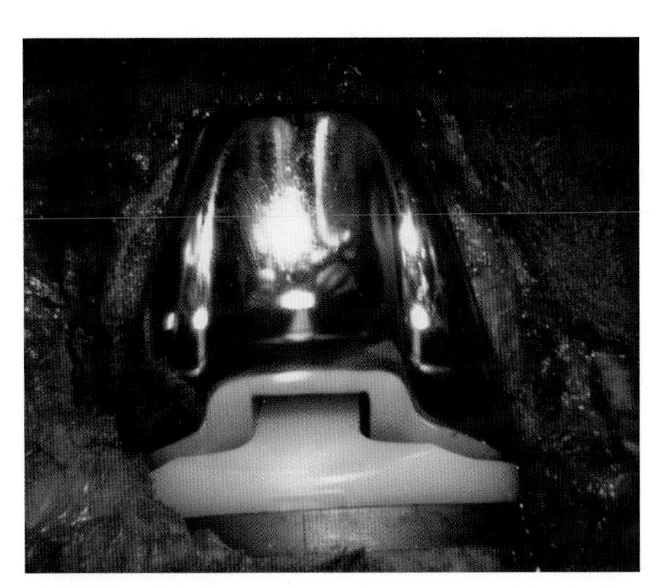

FIGURE 2–11. Tibiofemoral malalignment causes torsional stresses on the stabilizing post.

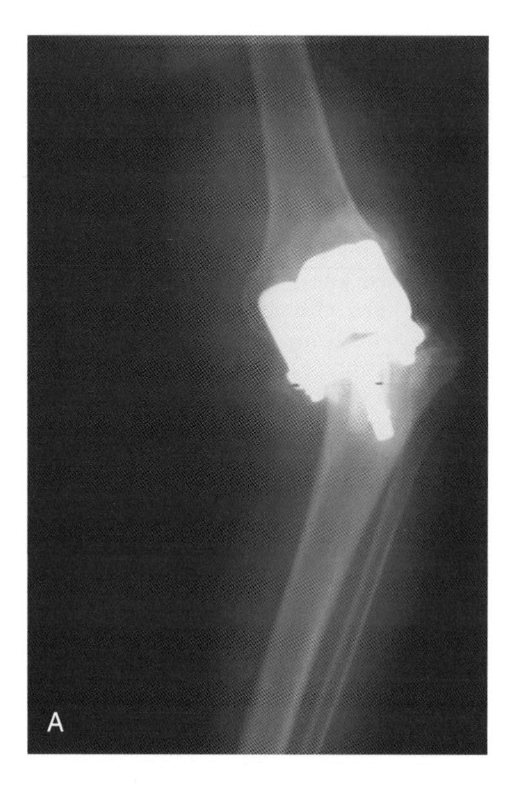

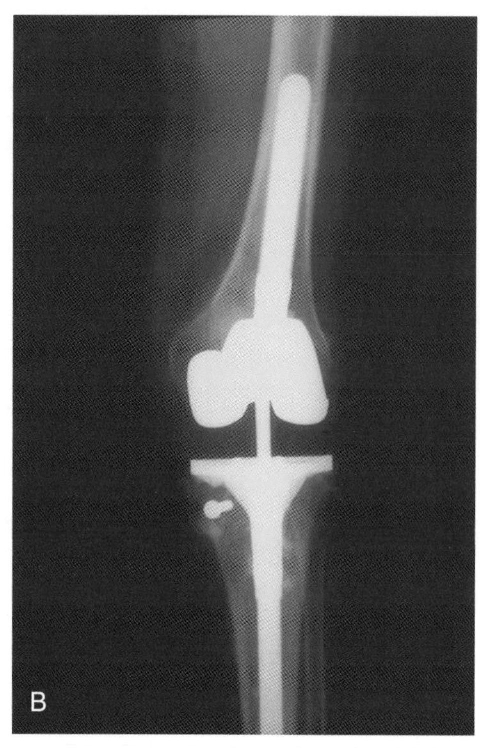

FIGURE 2–12. Many revisions require PCL substitution to restore stability.

is a buildup of scar tissue above the superior pole of the patella on the quadriceps tendon. This scar can become entrapped in the intercondylar housing of the stabilized femoral component in flexion, causing internal derangement as the knee is extended. When these symptoms are disabling, arthroscopic débridement of the scar tissue is necessary. The complication is minimized by removing all synovial tissue from the quadriceps tendon just above the superior pole of the patella at the time of the original arthroplasty and using a femoral component with a smooth transition from the trochlea into the intercondylar notch (Fig. 2–13).

A third disadvantage of PCL substitution is the removal of intercondylar bone stock for the housing of the femoral component. The amount of bone removed varies from design to design. More conservative prostheses save bone but have less constraint and therefore a higher potential for dislocation.

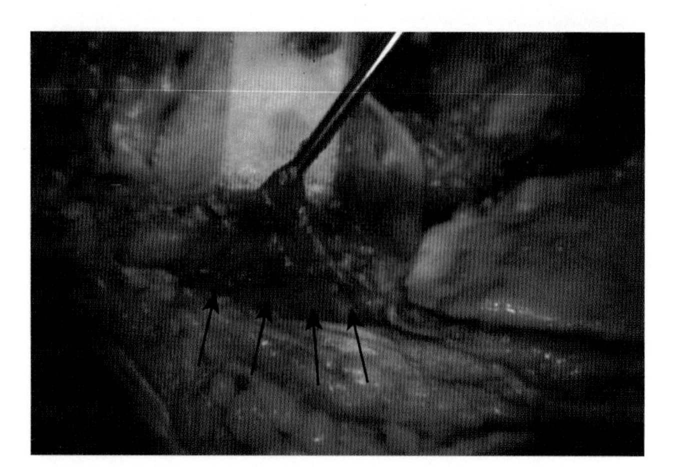

FIGURE 2–13. Retained synovium on the quadriceps tendon can be the nidus for the clunk syndrome.

Another design-related disadvantage is the inability of the posterior stabilized system to accommodate hyperextension of the knee without anterior impingement of the post on the housing (Fig. 2–14). Some current designs provide for no hyperextension, although most allow for approximately 10 to 12 degrees. Even with these more forgiving designs, the combination of femoral component flexion with posterior slope of the tibial component must be avoided. For example, 3 degrees of femoral flexion combined with 7 degrees of posterior slope might allow impingement to occur with little or no anatomic hyperextension of the knee.

Finally, the tibial post of stabilized designs is vulnerable to wear from rotational malalignment between the femur and the tibia that either is created by the surgeon at the time of arthroplasty or occurs dynamically because of the patient's gait or flexion pattern. Many surgeons arbitrarily align the rotation of the tibial component relative to a landmark on the tibial tubercle. The junction between the medial and middle thirds of the tubercle often is chosen. Although this may be appropriate for most knees, some others may require an alignment that is significantly internal or external to this landmark. Intuitively, the tibial alignment that is neutral with the femur will depend on the rotational alignment chosen by the surgeon for that specific knee. It also is influenced by the dynamics of the surrounding ligaments. I feel strongly that the rotational alignment of the tibia should be determined by extending the knee with the trial components in place and rotating the tibial component into a neutral position beneath the established femoral component. Rotating-platform mobile-bearing knees have the advantage of accommodating to malrotation created either by the surgeon or dynamically by the patient during functional activities (see Chapter 3).

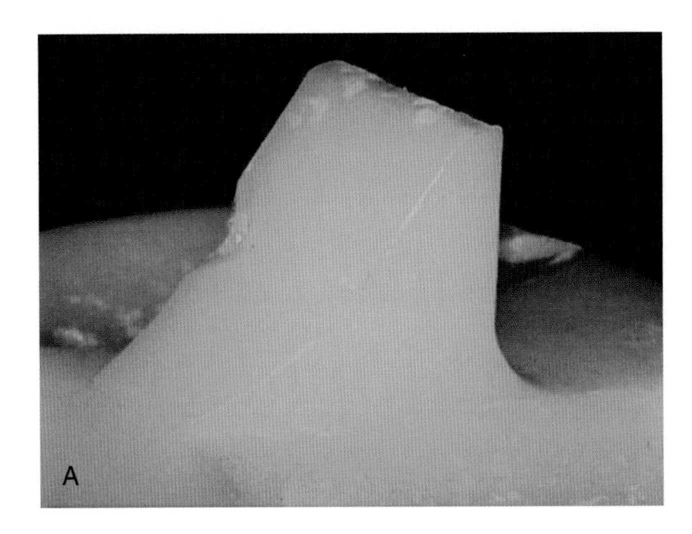

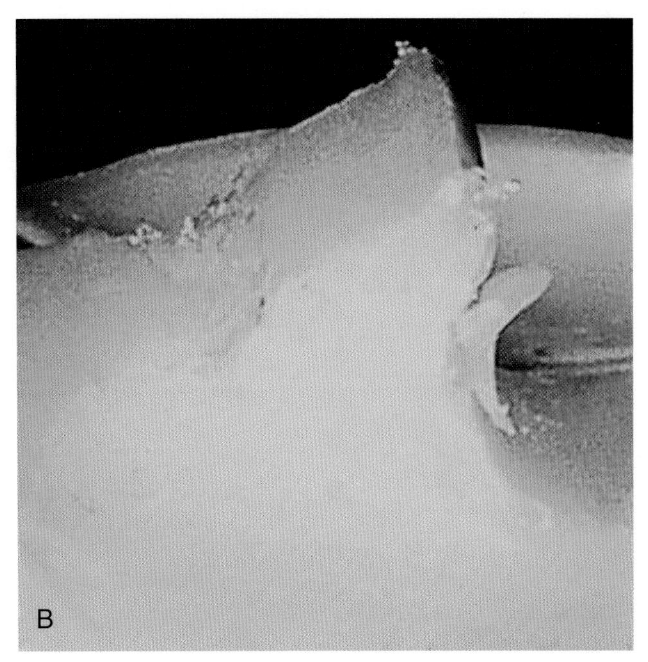

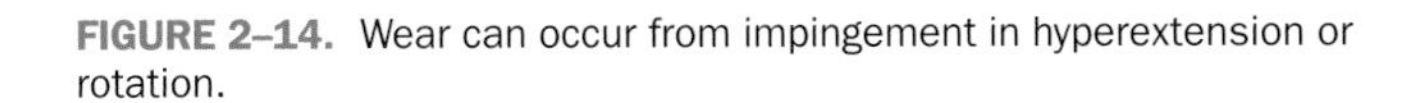

FIGURE 2–14. Wear can occur from impingement in hyperextension or rotation.

SUMMARY

Both posterior cruciate-retaining and -substituting techniques have been available for 30 years, and each technique has yielded excellent 10- to 15-year results. Each technique has advantages and disadvantages. Most prosthetic systems provide for either alternative, and surgeons can make their choice on what is comfortable for them based on their training and experience.

References

1. Scott RD, Volatile TB: Twelve years' experience with posterior cruciate-retaining total knee arthroplasty. Clin Orthop 1986;205:100–107.
2. Chmell MJ, Scott RD: Balancing the posterior cruciate ligament during cruciate-retaining total knee arthroplasty: description of the POLO test. J Orthop Tech 1996;4:12–15.
3. Scott RD, Thornhill TS: Posterior cruciate supplementing total knee replacement using conforming inserts and cruciate recession. Clin Orthop 1994;309:146–149.

CHAPTER 3

Mobile versus Fixed Bearings in Total Knee Arthroplasty

Mobile-bearing articulations for knee arthroplasty have been available for several decades. Nevertheless, they never gained great popularity and remained an alternative technique embraced by a small group of surgeons. However, recently there has been increased interest in mobile-bearing articulations, and almost every prosthetic company is pursuing a mobile-bearing design.

WHY CONSIDER A MOBILE-BEARING ALTERNATIVE?

Fixed-bearing knees, whether cruciate retaining or substituting, have a good track record at 10 to 15 years of follow-up. My own 10-year experience with fixed bearings demonstrates 100% survivorship of femoral components, tibial components, and all-polyethylene patellar components.[1] Reoperations were necessary in 5% of cases with metal-backed patellar components and 2% of cases without the patellar resurfaced; 4% of flat modular tibial inserts wore to a point where they needed to be exchanged by 10 years after surgery. Ironically, metal-backed patellar components are no longer used in most systems unless they are of mobile-bearing design.

Controversy persists regarding the need for universal patellar resurfacing. A 2% failure rate of unresurfaced patellae at 10 years still makes nonresurfacing a viable option for selected patients.[2]

The 4% incidence of tibial insert wear requiring reoperation is the problem that in theory might be addressed by mobile-bearing articulations. These were designed to allow high conformity between metal and plastic to minimize stresses and lower the potential incidence of wear. Stress on the polyethylene is related to conformity and can be related mathematically to the difference in the radius of curvature between one articulation and the other. The greater the difference, the greater the stress, and the smaller the difference, the less the stress on the polyethylene. Round-on-round and flat-on-flat articulations, therefore, would represent low-stress articulations, whereas round-on-flat articulations could create high stresses. By the mid-1990s, most knee system designers had abandoned round-on-flat articulations in favor of those with more conformity. I personally advanced to the use of curved inserts 100% of the time by the early 1990s.[3]

It must be remembered, however, that many factors other than conformity affect polyethylene wear (Table 3–1). These include the method of fabrication of the polyethylene, i.e., whether it is compression molded or bar extruded. The resin utilized also makes a difference, as does quality control. Other factors include the surface preparation, the thickness, the effect of gamma radiation on oxidation, dynamic forces such as sliding and shearing that are imparted by the individual patient, the opposing surface (the femoral side), and the undersurface (the back side).

At the time of this writing, back-side wear is receiving a lot of attention. Retrievals from virtually all modular total knee arthroplasty systems have been shown to have a vari-

TABLE 3–1 FACTORS THAT AFFECT POLYETHYLENE WEAR
Surface preparation
Thickness
Molecular weight
Fabrication method
Oxidation
Conformity
Contact area
Sliding and shearing forces
Opposing surface (femoral component)
Undersurface (back side)

able pattern and extent of back-side wear.[4] My experience with modular tibial inserts began in 1984. It was extremely rare to encounter back-side wear from inserts implanted from the mid-1980s to the early 1990s. It became more frequent among many total knee systems in the mid-1990s. Most likely a number of factors were involved; they might include the resins that were utilized, methods of polyethylene preparation, and sterilization methods, especially gamma radiation in the presence of oxygen. An important contributory factor also must be the increased conformity of the top side of the inserts that were then in use. With round-on-flat inserts, forces were dissipated at the top surface of the insert before they were transferred through the polyethylene to the insert-tray interface (Fig. 3–1). On the other hand, conforming inserts would transfer this stress directly to the back side. It does not seem to me to be a coincidence that I have some patients with bilateral knee replacements with a conforming insert on one side and a flat insert on the other, who suffer back-side wear on the conforming side and more benign top-side wear on the flat side.

Herein lies the first of several potential advantages of rotating-platform mobile-bearing knees. This type of articulation can provide high conformity on the top side to minimize surface wear without the adverse effects of constraint. Back-side wear is addressed by allowing the undersurface of the insert to move freely as determined by the dynamic forces across the knee on a flat-on-flat surface that provides the least amount of stress to the polyethylene. In addition to being a flat-on-flat articulation, the rotating-platform insert mandates unidirectional rather than multidirectional wear. Unidirectional wear also is favorable to the longevity of polyethylene.[5]

A second important advantage of a rotating-platform mobile bearing is the ability of the prosthetic articulation to accommodate to malrotation between the femur and the tibia that either is created at operation by the surgeon or occurs postoperatively during functional activities. This malrotation is what imparts torsional stresses through the conforming insert to the back side in fixed bearings. In a rotating-platform knee, the surgeon can choose optimal placement of the tibial tray on the proximal tibial bone and allow the insert to accommodate to the femur in all degrees of flexion (Fig. 3–2).

Yet another advantage of mobile bearings is maintenance of high contact area in high flexion. During high flexion in both the normal and replaced knee, the lateral condyle of the femur generally rolls posteriorly on the tibial plateau. In fixed bearings, this high rollback cannot occur in the presence of conforming sagittal topography. It can occur with round-on-flat articulations, but this often leads to catastrophic late posterior polyethylene wear. A mobile-bearing articulation allows posterior translation of the femur on the tibia to occur in high flexion while maintaining high conformity at the top-side articulation (Fig. 3–3).

DISADVANTAGES OF MOBILE BEARINGS

Mobile bearings without stops can subluxate, impinging on soft tissues, and even possibly dislocate. Bearings with stops, however, might be subject to wear because of repetitive impingement on the stop. To prevent impingement, most mobile-bearing inserts are slightly smaller than equivalent fixed-bearing inserts (Fig. 3-4). This allows a certain amount of rotation or translation to occur on top of the tray before soft tissue impingement can occur.

Mobile-bearing knees also are somewhat more sensitive to certain technical considerations while they are forgiving to others, such as malrotation. For rotating platform knees, the most significant technical complication is "spinout" of the bearing (dislocation), usually a result of flexion gap asymmetry. As a consequence of flexion gap asymmetry with or without posterior cruciate tightness, a mobile bearing could fail early with spinout. Fixed-bearing knees, however, may be able to tolerate flexion gap asymmetry for a much longer period of time, failing late as a result of progressive instability problems or polyethylene wear. The surgeon is implicated for the early mobile-bearing failure, whereas the natural course of events exonerates the surgeon in a fixed-bearing knee.

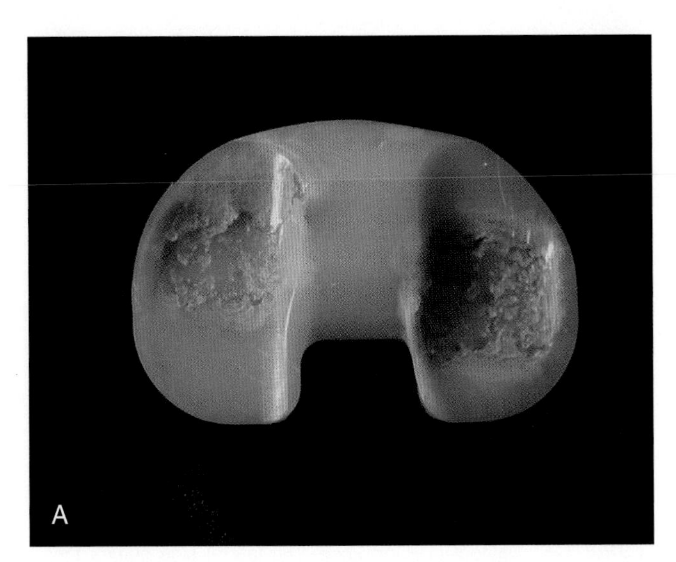

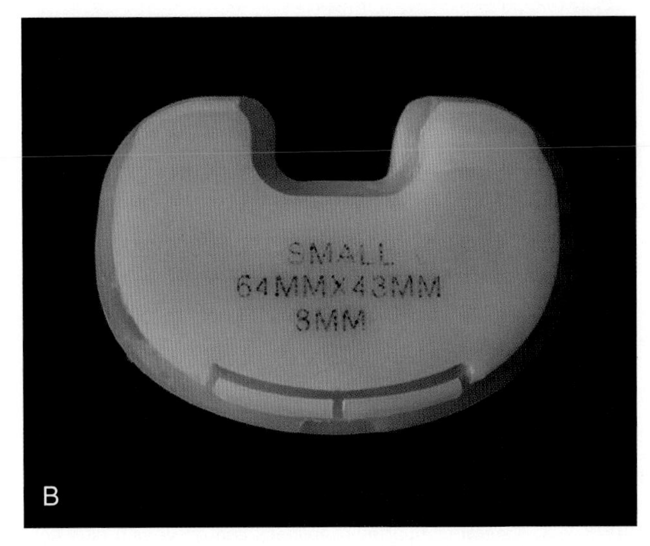

FIGURE 3–1. Postoperative retrieval of a flat insert after 15 years. Top-side wear (*A*) predominates over back-side wear (*B*).

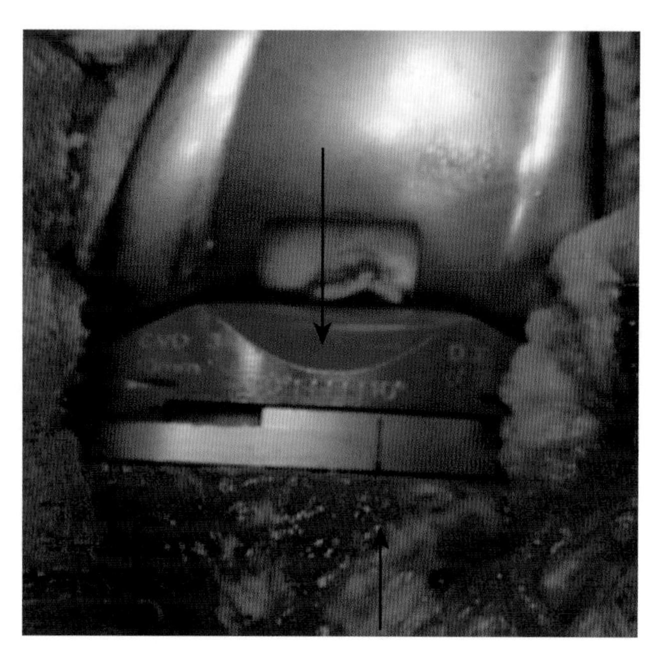

FIGURE 3–2. Fifteen degrees of malrotation between the center point of the insert and of the tray in a rotating-platform knee.

Avoiding Spinout

Rotating-bearing dislocation, or spinout, occurs in high flexion (Fig. 3–5). The lateral femoral condyle moves posteriorly, and the lateral half of the insert dislocates forward. The medial side maintains its articulation. A curved insert utilized for posterior cruciate retention is more vulnerable to spinout than a posterior stabilized insert. There are two reasons: (1) a tight posterior cruciate ligament (PCL) usually is the cause of spinout, and after the PCL has been released, this alone may cure the problem; (2) the intercondylar constraint of the posterior stabilized insert minimizes spinout potential.

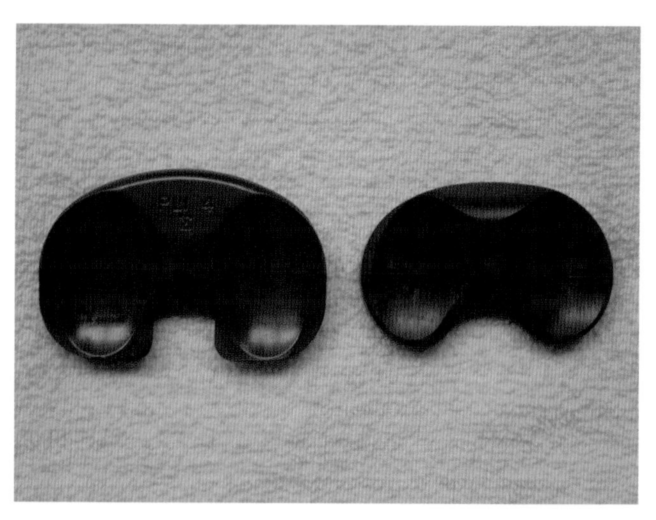

FIGURE 3–4. Rotating-platform (RP) bearings are smaller than fixed bearings.

What to Do If Spinout Occurs

The possibility of spinout should always be checked with the patella located. I have seen cases in which spinout occurred with the patella everted and disappeared with the patella located, and vice versa. If spinout persists with the patella located, a tight PCL should first be sought, since it is the most common cause. This can be seen under direct vision, or the tightness can usually be palpated. The release should be performed on the femoral side starting with the most anterior and lateral fibers and progressing to the more posterior and medial fibers. I have seen some cases in which merely 20% of the PCL needs to be released to eliminate spinout and others in which virtually the entire PCL has to

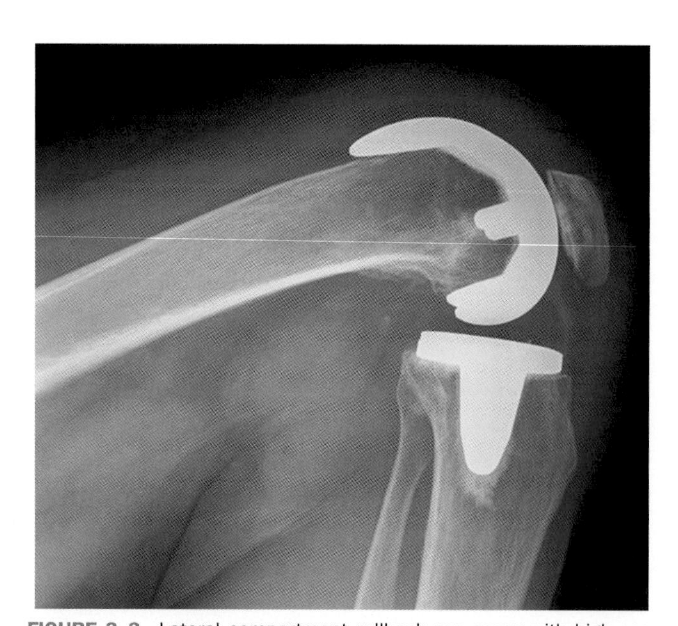

FIGURE 3–3. Lateral compartment rollback can occur with high congruency maintained.

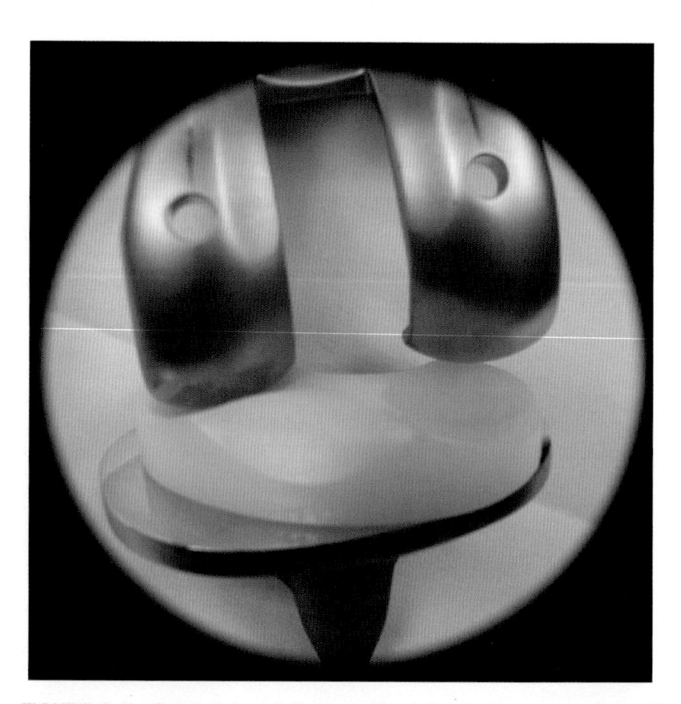

FIGURE 3–5. Spinout in a left knee. The lateral side comes forward while the medial side remains engaged.

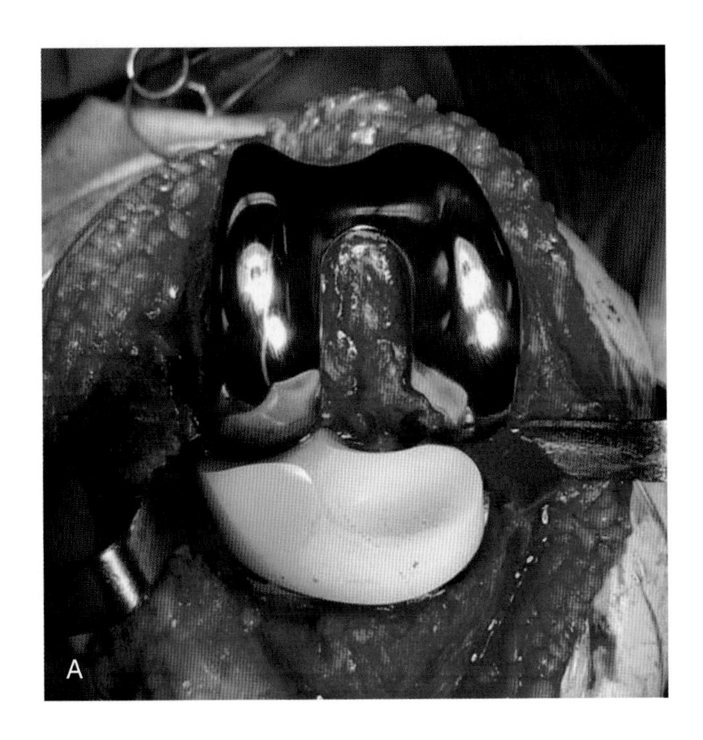

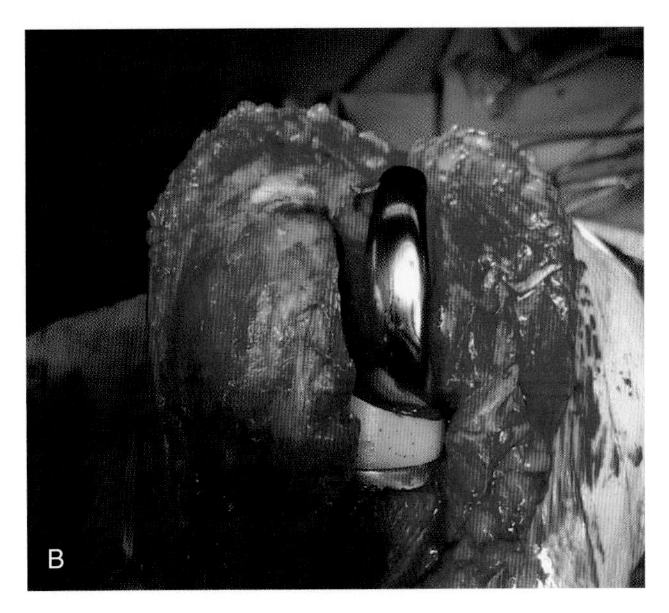

FIGURE 3–6. Medial spinout (*A*) usually disappears with the capsule closed or the patella located (*B*).

be cut. Even in the latter case, conversion to posterior cruciate substitution rarely is necessary.

If the spinout persists and the lateral side is coming forward, I would check for a tight popliteal tendon. I myself have never seen this to be the cause, but I suspect that it is possible. If lateral spinout still persists, I might try the next larger size (same thickness) of polyethylene bearing. The rationale for the larger size is that it will provide a longer anteroposterior dimension to the insert, inhibiting dislocation. Any given size of rotating-platform bearing is smaller than the same size of fixed bearing. The explanation for the difference is to allow a smaller tibial tray to be utilized with a larger femoral component. In matched femoral and tibial sizes, the matched insert allows 10 degrees of internal and external rotation before the insert protrudes over the edge of the metal tray. A larger insert on a smaller tray still allows 5 degrees of internal and external rotation without overhang. It does, however, result in a slight decrease in contact area. The difference is small though, and the resultant contact area is still greater than for nearly all fixed-bearing designs.

If, despite the above strategies, spinout still persists, the surgeon can switch to either a posterior stabilized insert or a fixed bearing.

Occasionally, when spinout occurs, the medial side comes forward (Fig. 3–6). This scenario almost always involves a severe varus knee in which an extensive medial capsular dissection has been performed for exposure. The medial spinout will nearly always disappear when the capsule is closed or the patella is located. One suture in the medial capsular closure at the joint line is all that is necessary to confirm that this will resolve the spinout. If it persists, a thicker insert will be necessary to stabilize the flexion gap and the lateral side will almost always be accepting. This thicker insert may limit terminal extension so that the distal femur may possibly have to undergo an additional 2 mm of resection to prevent flexion contracture.

CURRENT INDICATIONS FOR ROTATING-PLATFORM COMPONENTS

In my current practice, I am implanting rotating-platform components in younger, more active patients. I use the rough guideline of 65 years of age or younger. I also use rotating-platform components on all posterior-stabilized prostheses in primary knees to relieve torsional stresses on the post that might be transmitted to the back side of a modular insert. In elderly patients of approximately 75 years of age or older, I use all-polyethylene tibial components. For patients between the ages of 65 and 75 years, I may use either of the above-mentioned types or a modular fixed-bearing tibial prosthesis.

References

1. Schai PA, Thornhill TS, Scott RD: Total knee arthroplasty with the PFC system: results at a minimum of ten years and survivorship analysis. J Bone Joint Surg Br 1998;80:850–858.
2. Kim BS, Reitman RD, Schai PA, Scott RD: Selective patellar nonresurfacing in total knee arthroplasty: 10 year results. Clin Orthop 1999;367:81–88.
3. Scott RD, Thornhill TS: Posterior cruciate supplementing total knee replacement using conforming inserts and cruciate recession. Clin Orthop 1994;309:146–149.
4. Conditt MA, Stein JA, Noble PC: Factors affecting the severity of backside wear of modular tibial inserts. J Bone Joint Surg Am 2004;86:305–311.
5. McEwen HM, Barnett PI, Bell CJ, et al: The influence of design, materials and kinematics on the in vitro wear of total knee replacements. J Biomech 2005;38:357–365.

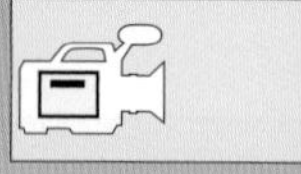

CHAPTER 4

Primary Total Knee Arthroplasty Surgical Technique

I have tried to make the surgical technique of primary total knee arthroplasty (TKA) as generic as possible. Obviously, TKA systems will vary in terms of instrumentation and nuances of surgical technique. Some differences will also exist between posterior cruciate ligament (PCL) retention and substitution.

POSITIONING OF THE PATIENT

Total knee arthroplasty is always performed with the patient in the supine position. The operating table should be level. The rare exception occurs when TKA is being performed below a fused or ankylosed hip.[1] In this case, the table is in the level position for the exposure and closure. During the arthroplasty, the patient is placed in the Trendelenburg position and the foot of the table is dropped; the uninvolved leg is supported on a separate stool or table.

I usually expose the knee in flexion, especially in obese patients or if a tourniquet is not utilized. I close the knee in extension except for placement of the most proximal sutures in the quadriceps mechanism, which is facilitated by a flexed knee and a proximal self-retaining retractor.

Placement of the Footrest

I prefer a commercially available cylindrical footrest that supports the knee in flexion during the arthroplasty. If this is not available, a satisfactory substitute is a towel or blanket rolled into a cylinder and taped into position. The optimal level for placement of this support is at the fattest part of the patient's calf (Fig. 4–1). This supports the knee in maximal flexion after satisfactory exposure has been achieved. The level for this support, therefore, is independent of the preoperative range of motion but reflects the flexion that will be achieved once the quadriceps mechanism is everted and the knee is mobilized.

PREPARATION OF THE LEG

Any shaving of hair around the area of the planned incision is done just prior to sterile preparation of the leg. I include the foot and prepare this part of the leg first and then hold the foot with a sterile towel as the remainder of the leg is prepared. A double-thickness sterile stockinette is then rolled from the foot to the level of the thigh tourniquet. The outer thickness of the double stockinette is cut and landmarks about the knee are palpated through the inner thickness. The appropriate proximal, middle, and distal landmarks are marked with a sterile pen through the stockinette. The inner stockinette is then cut, the incision is drawn, and three transverse lines are made to assist with wound alignment at the time of closure.

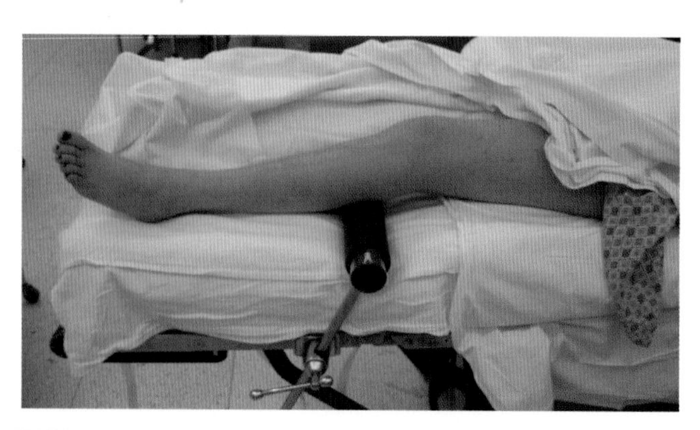

FIGURE 4–1. A transverse bar is placed at the bulkiest part of the calf to support the knee in flexion during the procedure.

Finally, the entire leg is wrapped in an adhesive plastic surgical drape. A betadine-impregnated drape is used at the surgical site. The foot is included with this wrapping so that the entire leg will remain dry and sealed off during any irrigation of the wound. Two adhesive drapes are necessary to complete this process. A smaller first drape seals off the foot, and the larger second drape seals the leg from thigh to ankle. Sometimes a third drape, cut into smaller strips, is necessary to seal off any uncovered areas.

The Tourniquet

I use a tourniquet for all total knee arthroplasties with essentially two exceptions. The first is in the obese patient, especially one with a short thigh. A tourniquet is often ineffective in these patients and compromises the proximal extent of the surgical field.

The second exception is a patient with known peripheral vascular disease and absent pulses confirmed by Doppler examination. These patients always have a consultation with a vascular surgeon preoperatively. Even if there has been successful bypass surgery, I do not use a tourniquet. The incision and initial exposure are made with the knee in flexion, which minimizes bleeding and allows the vessels to be coagulated as they are encountered.

The tourniquet pressure utilized is 275 mm Hg in most cases. Occasionally, pressure as high as 350 mm Hg is necessary to avoid a venous tourniquet effect. Maximum tourniquet time is 90 minutes with a 10-minute interval before reinflation is considered. I elevate the limb for 30 seconds prior to inflation of the tourniquet. I prefer not to exsanguinate the limb with an elastic bandage (Esmarch's bandage) so that some blood remains in the veins and they are easier to identify. The first dose of prophylactic antibiotics is given at least 10 minutes before tourniquet inflation (see Chapter 14).

THE INCISION

A standard incision is straight, vertical, and approximately 15 cm long. It is centered proximally over the shaft of the femur, in its mid portion over the mid third of the patella and distally just medial to the tibial tubercle (Fig. 4–2). There is a trend to make shorter incisions, and this can be done by lessening the proximal half of the skin incision. If the initial exposure and closure are done with the knee in flexion, the proximal quadriceps can be accessed through a shorter skin incision.

Skin incisions must be modified in the presence of prior incisions about the knee (see Chapter 15). I prefer to avoid elevating large skin flaps and creating dead space. The subcutaneous dissection heads directly toward the landmarks for a medial parapatellar arthrotomy. Elevation of skin over the dorsal surface of the patella is only the amount that is sufficient to safely apply a holding clamp for cementing the patellar component.

MEDIAL PARAPATELLAR ARTHROTOMY

I prefer a medial parapatellar arthrotomy for all primary knees. In the past 30 years, I have had experience with three alternative approaches to the knee: subvastus, mid-vastus, and lateral parapatellar. I certainly do not object to their use in selected patients. Each, however, has potential disadvantages. For example, the subvastus and mid-vastus approaches can be difficult in short, obese, and muscular individuals. If a medial advancement is necessary at the time of closure, it may be difficult to achieve with these approaches. The lateral approach for valgus knees may prevent the surgeon from safely everting the patella medially. It may also be difficult to seal the arthrotomy from the subcutaneous space just beneath the skin incision with this approach.

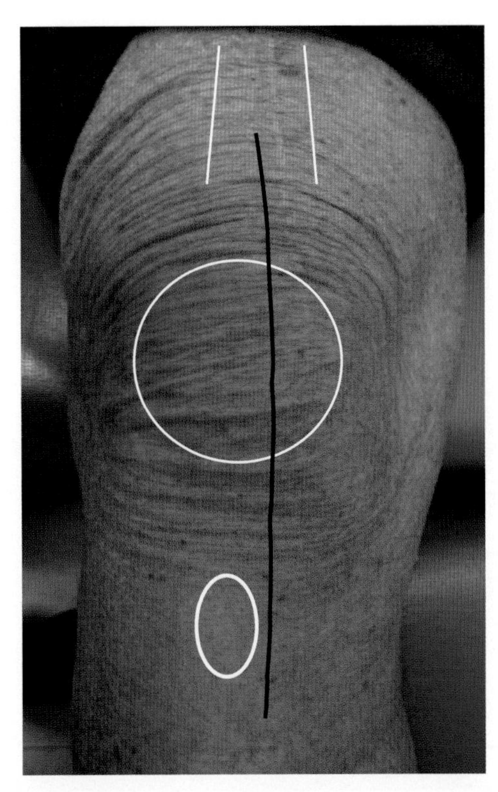

FIGURE 4–2. The incision is vertical, 13 to 15 cm in length, one third above and two thirds below the patella, centered above on the femoral shaft, over the medial third of the patella and ending just medial to the tibial tubercle.

The medial parapatellar approach can be used in virtually every case regardless of the preoperative deformity and range of motion. The three essential landmarks are the proximal medial border of the quadriceps tendon, a point halfway between the medialis insertion and the superior medial pole of the patella, and the medial border of the tubercle.

Two or three millimeters of the medial border of the quadriceps tendon are preserved proximally. At the superior pole of the patella, a soft tissue cuff is preserved to facilitate closure. At the tibial tubercle, a medial soft tissue cuff is carefully preserved for closure to the medial border of the patellar tendon. I mark the medial and lateral edges of the arthrotomy at the level of the superior pole of the patella to facilitate an anatomic closure at the end of the procedure (Fig. 4–3).

At the joint line, the arthrotomy severs the anterior horn of the medial meniscus. This facilitates eversion of the medial capsular tissue with the remaining meniscus attached for safe dissection of a subperiosteal anteromedial flap. Careful

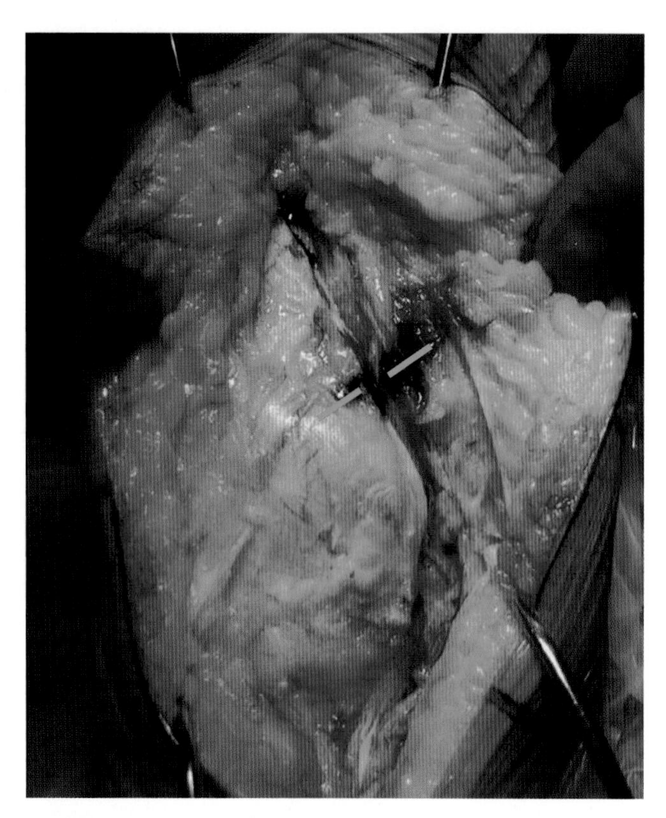

FIGURE 4–3. The medial and lateral borders of the arthrotomy are marked at the level of the superior pole of the patella to facilitate an anatomic closure.

preservation of this flap permits a secure distal closure at the end of the procedure. It also allows for the possibility of a side-to-side repair to the patellar tendon should the tendon's insertion be compromised (see Chapter 15).

The initial lateral dissection involves defining the infrapatellar bursa to the level of the patellar tendon insertion. A No. 10 blade is slid upside down into the bursa and tangential to the anterolateral tibial cortex. The scalpel is then passed coronally in this plane severing the coronary ligament and anterior horn of the lateral meniscus. In almost every case, the patella is then easily and safely everted. If eversion is difficult, I do not hesitate to perform a proximal release, as discussed in Chapter 8.

COMPLETING THE EXPOSURE

Before preparation of the bones is initiated, certain measures are taken to maximize exposure and mobilize the knee.

First, the patellofemoral ligament is released (Fig. 4–4). This is accomplished by putting a Z-retractor into the lateral compartment to tension this ligament. A curved hemostat is passed beneath its leading anterior edge, and a cutting cautery severs its fibers. This further mobilizes the patella and improves the exposure to the lateral compartment. Care must be taken to avoid inadvertently injuring the quadriceps tendon or placing the clamp so deeply as to involve the popliteus tendon or lateral collateral ligament.

Next, the Z-retractor is placed medially, and the anterior horn of the medial meniscus is excised. This gains access to

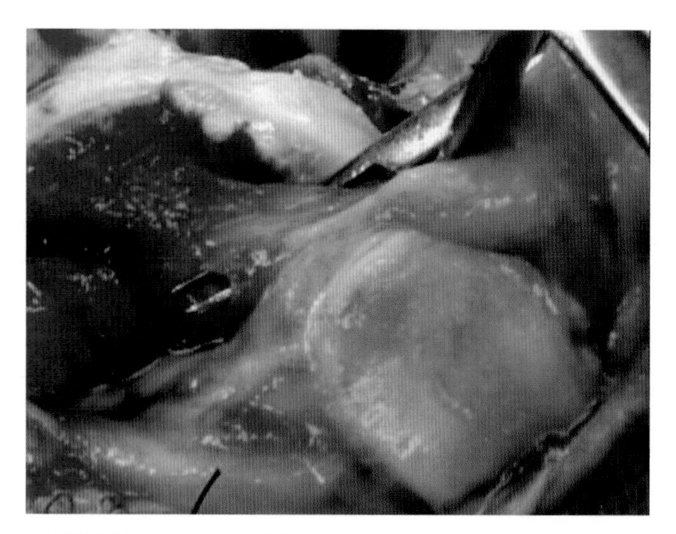

FIGURE 4–4. The patellofemoral ligament is identified and cut.

the plane between the deep medial collateral ligament and the superior border of the medial tibial plateau. A curved, 1-cm osteotome is inserted into this plane and tapped posteriorly until it dissects its way into the semimembranous bursa (Fig. 4–5). The anterior cruciate ligament, if intact, is completely sacrificed. The tibia can then be delivered in front of the femur by hyperflexing the knee, pulling the tibia forward, and externally rotating it.

Prior to removing the lateral meniscus, a scalpel is used to create a 1- to 2-cm slit just peripheral to the lateral meniscus at the junction between its anterior and middle thirds. Through this slit is placed a bent Hohman retractor, which will be used throughout the operation for lateral exposure.

The lateral compartment is now well exposed (Fig. 4–6). The entire lateral meniscus is removed with sharp dissection; I find it is easiest to start at the posterior horn and then return to the anterior horn and midsubstance until the resection is complete. The lateral inferior genicular artery will be encountered just peripheral to the meniscus during this dissection. The open lumen of both artery and vein are

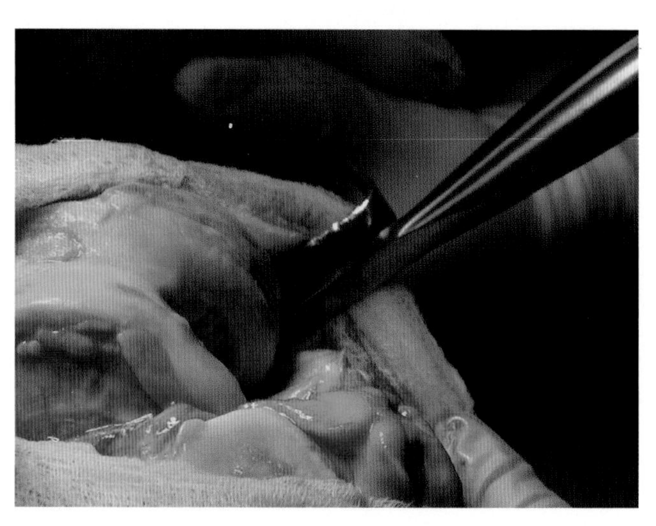

FIGURE 4–5. A curved, 1-cm osteotome dissects a plane between the deep medial collateral ligament (MCL) and proximal tibia.

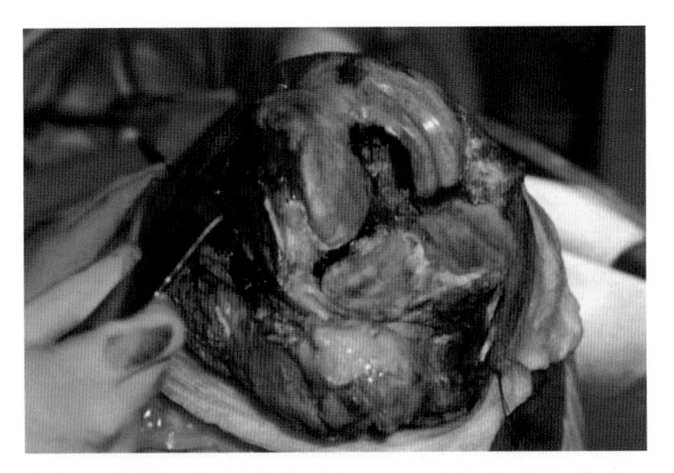

FIGURE 4–6. The tibia is delivered in front of the femur, and a bent Hohman retractor is placed just outside the lateral meniscus.

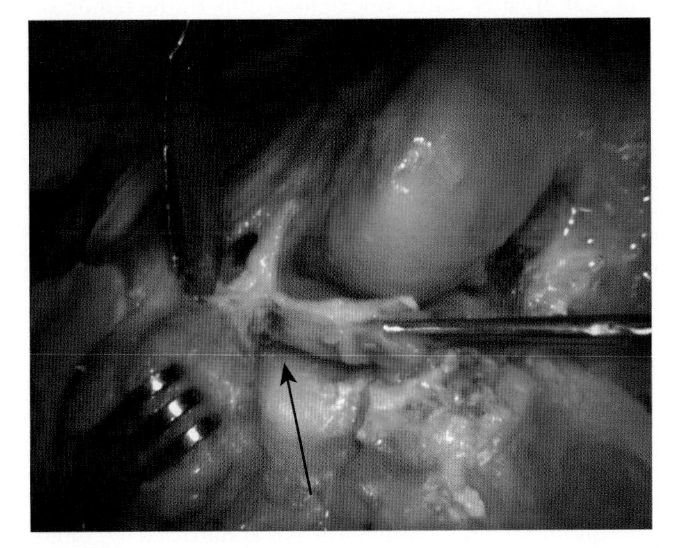

FIGURE 4–7. The lateral inferior genicular artery and vein are located and coagulated during excision of the lateral meniscus.

usually easily visualized in the posterior lateral corner of the knee and are coagulated to minimize postoperative bleeding (Fig. 4–7). Finally, the fat pad is dissected off the anterior proximal portion of the lateral tibial plateau to allow eventual placement of the tibial cutting jig. A small amount of the fat pad can be removed, if necessary, for better exposure.

PREPARATION OF THE FEMUR

To prepare the femur, it is important to first define the anatomy of the intercondylar notch and expose and define the PCL origin. Intercondylar osteophytes are removed with a $\frac{3}{8}$-inch osteotome and dissected free of the PCL (Fig. 4–8). The medullary canal of the femur is entered approximately 1 cm above the origin of the PCL and a few millimeters medial to the true center of the intercondylar notch (Fig. 4–9). The preoperative anteroposterior (AP) radiograph of the femur will help locate the entry point for the intramedullary alignment rod. This can be done by passing a line down the center of the shaft of the femur and seeing where it exits in the

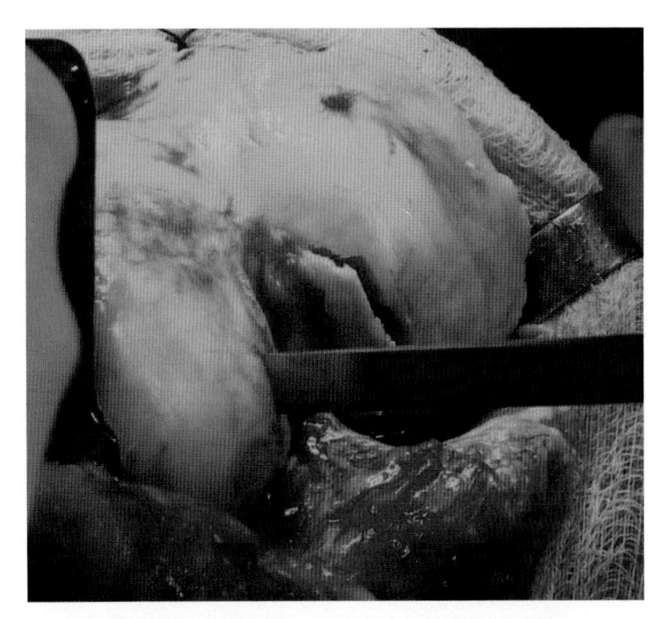

FIGURE 4–8. Intercondylar osteophytes are removed to define the PCL.

intercondylar notch (Fig. 4–10). As noted, it is usually several millimeters medial to the true center. If the canal were to be entered in the true center of the notch, the valgus angle chosen would be effectively increased by several degrees. I think this is the most common reason why surgeons inadvertently place the femoral component in too much valgus. They enter the canal in the true center of the notch and utilize a 7-degree valgus bushing. The actual angle of the distal femoral resection becomes 9 or 10 degrees of valgus.

Once the entry point is chosen, I prefer to use a small gouge to initiate the hole and allow the drill to subsequently precisely enter into the chosen spot. The drill hole should be larger than the diameter of the intramedullary alignment rod. I use a $\frac{3}{8}$-inch drill and a $\frac{1}{4}$-inch-diameter alignment rod. Some surgeons aspirate the fatty marrow from

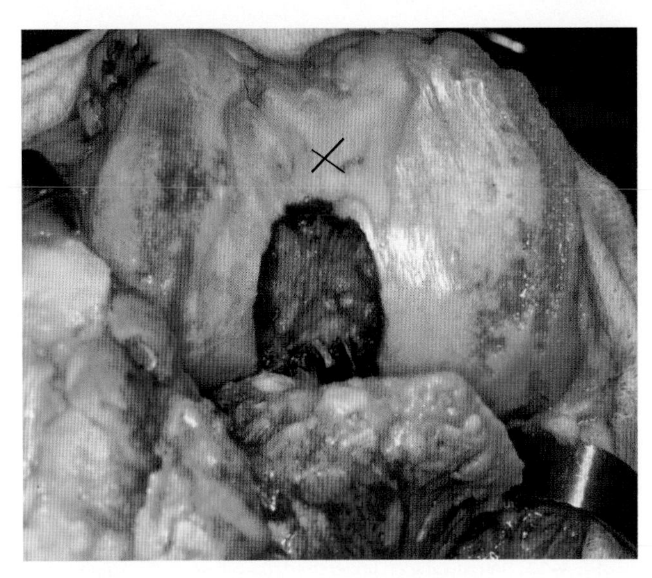

FIGURE 4–9. The entry point into the femoral canal is defined.

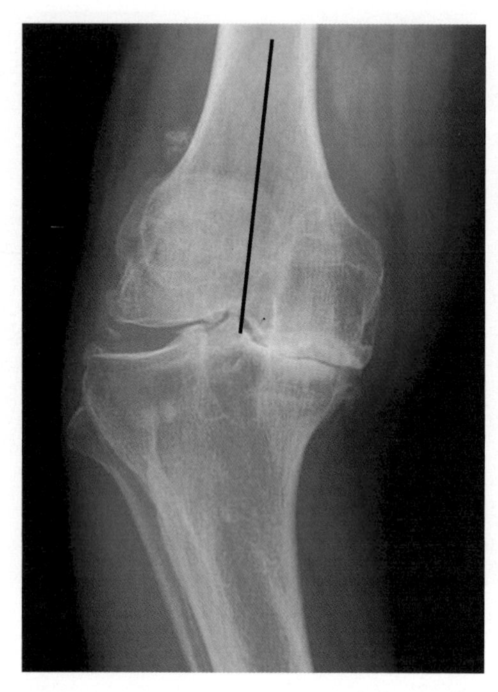

FIGURE 4–10. It is helpful to locate this entry point on the preoperative radiograph.

the distal femur and irrigate the canal. I have not found this to be necessary so long as the intramedullary alignment rod is smaller than the entry hole, fluted, and introduced slowly and gently. If there is any difficulty introducing the rod, the entry hole should be enlarged. On rare occasions when the rod fails to pass easily, I have found it helpful to first introduce an undersized rod to define the orientation of the canal. This method may reveal that the entry hole must be enlarged into one of four quadrants to allow easy passage (Fig. 4–11).

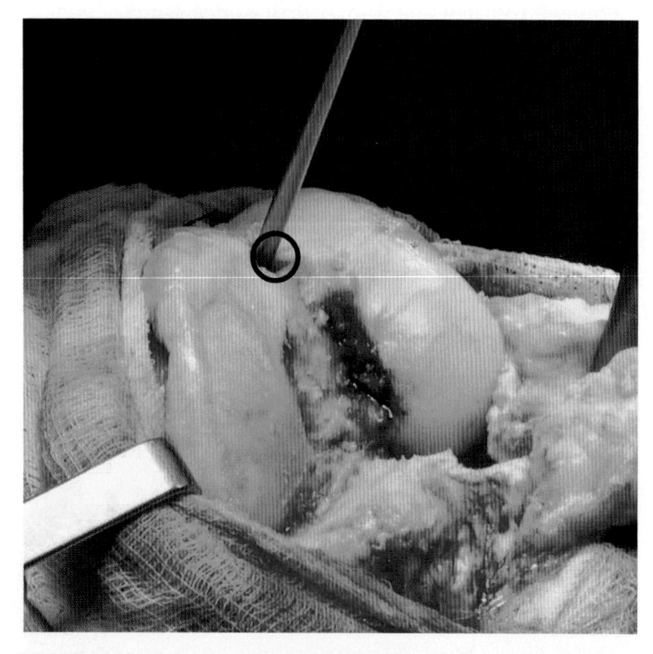

FIGURE 4–11. Introducing an undersized rod will show the surgeon how to reorient the larger rod for easier passage.

Distal Femoral Resection

The decision now has to be made about the amount of distal resection and the desired valgus angle. I think that many technique brochures are misleading concerning the amount of distal resection. They often recommend removing an amount of bone that is equivalent to the thickness of the metallic distal femoral condyle of the prosthesis. They should clarify that the amount of resection should also include the thickness of cartilage that was once present. Otherwise, the distal femoral resection will be approximately 2 mm more than a true "anatomic" amount. This would slightly elevate the joint line and possibly set up a knee that is looser in extension than in flexion (see Chapter 2).

In a PCL-preserving technique, the goal should be to restore the femoral joint line as precisely as possible and avoid a knee that is tighter in flexion than in extension. Erring toward underresecting the distal femoral condyle will achieve this goal. If, after initial preparation of both the femur and tibia, the knee is tighter in extension than in flexion, the distal femur can be revisited for 2 more millimeters of resection. This is quick and simple to accomplish. Excessive distal femoral resection is better tolerated in a PCL-substituting technique. Removing the PCL enlarges the flexion gap and allows the thicker polyethylene required to stabilize the knee in extension also to be tolerated in flexion.

In the presence of a preoperative flexion contracture, more than an anatomic amount of the distal condyle is resected to aid in correction of the contracture (see Chapter 9).

The Valgus Angle

The valgus angle chosen for the distal resection depends on preoperative templating and certain clinical factors. The goal in the majority of knee arthroplasties is to restore the mechanical axis to neutral. This is most efficiently achieved by creating a neutral mechanical axis at the distal femur and a neutral mechanical axis at the proximal tibia. To determine this angle, a long AP radiograph from the hip to the knee is taken in neutral rotation. A line is drawn from the center of the hip to the center of the knee. A perpendicular is then made at the knee to this line (Fig. 4–12). Finally, the angle formed by this line and a line of the center of the shaft of the femur can be measured. Usually the angle is between 5 and 7 degrees (Fig. 4–13).

Another advantage of this preoperative templating is to show the relative amounts of resection of the medial and lateral distal femoral condyles. Unless there is some sort of osteotomy, fracture, or dysplastic deformity, the amount of resection usually is slightly more medial than lateral. The line formed at the joint for a neutral mechanical axis will often be at the level of eburnated bone medially and intact cartilage laterally, or roughly 2 mm away from of the actual bone of the distal lateral condyle (Fig. 4–14). This information is useful when the distal cutting guide is applied and confirms what is shown on the preoperative templated radiograph. In severe valgus knees (see Chapter 6), this discrepancy can be quite considerable (see Fig. 6–8).

There are a few exceptions to attempting to accurately restore a neutral femoral mechanical axis. They all involve leaving the knee in slight (1 or 2 degrees) mechanical varus alignment. The reason would be to decrease stress on the

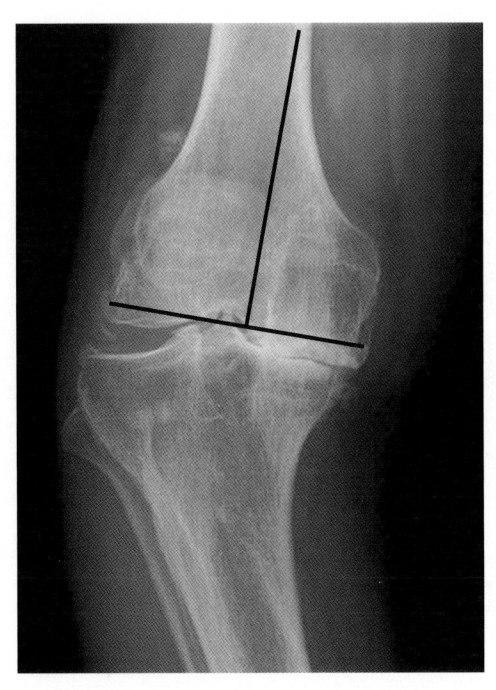

FIGURE 4–12. The angle of the resection is 90 degrees to a line from the center of the hip to the center of the knee.

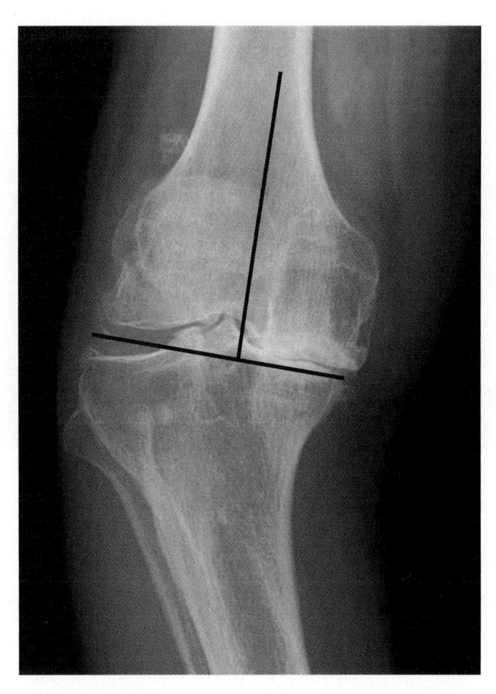

FIGURE 4–14. For most varus knees, a neutral mechanical axis at the joint line touches bone medially and intact cartilage laterally.

medial collateral ligament. The most common situation involves correction of a severe valgus deformity with an attenuated medial collateral ligament. By overcorrecting the alignment into a degree or two of mechanical varus, stress is taken off the medial side of the knee. Similarly, if there is inadvertent injury to the medial collateral ligament, some residual varus mechanical alignment will protect any surgical repair of the ligament (see Chapter 15).

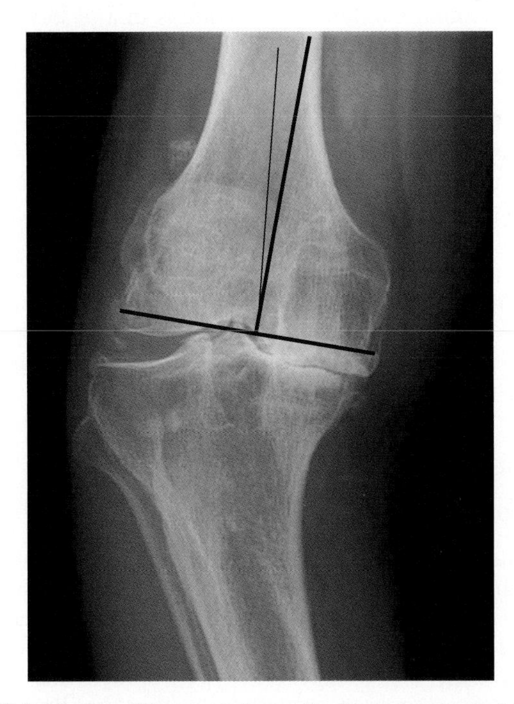

FIGURE 4–13. The difference between the lines representing the mechanical and anatomic axis is usually 5 to 7 degrees.

Although residual varus mechanical alignment is not to be encouraged in the routine primary knee, it is preferred for cosmetic purposes over residual mechanical valgus alignment in the obese patient with excessive medial soft tissues. Clinically, these patients appear to be in much more anatomic valgus than that represented by their radiographic alignment. Slight residual mechanical varus improves their cosmetic appearance. If a neutral mechanical axis is chosen for these patients, they should be forewarned of the apparent valgus appearance of the limb.

Sizing the Femur

I prefer to size the femur from posterior upward. This method is the most reliable to restore the joint line in flexion, balance the PCL, and minimize the chance for mid-flexion laxity. Two skids slide under the posterior condyles and a moveable stylus measures the AP dimension of the femur based on the anterior cortex just superior to the trochlea. If the measurement shows a dimension at a half size or larger, I will use the larger size. An exception to this rule would be a patient with poor preoperative flexion where an attempt is made to make the prosthetic trochlea as flush with the anterior cortex as possible to increase quadriceps excursion. Another exception would be the patient (usually female) whose medial lateral dimension is proportionally smaller than their AP dimension. Using the larger size would cause too much mediolateral overhang. Thus, the smaller size is chosen (see Chapter 15).

For half sizes and smaller, I choose the smaller size. The two options that allow downsizing without notching the anterior cortex are to make the distal femoral resection in a few degrees of flexion or to size the femur from anterior downward. See Chapter 15 for the techniques and consequences of using these two methods.

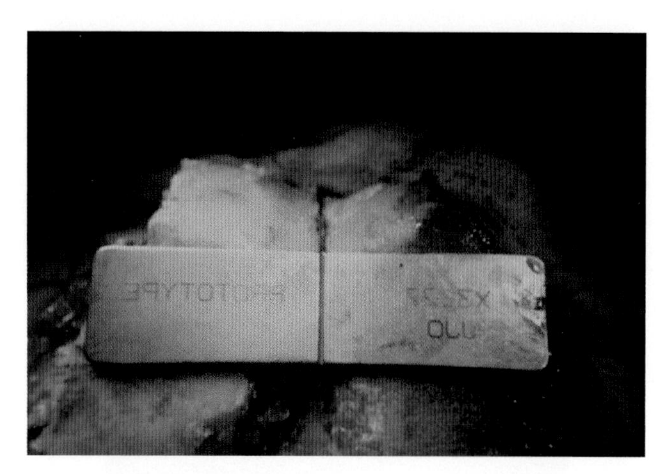

FIGURE 4–15. The Whiteside line is perpendicular to a line down the deepest part of the trochlear groove.

Determining the Rotational Alignment of the Femoral Component

After the femoral component has been sized, its proper rotational alignment must be determined. As discussed in Chapters 7 and 15, at least four methods are popularly used to determine femoral component rotation. These include the Whiteside line (the trans-sulcus axis) (Fig. 4–15), the transepicondylar axis (Fig. 4–16), 3 degrees of external rotation off the posterior condyles (Fig. 4–17), and rotational alignment that yields flexion gap symmetry (Fig. 4-18*A* and *B*). During surgery, I assess all four methods, but my primary consideration is flexion gap symmetry.[2] The sizing guide I use provides for the placement of pinholes for the subsequent cutting guides that can automatically build in 3 degrees of external rotation (see Fig. 4–17). I use these to set my preliminary rotation and then add more external rotation as needed to achieve a rectangular flexion gap. To build in more external rotation for the cutting guide, I must either move the medial pinhole upward or the lateral pinhole downward. A convenient instrument for this purpose is a navicular gouge. This is tapped into the new location for the pinhole at the same time displacing the bone from this new position to fill the defect present at the original pinhole.

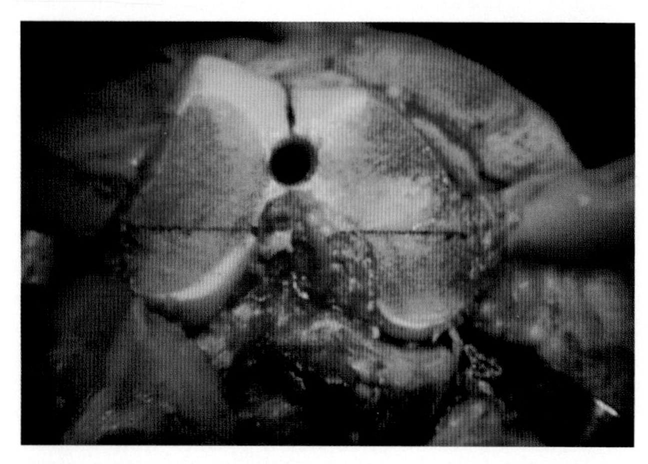

FIGURE 4–16. The transepicondylar axis is usually parallel to the Whiteside line.

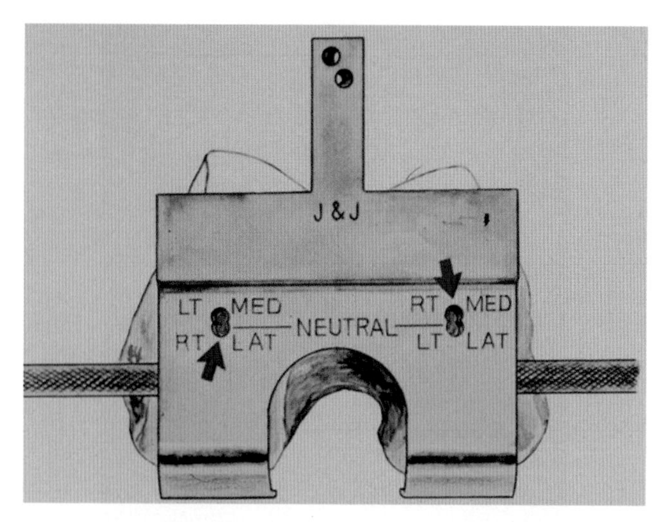

FIGURE 4–17. Most total knee systems provide a way to build in 3 degrees of external femoral rotation off the posterior condylar axis. In this system, the upper hole is pinned medially and the lower hole is pinned laterally.

For varus knees, the medial pinhole is almost always moved upward to provide more medial space in flexion. For valgus knees, owing to the hypoplastic lateral femoral condyle, the lateral hole is usually moved downward (Fig. 4–19*A* and *B*). An exception occurs when the size of the femoral component chosen is already flush with the anterior femoral cortex. If the lateral side is moved downward in this case, the anterior cortex will be notched. Instead, the medial hole is moved upward.

It is rare for a knee to require internal rotation off the posterior condylar axis to achieve flexion gap symmetry. I have encountered this in only two situations. The first is in a severe varus knee that has suffered erosion of the posterior medial femoral condyle. The second is in a postosteotomy knee in which the tibial joint line is now in excessive valgus (see Chapter 10).

PLACEMENT OF THE AP CUTTING JIG

Most AP cutting jigs have spikes that will fit into the holes created through the initial sizing guide. The guide is seated flush with the distal condylar resections. The proper contact of the jig with the bone should be assessed by viewing it directly from the side. Some jigs provide ancillary pins that will further secure the cutting jig on the end of the distal femur (Fig. 4–20).

Completing the Femoral Cuts

Trochlear Resection

The anterior or trochlear cut is made first. The main concern with this cut is to be certain to avoid notching the anterior cortex. The amount of resection for each individual case can be gauged by reviewing the preoperative lateral radiograph. Occasionally, the trochlea is hypertrophic with a large amount of osteophyte formation creating the illusion that the trochlea resection will be excessive. At the opposite end

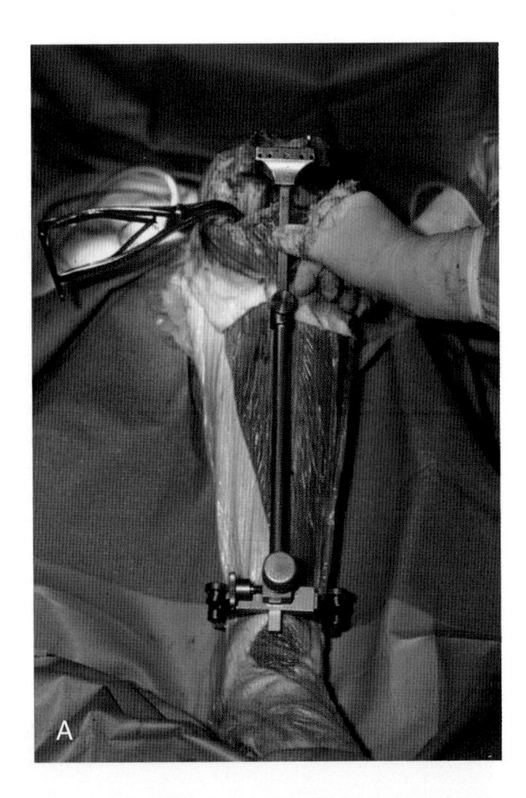

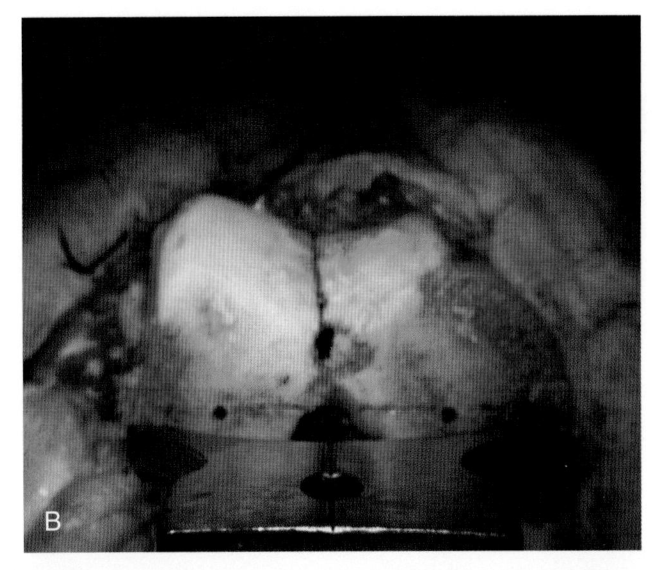

FIGURE 4–18. *A*, A rectangular flexion gap can be established by tensing the medial and lateral tissues and relating the femoral rotation to the external tibial alignment jig. *B*, The pinholes should be parallel to the alignment jig.

of the spectrum is the "hypoplastic" trochlea seen in patients with patella alta and patellofemoral dysplasia (Fig. 4–21). If there is ever concern that the trochlear resection might be excessive, a conservative initial resection is made approximately 2 mm proud of the cutting jig.

This cut will expose the proximal junction between the trochlea and the anterior cortex of the femur and allow a more accurate assessment to be made concerning the potential for notching the anterior cortex. I would recommend against the practice of many surgeons who remove the fat overlying the anterior cortex and incise the periosteum. I believe that this action predisposes the knee to form heterotopic bone in this area, which could limit postoperative quadriceps excursion (see Chapter 8). If it appears that the planned trochlear resection would, in fact, notch the anterior cortex, the femur should be recut in a few degrees of flexion (see Chapter 15), or the pinholes for the cutting jig should be displaced the appropriate distance anteriorly by means of the navicular gouge technique.

Posterior Condylar Resection

The posterior condylar cuts are next completed. The medial collateral ligament is in jeopardy during the medial posterior condylar resection (see Chapter 15). It is important to have a well-placed medial retractor to protect the ligament from the medial excursion of the saw blade (see Fig. 15–5). If a wide saw blade is initially utilized, the cuts are best completed with a narrower saw blade or an osteotome.

Chamfer Cuts

The chamfer cuts are next completed. Most systems provide an AP cutting guide with slots for the chamfer cuts

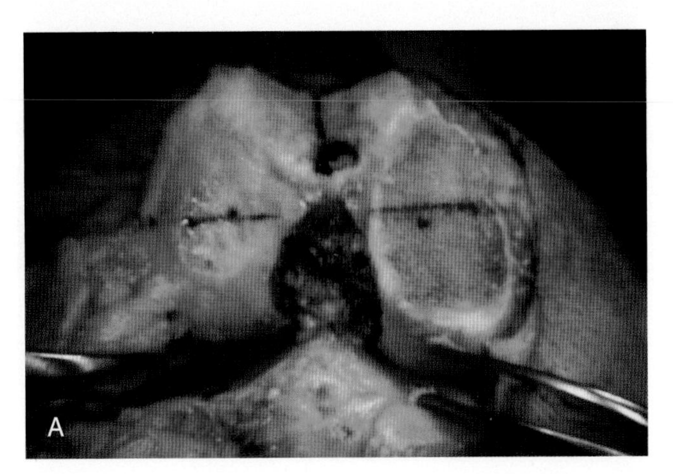

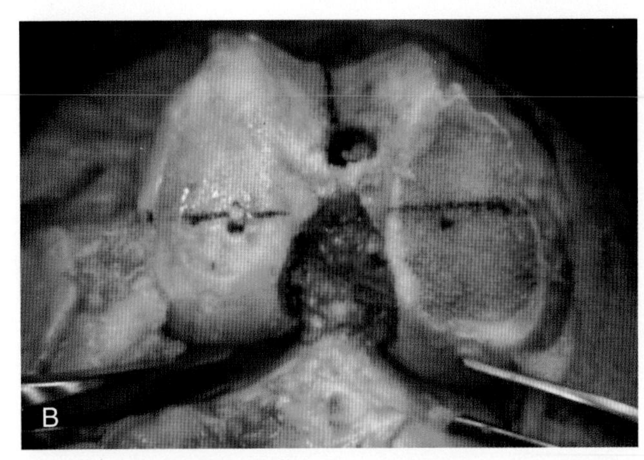

FIGURE 4–19. *A*, In this valgus knee, more external rotation of the pinholes is necessary for flexion gap symmetry. *B*, To increase the external rotation, the lateral pinhole is lowered with a navicular gouge.

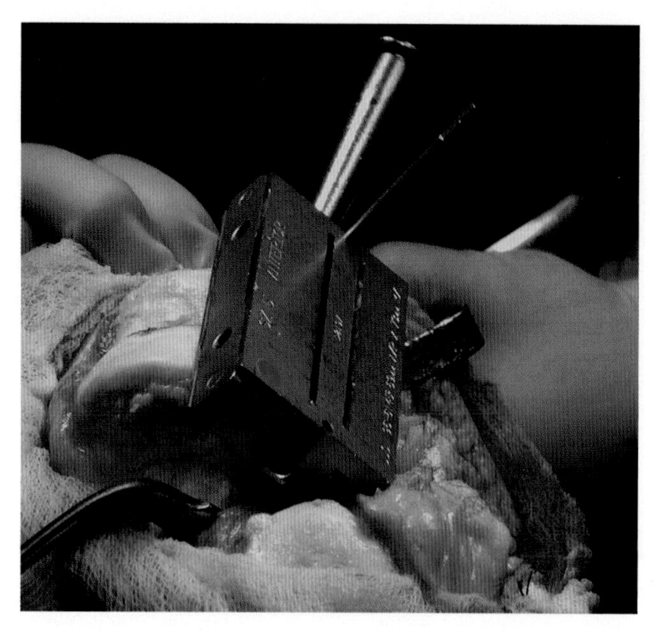

FIGURE 4–20. Placement of the AP cutting jig.

(Fig. 4–22*A*). Despite this, I like to revisit the chamfer cuts with a separate chamfer guide. I do this because sometimes the AP cutting block is not fully or symmetrically seated or may lift off slightly from the end of the femur. Redoing the chamfer cuts with the isolated block ensures that they are accurate (Fig. 4–22*B*).

Final Preparation of the Femur

Final preparation of the femur is accomplished after tibial preparation when there is greater posterior exposure. The trial femoral component is applied for the first time. I use a femoral inserter that holds the component rigidly so that I can apply an extension force as the trial is seated (Fig. 4–23). Femoral components tend to go into flexion when they are first applied. There are two reasons for this. The first is a trochlear cut that diverges slightly more than dictated by the anterior cutting guide. The second is due to underresection of a posterior condyle, almost always on the medial side. The hard medial bone deflects the saw blade into a diverging pathway.

Both situations can be assessed and remedied by reapplying the AP cutting guide when the chamfer cuts have been completed. Slight divergence of the saw blade that is not apparent with the chamfer cuts intact becomes obvious when they are missing.

Once the trial femoral component is seated, it must be properly positioned in the medial-lateral dimension. Medial or lateral overhang of the prosthesis must be avoided and is most commonly seen in the female patient (see Chapter 15). The optimal mediolateral position for the component is flush with the lateral distal femoral cortex at the level of the trochlea and distal condyle (Fig. 4–24). The ability to achieve

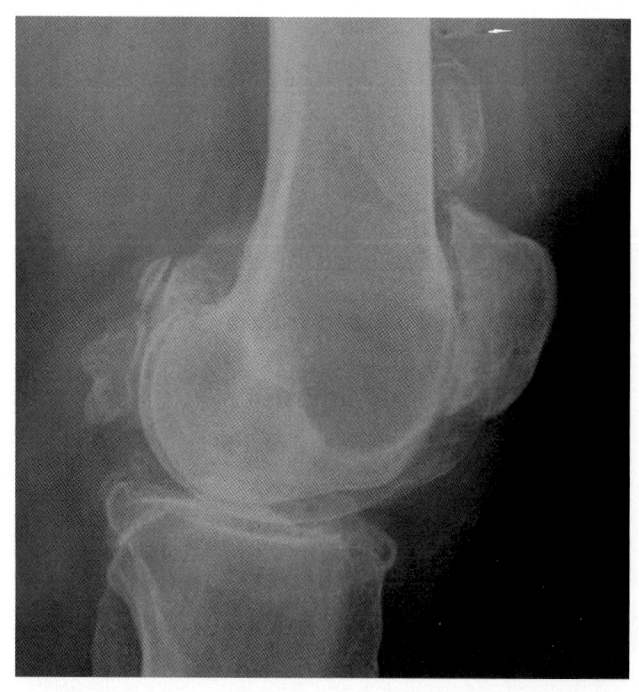

FIGURE 4–21. Lateral radiograph of a femur with a "hypoplastic" trochlea.

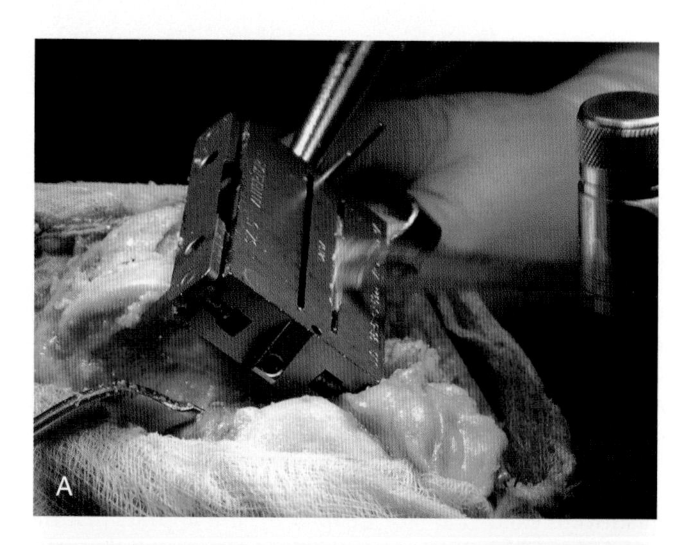

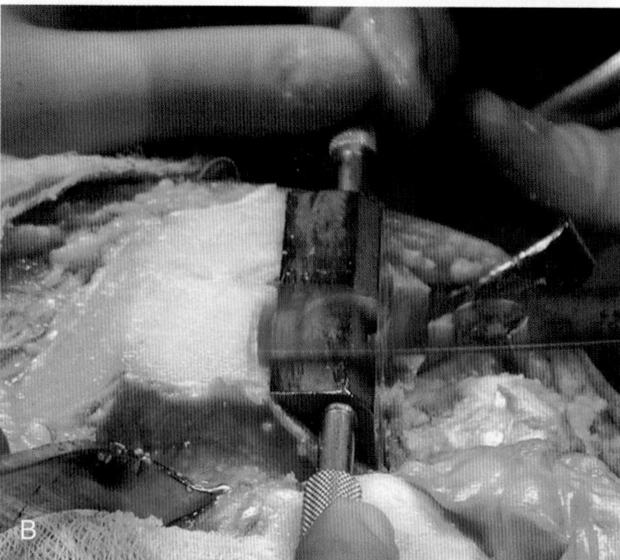

FIGURE 4–22. *A*, Making the chamfer cut through a slotted guide. *B*, Confirming the accuracy of the chamfer cut with an open guide.

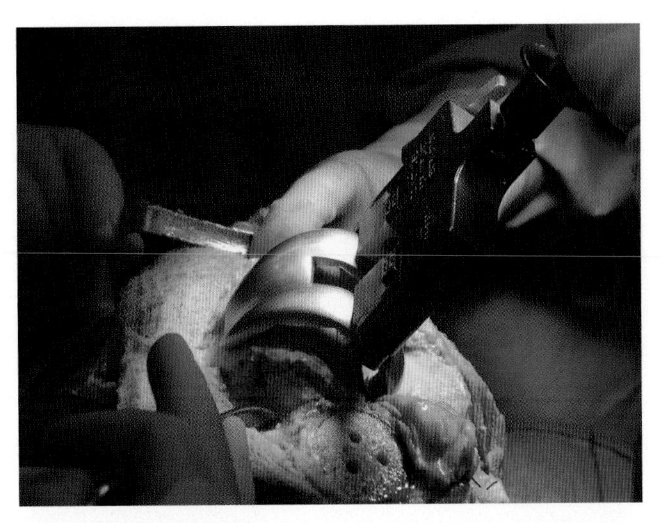

FIGURE 4–23. Applying the trial femoral component for the first time while applying an extension force.

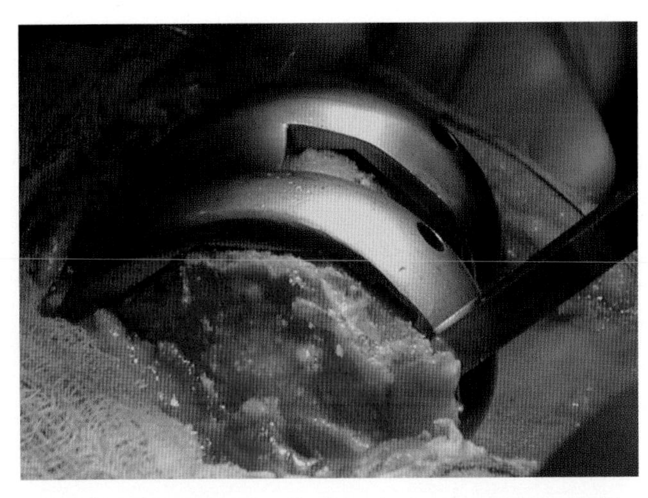

FIGURE 4–25. Any overhanging lateral osteophytes are removed.

this position varies with the prosthetic design. Only asymmetric femoral components can optimally cap the cut trochlear surface of the femur. Symmetric components that come flush with the medial cortex at the level of the trochlea cannot possibly fully cap the cut surface of the trochlea. Intuitively, this will compromise patellar tracking in the first 30 degrees of flexion.

After the femoral component has been moved laterally to be flush with the lateral cortex, any remaining peripheral osteophytes are removed. It is most important to achieve this at the level of the origin of the popliteus tendon to prevent a possible popliteus impingement syndrome[3] (Fig. 4–25; see Chapter 15). Any overhanging medial osteophytes are also removed flush with the femoral component.

Finally, it is important to remove posterior condylar osteophytes and any uncapped posterior condylar bone. This is best achieved with the trial femoral component in place and the tibial resection completed. While an assistant elevates the femur using a bone hook in the intercondylar

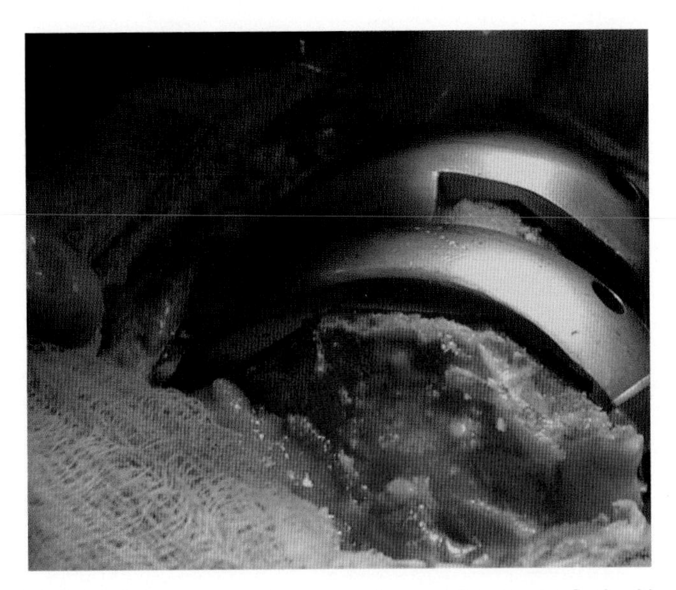

FIGURE 4–24. The femoral component is positioned to be flush with the lateral cortex.

notch, a curved $\frac{3}{8}$-inch osteotome is passed tangentially along all the borders of both posterior condyles to outline the posterior osteophytes and uncapped posterior condylar bone (see Fig. 9–4*A*). The trial is then removed, and the outlined bone is resected (see Fig.9–4*B*). The surgeon's finger can be used to palpate the posterior recesses for any retained bone or loose bodies. The ability to easily pass an index finger into these recesses usually indicates that the flexion gap is large enough to receive a 10-mm-thick composite tibial component.

ASSESSING THE POTENTIAL FOR CEMENTLESS FEMORAL FIXATION

The use of cementless femoral fixation remains controversial. Most surgeons familiar with cementless femoral fixation report excellent results with this technique. Success is obviously dependent on the initial primary fixation of the component. My own experience with the use of cementless porous-ingrowth femoral components has been excellent and equivalent to results with cemented fixation (see Chapter 16).

I have collected some data on bilateral simultaneous knee arthroplasties with a cementless femur on one side and a cemented one on the other. Fluoroscopically controlled evaluation of the lateral radiograph of these patients indicates that the femoral zone IV interface of the cementless components is more favorable than the zone IV interface in cemented components (Fig. 4–26). This finding has implications for long-term survivorship, since zone IV lucency may predispose the knee to late femoral component loosening[4] or allow ingress of wear debris and subsequent osteolysis. For this reason, I still advocate consideration of cementless femoral fixation in younger patients. (The zone system was developed by the Knee Society.[5])

The intraoperative criterion for cementless fixation combines the assessment of the precision of the fit as viewed from the side and of the force required to disimpact the trial from the femoral bone. The disimpaction test is admittedly crude but appears to be effective in screening patients. If the trial femoral component can be removed by hand or with a very light tap of the slap hammer of the insertion/extraction

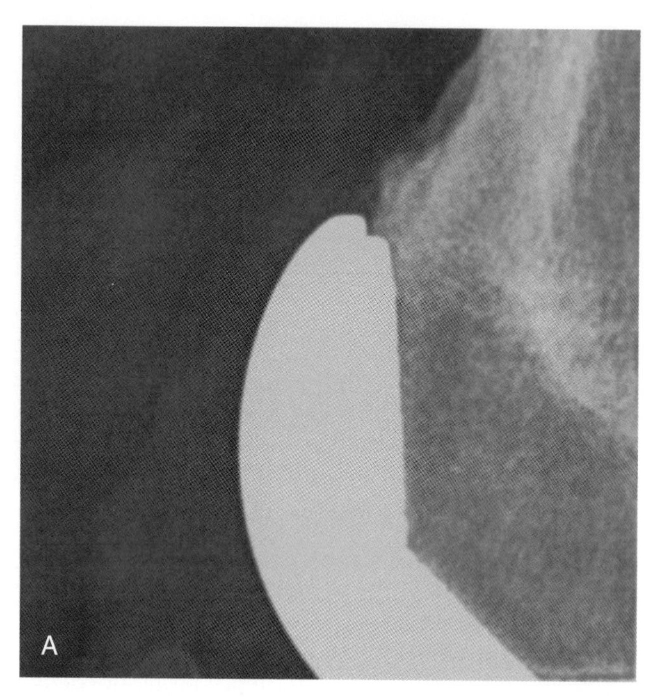

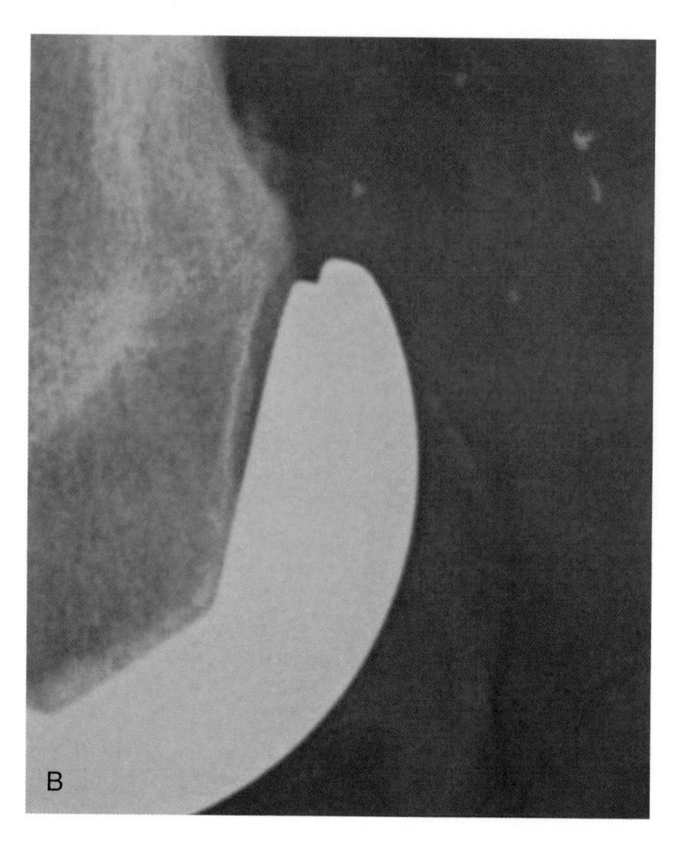

FIGURE 4–26. *A*, The uncemented side of a bilateral case shows no zone IV lucency. *B*, The cemented side of a bilateral case shows zone IV demarcation.

device, the femoral component always is cemented. If it takes multiple taps of the slap hammer and trial extraction is difficult, cementless fixation is appropriate. In borderline cases, the femur should be cemented.

The precision of the cuts as viewed from the side does not appear to be as critical to the success of cementless fixation. If there are large gaps, the femur should obviously be cemented. If there are small gaps, they can be filled with bone slurry, and clinical success of the technique can be expected if the component passes the disimpaction test.

On follow-up lateral radiographs of cementless femoral components, variations in the bone density pattern are sometimes seen depending on the intimacy of contact between the femoral component and the bone in any specific area (Fig. 4–27).

PREPARATION OF THE PATELLA

Clearing the Quadriceps Tendon

Any residual synovial tissue on the quadriceps tendon just above the superior pole of the patella should be removed to avoid the potential for postoperative soft tissue crepitus in a PCL-retaining technique or the clunk syndrome in a PCL-substituting design (see Fig. 2–13 and Chapter 2).

Measuring Patellar Thickness and Applying a Cutting Jig

Patellar thickness is measured prior to preparation. Female patellae usually are 22 to 24 mm thick and male patellae 24 to 26 mm.[6] If available, a patellar cutting jig is applied (Fig. 4–28). It should be set to allow a bone remnant that amounts to the precut patellar thickness minus the thickness of the prosthetic patellar button. Preoperative templating can help plan the resection, especially in dysplastic cases (see Figs. 7–19, 7–20, and 7-21).

Cutting the Patella

I prefer to cut the patella from medial to lateral and from chondro-osseous junction to junction. On the lateral side, all remaining cartilage should be removed down to a sclerotic

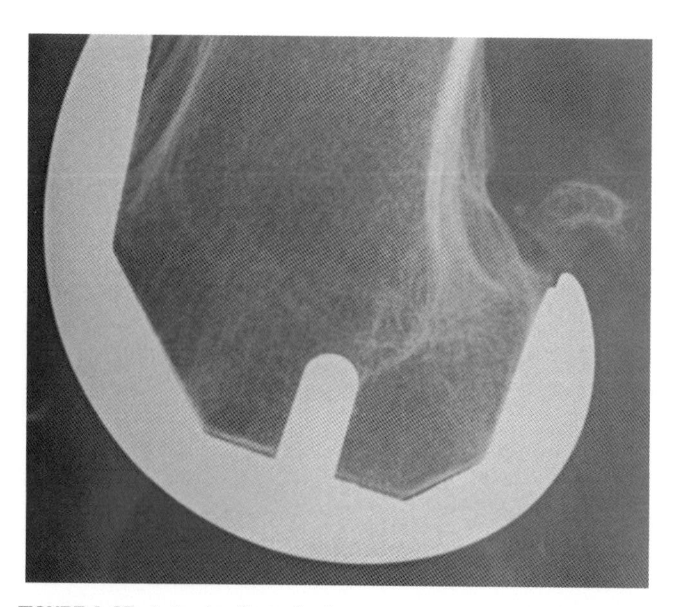

FIGURE 4–27. Lateral radiograph of an asymptomatic cementless femoral component shows zones of osteopenia where contact was incomplete.

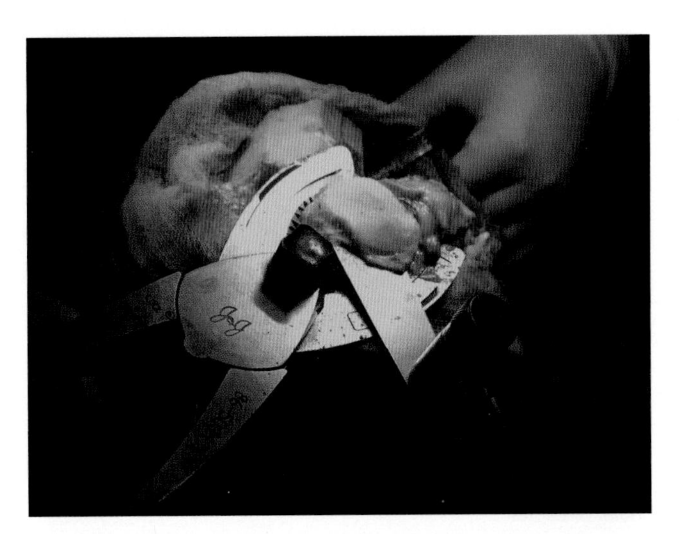

FIGURE 4–28. A patellar cutting jig can facilitate the resection.

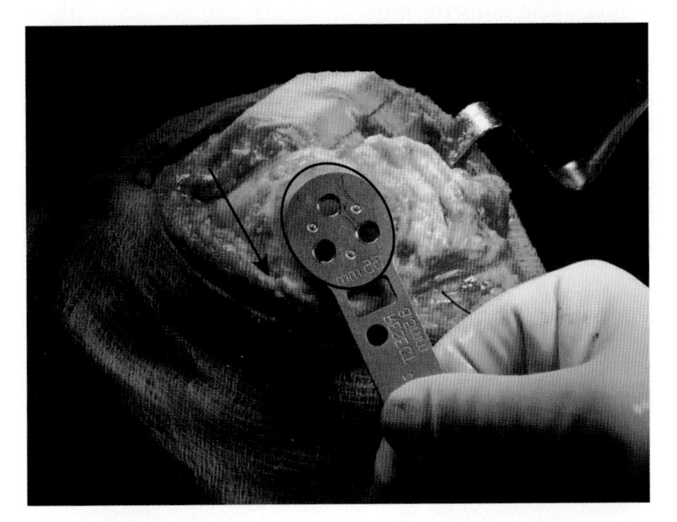

FIGURE 4–29. Medial placement of the patellar template.

bone surface. The thickness of the patellar remnant can be measured off the resected medial side. Avoid oversizing the patella in both the anteroposterior and mediolateral dimensions. If undersized, the patellar prosthesis should be displaced medially to facilitate patellar tracking (Fig. 4–29). The uncapped lateral bone should be outlined and then chamfered to relieve possible bone impingement on the metal trochlea (Fig. 4–30). The composite thickness should be measured after preparation to avoid "overstuffing" the patellofemoral compartment. After the patella is properly sized, lug holes are drilled through the appropriate template.

PREPARATION OF THE TIBIA

Either the femur or the tibia can be prepared first for TKA. I prefer femur first in primary surgeries because after femoral resection has been completed, the tibial exposure is facilitated. In revision surgery, however, I always prepare the tibia first. In a primary procedure, the amount of femoral and tibial bone resection and the alignment angles are independent of each other if the surgeon's goal is to perform

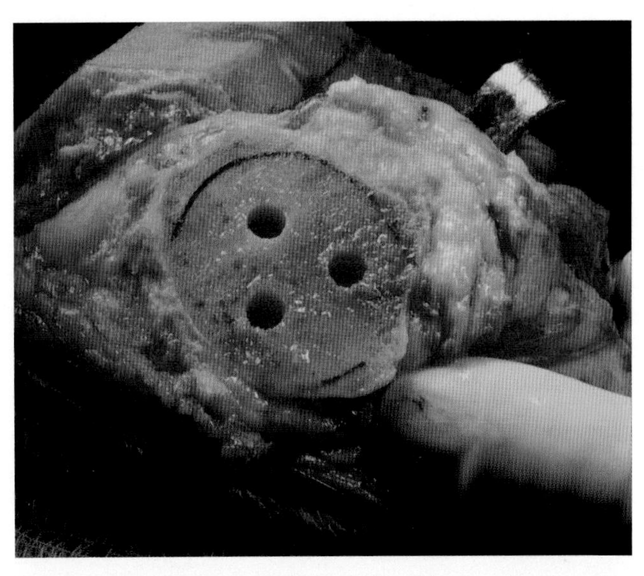

FIGURE 4–30. Uncapped patellar bone should be chamfered to relieve potential impingement of the metal trochlea.

measured resections based on thickness of components and maintenance of the joint line. The only bone cuts that are dependent on one another are those that determine the rotational alignment of the femoral component. Tibia-first surgeons create flexion gap symmetry by using spacer blocks. Femur-first surgeons can establish flexion gap symmetry by relating the femoral component rotation to an external tibial alignment device.

Determining the Amount of Tibial Resection

As for the femur, I prefer a measured resection technique based on the thickness of component to replace the resected tissue. For a prosthesis with a composite thickness of 8 mm, 8 mm would be removed from the more prominent plateau, almost invariably the lateral side. This measurement would include any residual cartilage.

If a metal-backed component is being used, a composite thickness as much as 10 mm may be required to allow for the minimum 6 mm of polyethylene required by the FDA (depending on the thickness of the metal tray). Most total knee systems apply a stylus to assess this thickness (Fig. 4–31).

Alternatively, the amount of resection can be based on removing 0 to 2 mm from the deficient side. This method should not be used if it means that more than 12 or 13 mm will be removed from the lateral side. In these cases, the deficient side will require some form of augmentation (see Chapter 12).

Intramedullary versus Extramedullary Alignment

Most total knee systems provide the option of intramedullary or extramedullary tibial alignment devices. I prefer the extramedullary method for several reasons. Unlike the assessment of alignment on the femoral side, proximal and distal anatomic landmarks are readily visible on the tibia. Using extramedullary alignment avoids instrumentation of the medullary canal of the tibia with its potential for generating fat embolization and for propagating the extent of any po-

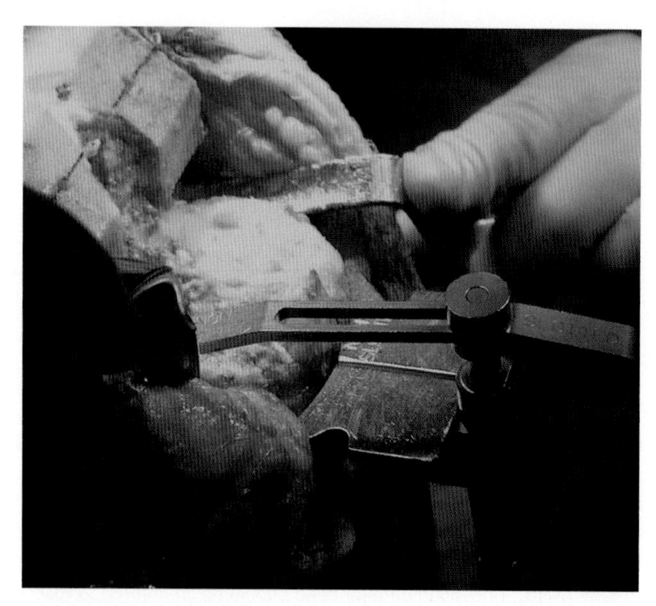

FIGURE 4–31. A stylus can measure the amount of tibial resection from either the high or the low side.

tential postoperative infection. In addition, many tibias have a valgus bow, especially in the patient with a constitutional valgus alignment (see Chapter 6).

In these patients, long films are required to fully evaluate the bowing and guide the surgeon as to where to enter the medullary canal at the level of the tibial plateau. In some tibias, the bow is so excessive that an intramedullary alignment rod cannot be accommodated. If the surgeon insists upon its use, the tibial resection will be prejudiced into significant valgus. In knees undergoing revision where the surgeon is using a long-press-fit intramedullary tibial extension, intramedullary alignment devices are appropriate. In some cases of bowed tibias, offset stems may be necessary.

Determining Alignment of the Tibial Resection with Extramedullary Devices

Several maneuvers are helpful in increasing the accuracy of an extramedullary alignment device. Proximal and distal landmarks are readily available. Proximally, the resection guide ideally should be centered between the medial and lateral tibial cortices. In reality, this is difficult to achieve because an external alignment device is usually displaced several millimeters medial to the true center because of the tibial tubercle, patellar tendon, and fat pad (Fig. 4–32). As long as the surgeon is aware of this and compensates for it, it will not prejudice the cut into varus. The distal anatomic landmark for an extramedullary device is the readily palpable sharp anterior crest of the tibia.

I do not use the foot, specifically the second metatarsal, as a distal landmark, since any rotational foot abnormality will distort this measurement. The sharp anterior crest of the tibia at the level of the malleoli is an anatomic landmark that is independent of any foot or ankle deformity and is readily palpable, even in obese patients. Some surgeons suggest bisecting the inter-malleolar distance or the soft tissue girth at the ankle. We have documented that the true center of the ankle is approximately 3 mm medial to these two

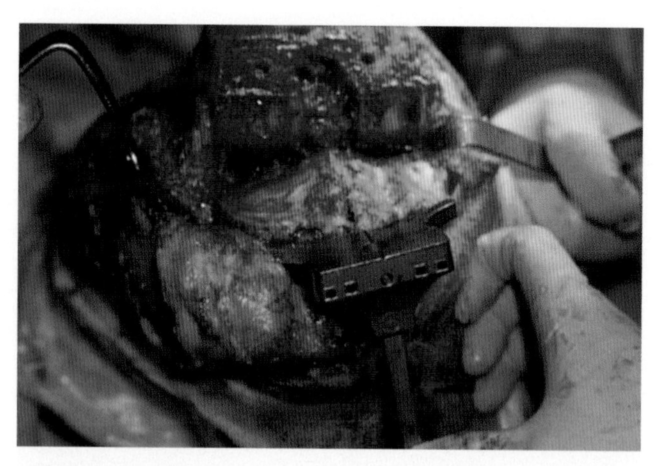

FIGURE 4–32. Extramedullary tibial guides are usually applied slightly medial of center.

points.[7] The surgeon must therefore compensate with an adjustment at the ankle.

The most effective way to compensate for the potential alignment distortions that exist proximally and distally is to have a moveable ankle device that can be displaced medially (Fig. 4–33). Six millimeters of medial displacement will usually compensate for the 3 mm occurring proximally and the 3 mm occurring distally, avoiding varus malalignment of the tibial resection.

Posterior Tibial Slope

Posterior tibial slope in the "normal" knee can be quite variable. I have seen it be anywhere between 0 and 15 degrees.

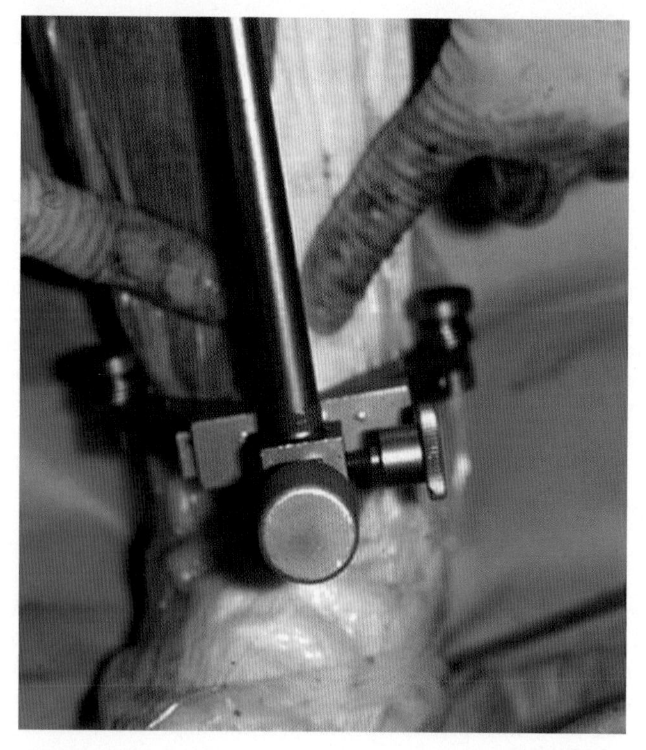

FIGURE 4–33. The distal ankle adjustment should be translated medially up to 6 mm and centered over the distal tibial anterior crest.

In arthroplasty, posterior slope has both advantages and disadvantages. Advantages include opening up the flexion gap to make PCL balancing easier and enhancing metal-to-plastic contact in maximum knee flexion.

Disadvantages include the promotion of too much rollback of the femur on the tibia in a nonconforming design and mandating that the articulating surfaces must hyperextend on one another when the limb itself is in full extension. I like to apply some posterior slope to the tibial resection but avoid an excessive amount. Generally I use approximately 5 degrees. I achieve this using an external alignment device by moving the ankle adjustment anteriorly away from the ankle. Depending on the length of the limb, 1 or 2 degrees of posterior slope is applied for every 5 mm of anterior displacement of the jig. The effect will obviously be greater for short limbs and smaller for longer limbs.

There are at least three situations in which no posterior slope should be applied. The first is in the presence of a severe preoperative flexion contracture. Increased anterior (vs. posterior) tibial resection aids in the correction of a flexion contracture (see Chapter 9). The second situation is in the presence of a tibia with an abnormal upward rather than downward slope. This is most commonly seen after high tibial osteotomy or in the presence of a healed proximal tibial fracture (Fig. 4–34). The third situation occurs when using a knee system that allows limited hyperextension between the articulating surfaces. This is most commonly seen in posterior stabilized designs where the stabilizing post will impinge on the anterior aspect of the intercondylar housing for the peg (see Fig. 2–14). Specific designs vary in their forgiveness, and surgeons must be aware of the limitation of the system they are using (see Chapter 2).

PERFORMING THE TIBIAL RESECTION

When the proximal tibial resection is being performed, it is important that the surgeon's arm is braced against the tibia so that the saw blade is prevented from accidentally cutting out of sclerotic bone and possibly injuring adjacent soft tissues. I brace my left fist up against the proximal tibia while controlling and aiming the saw with my right hand. It is extremely important that the medial collateral ligament (MCL) be protected during the resection by placement of a metallic retractor between the ligament and the medial border of the proximal tibia (see Fig. 15–6).

There are several ways to protect the PCL during the resection. One is to create a small slot in front of the PCL using an oscillating saw and then insert a 1-cm-wide osteotome into the slot to protect the posterior tissues from the excursion of the oscillating saw. A second way is to preserve a wedge-shaped island of tibial spine in front of the ligament by outlining this with an oscillating saw or reciprocating saw. I prefer the latter method and use a wide blade to initiate the tibial resection to the mid-coronal plane and then outline the saved wedge of tibial spine with the saw blade. I then switch to a narrow blade and complete the medial and lateral resections. The preserved island can be denuded of soft tissue in situ with the oscillating saw and severed just in front of the PCL to be used as a bone plug to seal off the femur where the hole was made for the intramedullary femoral alignment device. The tibial surface is best exposed by placement of a Z-retractor medially, a bent Hohmann retractor laterally, and a forklike retractor posteriorly that straddles the PCL tibial insertion (Fig. 4–35).

Sizing the Tibia

Once the tibial resection has been completed, the tibia can be sized. Most systems allow independent sizing of the femur and the tibia so that one size larger or smaller on either side is compatible. I have rarely seen a two-size discrepancy. This might occur if one bone is affected with Paget's disease or if

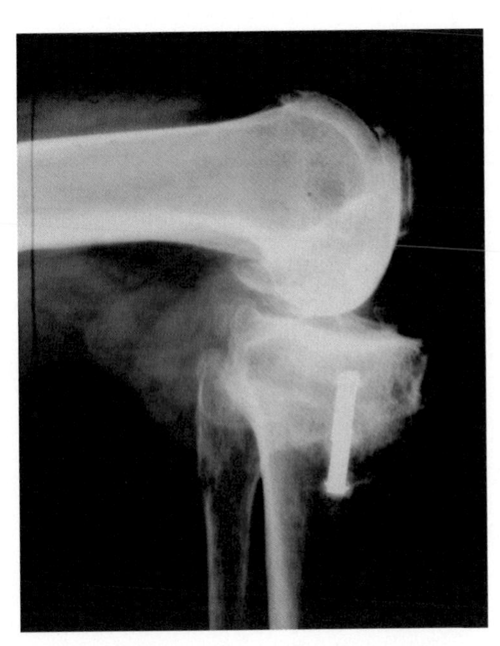

FIGURE 4–34. No posterior slope should be applied when there is pathologic upslope from a healed osteotomy or fracture.

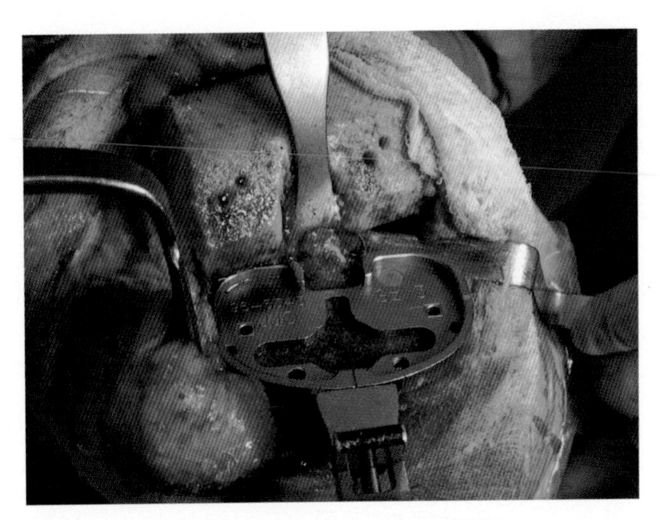

FIGURE 4–35. Excellent exposure can be achieved for sizing the tibial component in both PCL-retaining and -substituting techniques.

its size influenced by the specifics of a healed fracture. The goal of sizing the tibia is to maximally cap the bone while avoiding significant tray overhang. Any overhang anterior to the mid-coronal plane of the tibia can be symptomatic, causing a painful soft tissue inflammation (Fig. 4–36). Posterior overhang is frequent on the lateral side because this dimension is generally shorter than the AP dimension on the medial side. Slight posterior overhang (several millimeters) appears to be well tolerated and rarely symptomatic. Overhang of more than a few millimeters could conceivably cause popliteus impingement (see Chapter 15).

When I have to choose between tibial sizes, I prefer to use the smaller size to avoid the possibility of symptomatic overhang. In the presence of a severe varus deformity requiring release of medial structures, I intentionally undersize the tray and shift it laterally. The uncapped medial bone is outlined and removed effectively, accomplishing a medial release by shortening the distance between the origin and insertion of the medial collateral ligament (see Chapter 5).

Determining the Rotational Alignment of the Tibial Component

At least four ways have been described to orient the rotational alignment of the tibial component. An older method no longer in use involved a trial tray that hooked onto the posterior cortex of the medial and lateral plateaus.

A second method is to use an asymmetric tray that mimics the cut surface of the tibia and apply the tray anatomically. Although this method can possibly achieve maximal capping of the tibia, there are two difficulties with its use. The first involves the fact that it ignores the linkage of the tibial rotation to that of the femur when the knee is in extension and the articulation is maximally loaded during walking. The second problem is related to the first in that if the surgeon wishes to change the tray rotation for better articular congruency with the femur, rotating the asymmetric tray will accentuate any anterior or posterior overhang.

A third way to align the tibial rotation is to base it on the tibial tubercle. The most commonly used landmark is the junction between the medial and central thirds of the tubercle. This method, like the others, ignores the attempt to establish articular congruency between the femur and the tibia for each individual knee when it is extended and loaded. These first three methods can only be successful in the presence of a rotating platform type of articulation that allows the insert to automatically accommodate to the femur throughout the arc of motion (see Chapter 3).

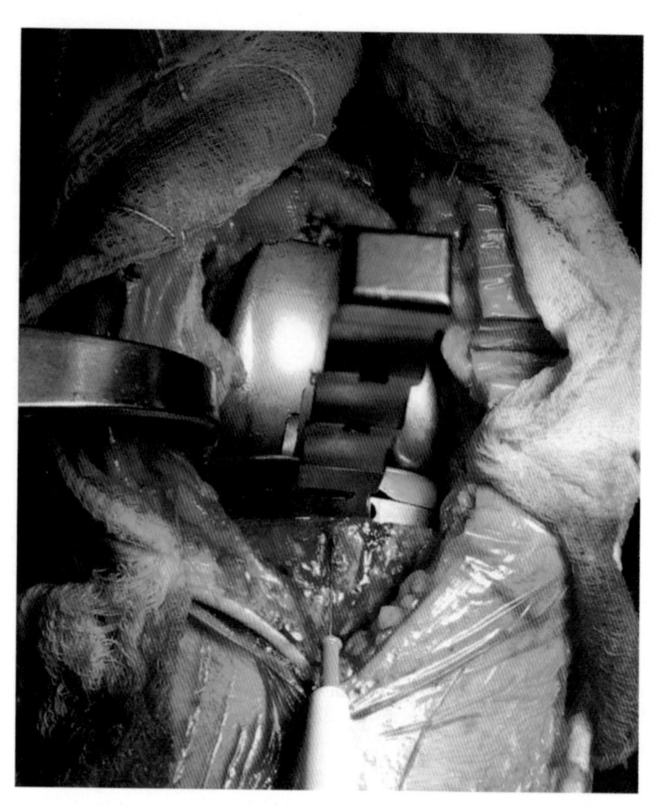

FIGURE 4–37. In fixed-bearing knees, tibial component rotation should be correlated with the femoral component rotation with the knee in full extension.

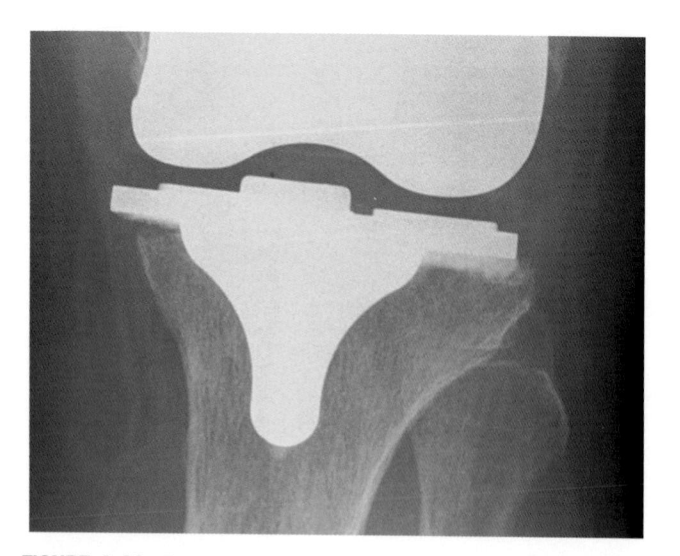

FIGURE 4–36. Tray overhang anterior to the mid-coronal plane of the tibia must be avoided.

The fourth method is the one I believe must be used for fixed-bearing components. This is to first establish the femoral rotation properly and then correlate the tibial rotation with the femur when the knee is in extension (Fig. 4–37). Systems vary as to how forgiving they are to the amount of rotational mismatch that will not create significant torsional forces on the articulation that would then be transferred to the insert tray interface and then possibly to the prosthesis-cement or bone-cement interface. Articulations with high conformity on the top side are the least forgiving and the most likely to be responsible for generating backside wear (see Chapter 3).

LIGAMENT BALANCING

Preliminary (and often final) ligament balancing is accomplished during initial exposure prior to final preparation of the femur and tibia (see Chapters 5, 6, and 9). Varus/valgus stability in flexion is achieved via femoral component rotation. Fine-tuning of all aspects of ligament balancing is done after placement trial of the trial components.

COMPONENT TRIALS

In a PCL-retaining technique, the tibial trial component must always be placed first. I believe that if the surgeon is able to insert the femoral component followed by the tibial component, the flexion gap is probably too lax unless the trial is a flat articulation with no sagittal conformity (see Chapter 2). In a PCL-substituting technique, however, the femoral component can be inserted first, and in fact this is often recommended.

The initial thickness of tibial trial chosen is the thinnest composite available for the system unless it is obvious that the flexion and extension spaces will require a thicker size.

Flexion stability is assessed first. This is done by applying the POLO test (see Chapter 2). With the knee at 90 degrees of flexion, the surgeon attempts to pull the tibial trial out from underneath the femoral component. In essence, this is a flexion distraction test, which depends on the height of the posterior lip of the tibial trial relative to the bottom of its sagittal curvature. This difference indicates how much the flexion gap must open up to allow the tibial trial to be pulled out from underneath the femoral component. I generally use a trial that has a posterior lip with a height of approximately 3 mm so I am performing a 3-mm distraction test. A corollary of this test is the inability to push in the tibial trial underneath the femur with the knee in 90 degrees of flexion.

If pullout is not possible, the flexion gap is not too loose and now must be assessed to see if it is too tight. This is done by observing lift-off of the tray from the anterior tibial cortex when the knee is flexed between 80 and 100 degrees.

This lift-off is the result of a tight PCL forcing the femur posteriorly so that it impinges on the posterior lip of the tibial component, pushing the tray down in back with corresponding lift-off in front. If the sagittal tibial topography is flat, excessive rollback can occur without lift-off. The extent of this rollback is best observed with the patella relocated. This is because an everted patella and quadriceps mechanism will artificially pull the tibia into external rotation during flexion, promoting excessive rollback on the medial side. This may also create an artificially positive lift-off test with a curved insert. Positive lift-off, therefore, should always be confirmed with the patella relocated. The PCL can also be observed and palpated for its tension. Another common observation with a tight PCL is movement forward or distally of a femoral trial in flexion beyond 90 degrees. This is because ligament tension is forcing rollback and an imprecisely fitting trial compensates by moving forward or distally to remain congruent with the sagittal conformity of the trial insert.

When I am assessing the flexion gap in a PCL-substituting knee, I adhere to the pull-out test to avoid excessive laxity and total dependence on the prosthetic constraint.

Adjusting Flexion/Extension Gaps

After the trial components are inserted, the flexion and extension gaps are assessed starting with the thinnest composite thickness of tibial component. Each gap can be too loose, too tight, or of appropriate tension. The level of the distal femoral resection influences the extension gap. The level of the posterior condylar resection influences the flexion gap. The level of the tibial resection influences both the flexion and the extension gap.

If both flexion and extension gaps are too loose, a thicker tibial component is required. If both gaps are too tight, more tibial resection is necessary. Proper spacing of the flexion gap takes place first, and any residual tightness or laxity in the extension gap is corrected secondarily.

The easier mismatch to fix is when the extension gap is tighter than the flexion gap. This is treated by increasing the distal femoral resection (see Chapter 9). The more difficult mismatch to resolve is when the flexion gap is tighter than the extension gap and the PCL is being preserved. There are four ways to deal with a tighter flexion gap. The first is to increase the posterior slope of the tibial cut but to avoid a posterior slope greater than 10 degrees. The second is to release the PCL. I prefer to do this from its femoral attachment (see Chapter 2). The third is to downsize the femoral component to one with a smaller anteroposterior dimension as long as notching of the anterior femoral cortex is avoided. This downsizing will require more posterior condylar resection and will therefore increase the flexion gap without affecting the extension gap.

The fourth method is to stabilize the flexion gap with the appropriate tibial resection and thickness of tibial component and treat the lax extension gap by cementing the femoral component proud of the bony cuts to a level that achieves extension stability. Several tricks can be used to accomplish this. One is to use distal femoral metallic augments if available for the system being implanted (see Chapter 12). A second is to underdrill the femoral lug holes if lugs are present on the femoral component (Fig. 4–38). This will allow the lugs to bottom out at the level of the depth of the drilling and prevent the femoral component from becoming fully seated. Confirmation that this method will be appropriate can be obtained by using the real femoral component as if it were a trial. This method of underdrilling a lug hole can also be used to cement a femoral component asymmetrically proud and adjust the varus/valgus alignment of the femoral component if necessary. It must be remembered that if the femoral component is cemented proud of the distal resections, some posterior

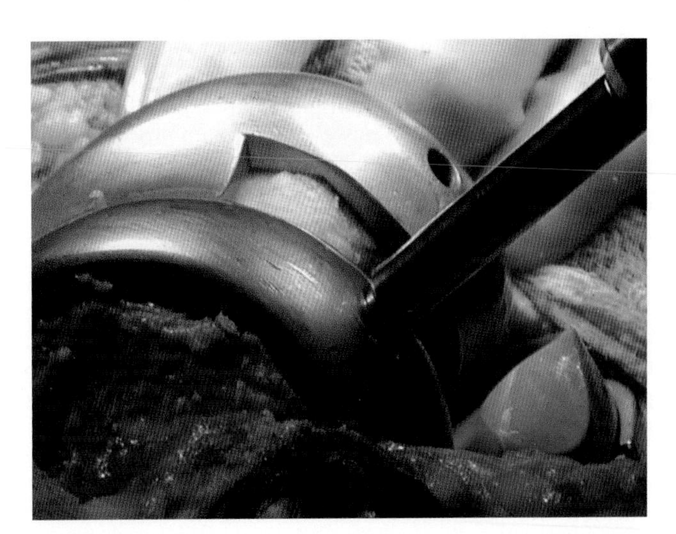

FIGURE 4–38. Underdrilling a femoral lug hole can allow the real component to be cemented proud of the resection.

condylar bone may be uncapped to the extent that the component is proud of the cuts. If so, this anatomic area should be revisited to remove any uncapped posterior condylar bone and relieve potential impingement with the posterior lip of a tibial component.

ASSESSMENT OF PATELLAR TRACKING

At the time of testing components, patellar tracking is also assessed (see Chapter 7). I use the so-called "rule of no thumb" test for this assessment.[8] In this maneuver, the patella is returned to the trochlear groove and the knee is flexed without the surgeon's thumb or without clamps or sutures securing a capsular closure. If the patella tracks congruently when the knee is flexed, with good contact between the medial facet of the patellar prosthesis and the medial aspect of the trochlear groove, no lateral release need be contemplated. However, if the patella dislocates, partially dislocates, or tilts laterally, a lateral release may be indicated. It is reasonable to repeat the "no thumb" test with the tourniquet deflated to be certain that restricted quadriceps movement is not responsible for a positive test. I would also repeat the test with one suture closing the capsule at the level of the superior pole of the patella. If tracking is now congruent and the tension on the suture is not excessive, no lateral release is necessary. My preferred technique for lateral release for patellar tracking is described in Chapter 7.

FINAL PREPARATION PRIOR TO CEMENTING OF COMPONENTS

Final preparations are made to insert the real prosthetic components. The lug holes for the femoral component are now completed.

I delay this step until the end in case the femoral resection has to be increased or modified. In the system I use, the spikes that hold the cutting jigs are smaller than the component lugs and would not allow reapplication of these jigs to be secure and accurate.

All bone surfaces are now cleansed with pulsatile lavage. An exception occurs when cementless fixation is being utilized on the femoral side. If there is sclerotic medial tibial bone (as is common in a preoperatively varus knee), I use a punch or drill to make multiple small holes for cement penetration. At this time, however, I have no proof that this makes for a better bone-cement interface and longevity.

CEMENTING COMPONENTS

The tibial component is cemented first. Cement is placed into the metaphysis for the stem or keel of the prosthesis and then onto the tibial plateau. The component is tapped into position. Any extruded cement is removed. If the knee is modular, the tibial insert is not yet applied.

Next, the femoral component is cemented. Cement is placed on all the femoral surfaces except only a thin film is smeared and pressurized onto the posterior condylar surfaces. This is to prevent extrusion of cement to the back of the knee where it is hard to access. Cement is also placed into the recesses of the prosthetic posterior condyles and chamfers. With this technique, any extruded cement will come forward and can be removed. After the femoral component is partially impacted into position, the trial modular insert is placed into the tray and femoral impaction is completed. Finally, the knee is brought to full extension to pressurize the bone-cement interface during polymerization. If the knee was in varus preoperatively, I prefer to apply a gentle valgus stress in full extension as the cement polymerizes. This is to avoid the possibility of inadvertently applying a varus stress that could cause lift-off of the lateral side of the prosthesis and possibly adversely affect the lateral bone-cement or prosthesis-cement interface.

When the knee is maximally extended, more cement always extrudes from beneath the femur and sometimes anteriorly around the tibial tray. I flex the knee 30 to 45 degrees after the initial extension of the knee to gain access to remove this extruded cement. The knee is then extended for a final time to pressurize the bone-cement interface. I leave a little extruded cement anteriorly to determine when polymerization is complete.

After full polymerization, the knee is flexed, the tourniquet is deflated, and a second dose of antibiotic is administered. This is to assure maximum concentration of antibiotic in the postoperative joint hematoma. Bleeding is controlled via electrocautery. The most common vessels encountered are the medial superior geniculate in the capsular incision just above the patella and the medial inferior geniculate at the level of the fat pad.

The trial insert is then removed. The entire periphery of both the femoral and tibial components is checked for any additional extruded cement. The femur is lifted with a bone hook, and the posterior condyles are inspected and palpated for cement extrusion. Finally, the real insert is placed.

Prior to initiating closure, I like to pass an instrument such as a pituitary rongeur along the medial and lateral gutters at the level of the joint line and medially and laterally in the intercondylar notch. This is to assure that no osteophytes remain that might impinge on the polyethylene.

DRAINING AND CLOSING THE WOUND

I prefer to drain the knee after an arthroplasty. I place two small suction drains laterally and bring them out through separate stab wounds. I leave about 5 cm of the drain inside the knee. The drains are always removed the morning after surgery. I believe their most important function is to decompress the wound during the first hour or so after deflation of the tourniquet and wound closure. If drainage is excessive after this period of time, I would consider clamping the drains or even removing them (see Chapter 15).

I close the fat pad separately with several No. 2-O resorbable sutures. The capsule is closed with interrupted No. 1 monofilament resorbable sutures. I do not consider it necessary to perform the closure in flexion. The closure is initiated at the superior pole of the patella where medial and lateral marks have been made at the time of the initial arthrotomy to aid in lining up the closure at the end of the procedure. The closure is always anatomic unless the patient had a severe preoperative flexion contracture. In that case, the medial capsule is advanced distally on the lateral capsule

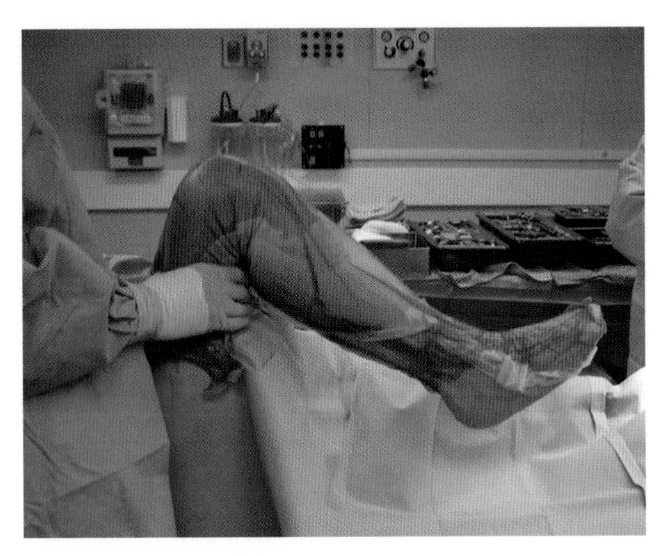

FIGURE 4–39. Flexion against gravity after capsular closure is the best predictor of postoperative range of motion.

to take the laxity out of the quadriceps mechanism and minimize a postoperative extensor lag (see Fig. 8–5 and Chapters 8 and 9). The subcutaneous tissue is closed in layers with No. 2-O resorbable sutures superiorly and No. 3-O inferiorly and for the more superficial tissues superiorly. I use No. 3-O interrupted nylon closure for the skin. The knots are initiated medially, and the suture is a vertical mattress type that is subcuticular on the lateral side. An interrupted closure eliminates the abnormal tension that would occur across a continuous subcuticular closure in maximal knee flexion. It also allows treatment of a minor wound healing problem if one or two sutures have to be removed for débridement and irrigation.

After the capsule is closed, the knee is flexed against gravity to measure the patient's quadriceps excursion and potential final flexion[9] (Fig. 4–39; see Chapter 8). The wound is dressed with nonadhesive gauze, sterile pads, and an elastic bandage from the foot to the thigh.

If the skin edges are oozing at the time the dressing is to be applied, I have found that taking 5 minutes to hold pressure on the incision will inevitably stop the bleeding and relieve postoperative concerns of draining incisions and stained dressings.

Immediately after surgery, the knee is placed in a continuous passive motion (CPM) machine set for 90 degrees of flexion if this range was achieved with the capsule closed. If there are concerns about the wound, a knee immobilizer is used for the first day or two until these concerns have passed (see Chapter 15).

PERIOPERATIVE MANAGEMENT

Anticoagulation

The ideal anticoagulation regimen following TKA remains controversial. For 3 decades I have been using warfarin prophylaxis transitioning to aspirin. I have no data on the true incidence of deep vein thrombosis (DVT) and nonfatal pulmonary embolus (PE) among my patients. Fatal PEs, however, over the last 3000 arthroplasties have been extremely rare with none, in fact, known to me. The most serious complication I have seen using warfarin has been one case of "warfarin necrosis" involving the breast and requiring emergency mastectomy.

I use low-molecular-weight heparin when warfarin is contraindicated but have been discouraged by a high incidence of postoperative bleeding.

I start patients on warfarin the night before surgery. The initial dose varies between 5 and 10 mg depending on the patient's age, weight, and medical status. The next dose of 3 to 5 mg is given on the evening of surgery, and the dose is then adjusted daily based on the international normalized ratio (INR) value, with a goal of 1.8 to 2.2.

Prior to discharge, patients are stratified into high- and low-risk categories. High risk includes bilateral cases (see Chapter 13), a prior history of DVT, estrogen therapy, a recent history of cancer, and other known high-risk factors. These patients remain on adjusted-dose warfarin for 4 to 6 weeks and transition to 81 mg of aspirin daily for a minimum of 6 more weeks.

Low-risk patients who are totally free of clinical signs of DVT obtain bilateral lower extremity ultrasound examinations prior to discharge. If their examination is negative for thrombus, they transition to aspirin, 81 mg per day, for 6 weeks. Those patients with calf clots remain on warfarin for 6 to 8 weeks and then have a repeat ultrasound examination. If there is no propagation of clot, they transition to aspirin. If the calf clot has propagated, vascular consultation is obtained. Those patients with a thigh clot on their initial ultrasound examination receive heparin therapy and vascular consultation.

Other perioperative measures thought to decrease the incidence of DVT include pulsatile stockings, a CPM machine, active ankle exercises, and ambulation within 24 hours.

Rehabilitation Protocol

Rehabilitation protocols continue to evolve and accelerate. After surgery, the knee is placed in a CPM machine in the recovery room at 90 degrees of flexion (if tolerated). The machine is used for a total of 6 to 8 hours per day. A knee immobilizer is often applied at night to maintain extension and provide comfort for transfers and initial ambulation the day of surgery. Depending on their social situation, patients can be discharged home on the third day after surgery or to a rehabilitation or skilled nursing facility.

Weightbearing for distances is protected with crutches or a walker for 4 weeks, but I permit full weightbearing as tolerated at home with the protection of a cane, crutch, wall, sink, counter, or furniture. Home visits by a physical therapist occur twice a week for several weeks.

If the left knee has been replaced, the patient can resume driving if comfortable and off narcotics. For the right knee, driving is delayed for 4 weeks from surgery.

All support is discontinued at 4 weeks except for a cane for distances at the patient's discretion.

Follow-up Appointments

The initial postoperative visit occurs approximately 4 weeks after surgery. Sutures have been removed at 10 days after surgery by a visiting nurse or at the rehabilitation facility.

The wound is checked along with range of motion and ambulatory ability. Postoperative radiographs including a standing AP, lateral, and skyline view are obtained and reviewed with the patient and family along with a prosthesis similar to their own implant. Further expectations are reviewed and printed information given regarding antibiotic prophylaxis.

I ask my patients to send in a written progress report at 3 months and to see me for an examination and radiograph at 1 year. Future examinations will occur at 2, 5, 7, 10, 12, and 15 years postoperatively assuming no worrisome symptoms appear during the intervals.

References

1. Masini MA, Madsen-Cummings N, Scott RD: Ipsilateral total knee arthroplasty after arthrodesis of the hip. J Orthop Tech 1995;3:1–5.
2. Olcott CW, Scott RD: The Ranawat Award: femoral component rotation during total knee arthroplasty. Clin Orthop 1999;367:39–42.
3. Barnes CL, Scott RD: Popliteus tendon dysfunction following total knee arthroplasty. J Arthroplasty 1995;10:543–545.
4. King TV, Scott RD: Femoral component loosening in total knee arthroplasty. Clin Orthop 1985;194:285–290.
5. Ewald FC: The Knee Society total knee arthroplasty roentgenographic evaluation and scoring system. Clin Orthop 1989;248:9–12.
6. Chmell MJ, McManus J, Scott RD: Thickness of the patella in men and women with osteoarthritis. Knee 1996;2(4):239–241.
7. Rispler DT, Kolettis GT, Scott RD: Tibial resection in total knee arthroplasty using external alignment instrumentation based on the true center of the ankle. J Orthop Tech 1994;2(2):63–67.
8. Scott RD: Prosthetic replacement of the patellofemoral joint. Orthop Clin North Am 1979;10:129–137.
9. Lee DC, Kim DH, Scott RD, Suthers K: Intraoperative flexion against gravity as an indication of ultimate range of motion in individual cases after total knee arthroplasty. J Arthroplasty 1998;13:500–503.

CHAPTER 5

Total Knee Arthroplasty in Severe Varus Deformity

THE TYPICAL PATIENT

Severe varus deformity appears to have no predilection for male or female patients. Typically, patients report that they have had some varus alignment in their knees since childhood. There may be a history of a medial meniscectomy. The deformity gradually progresses, and the patient may have severe deformity any time after the age of 50 years. Lateral subluxation of the tibia on the femur is not uncommon. The source of the varus deformity is the tibial side of the joint, in contrast to the valgus knee, for which the femoral side of the joint is responsible (Fig. 5–1).

EXPOSURE

The knee is exposed through a standard median parapatellar arthrotomy. Routine exposure proceeds with excision of the anterior horn of the medial meniscus. This provides access to the plane between the proximal tibial plateau and the deep medial collateral ligament (MCL). Into this plane a 1-cm curved osteotome is passed posteriorly to the level of the semimembranous bursa. This accomplishes an initial release of the deep MCL. If present, the anterior cruciate ligament (ACL) is resected. The tibia is now manipulated into external rotation and delivered in front of the femur (Fig. 5–2). Peripheral femoral and tibial osteophytes are removed to further release the medial structures that were tented over them (Fig. 5-3).

MEDIOLATERAL BALANCING

Unlike in the valgus knee, ligament balance in flexion and extension are interrelated. The valgus knee can be balanced in flexion prior to any releases by proper rotational alignment of the femoral component (see Chapter 6). In the varus knee, however, the knee should be balanced in extension before it is balanced in flexion via proper femoral component rotation.

Medial Release in Extension

As noted above, routine exposure of the knee and removal of femoral and tibial osteophytes accomplishes an initial

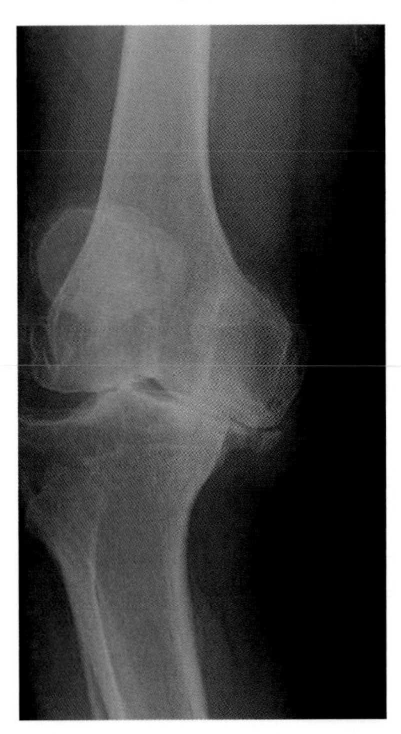

FIGURE 5–1. The varus deformity is usually due to deficiency of the medial tibial plateau, and often there is lateral subluxation of the tibia.

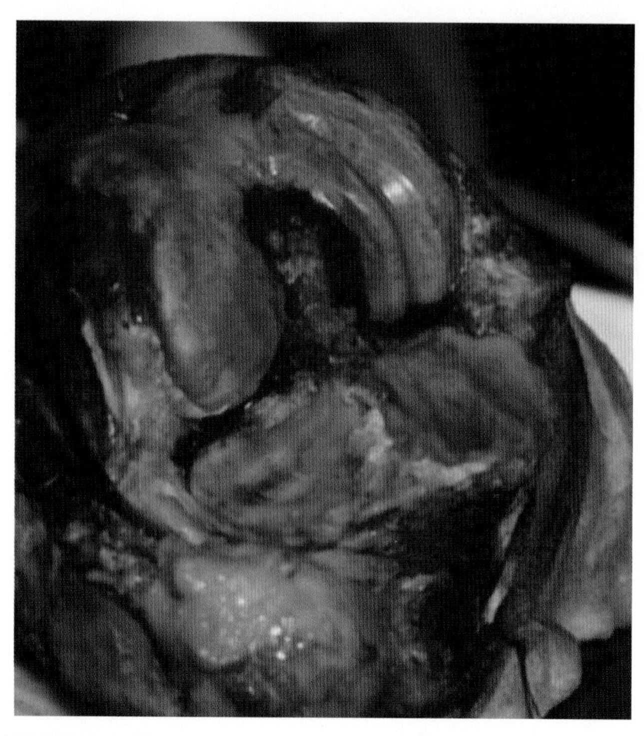

FIGURE 5–2. The tibia is delivered in front of the femur for the initial tibial resection.

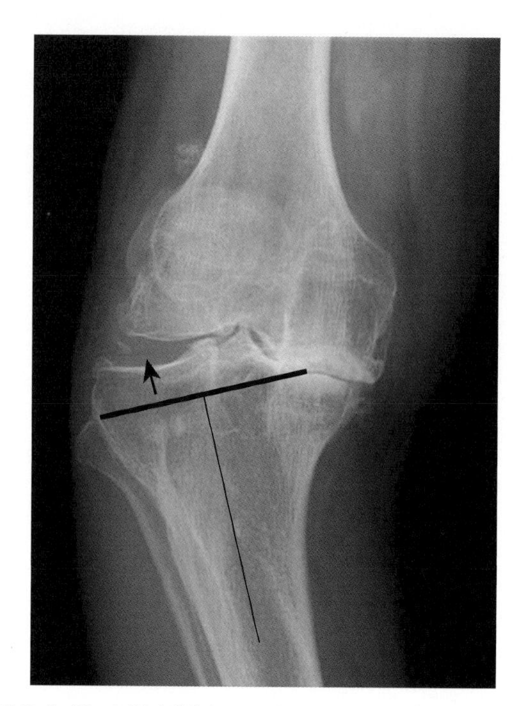

FIGURE 5–4. The initial tibial resection involves removal of 10 mm including cartilage from the intact lateral side.

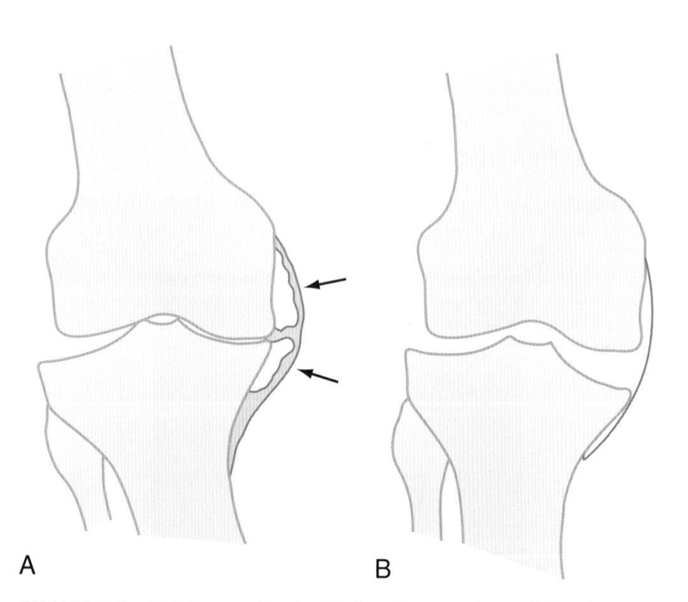

FIGURE 5–3. Initial correction is obtained by removing peripheral osteophytes from the femur and tibia that tent up the MCL.

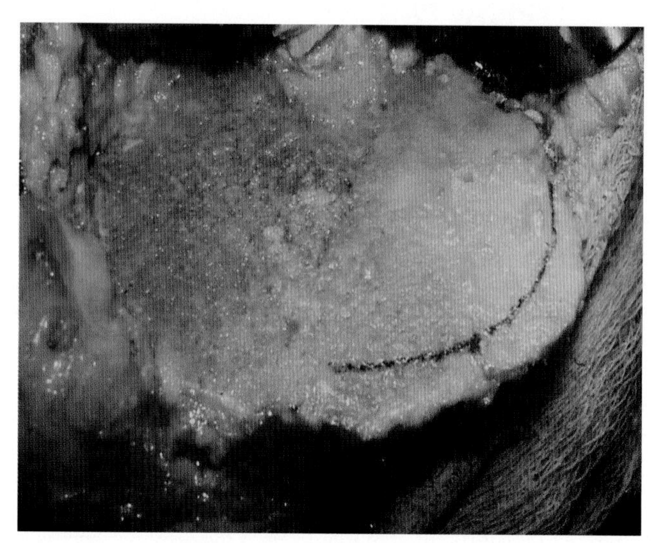

FIGURE 5–5. Uncapped tibial bone is outlined and resected to release the MCL.

medial release. For many varus knees, this is sufficient to achieve mediolateral balancing in extension. For severe varus knees, however, an additional release is necessary. I believe this is most successfully and safely achieved by the "shift and resect" technique.[1]

Shift and Resect Technique

After the tibia has been delivered in front of the femur, an initial conservative tibial resection is performed. The level of resection is based on the intact lateral side. The amount of lateral resection is approximately 10 mm including any residual cartilage (Fig. 5–4).

The angle of the resection is perpendicular to the long axis of the tibia and has a 3- to 5-degree posterior slope (see Chapter 4 for exceptions to this amount of posterior slope). The tibia is next measured for the size of tray. One size smaller is then chosen and shifted laterally to the edge of the cut surface of the lateral plateau. Preliminary tibial rotation of the tray is based on alignment with the medial third of the tibial tubercle. A marking pen is used to outline the uncapped portion of the medial tibial plateau (Fig. 5–5). This bone is removed with an angle of resection that is perpendicular to the tibial resection (Fig. 5–6). The MCL has been

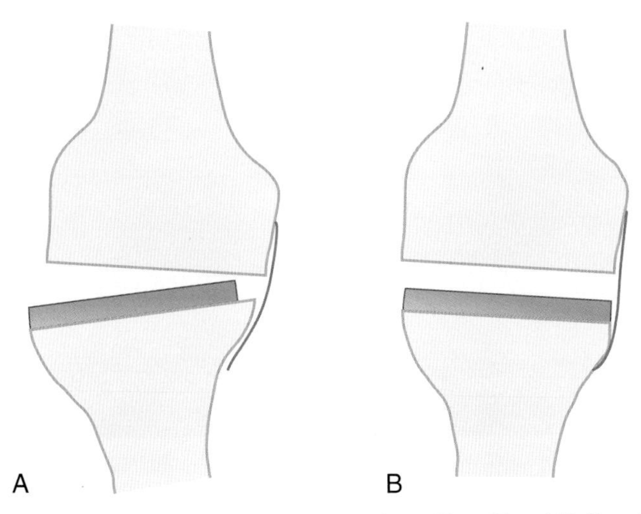

FIGURE 5–6. The shift and resect technique. (From Dixon MC, Parsch D, Brown RR, Scott RD: The correction of severe varus deformity in total knee arthroplasty by tibial component downsizing and resection of uncapped proximal medial bone. J Arthroplasty 2004;19:19–22.)

freed of its attachment to this resected bone prior to its removal, and the ligament should be carefully protected during the resection. The resection can be accomplished with a rongeur, a saw, or an osteotome. It is sometimes helpful to define the resection with multiple small drill holes that perforate the sclerotic medial bone.

Formal MCL Release from the Tibia

It is extremely rare for me to perform a formal distal MCL release. Should this be necessary, I would perform a subperiosteal dissection of the tibial attachment, progressing distally in stages until adequate release was obtained. I avoid this type of release if possible because it carries the danger of catastrophic loss of medial support at the time of the surgical release or in the future secondary to minor trauma.

DISTAL FEMORAL RESECTION

Distal femoral resection is planned in a routine fashion. A preoperative long anteroposterior (AP) radiograph that includes the hip and knee is helpful in planning the resection. Some severe varus knees are associated with a varus angle in the femoral shaft or proximally in the neck-shaft angle. These knees, therefore, may require that the distal femoral resection be made in slightly more valgus than is customary. Since the deformity usually is in the tibia, however, a standard distal femoral resection angle of 5 to 7 degrees generally is indicated. The resection should be drawn on the preoperative radiograph so that relative amount of medial versus lateral condylar bone to be removed can be estimated (Fig. 5–7). Despite the varus limb alignment, the resection usually calls for a millimeter or more removal of medial distal condyle versus lateral distal condyle. In general, the distal femoral resection guide will rest on eburnated bone medially and intact cartilage laterally (Fig. 5–8). The amount of distal femoral resection is correlated with the thickness of the metallic femoral component (see Chapter 4). In the

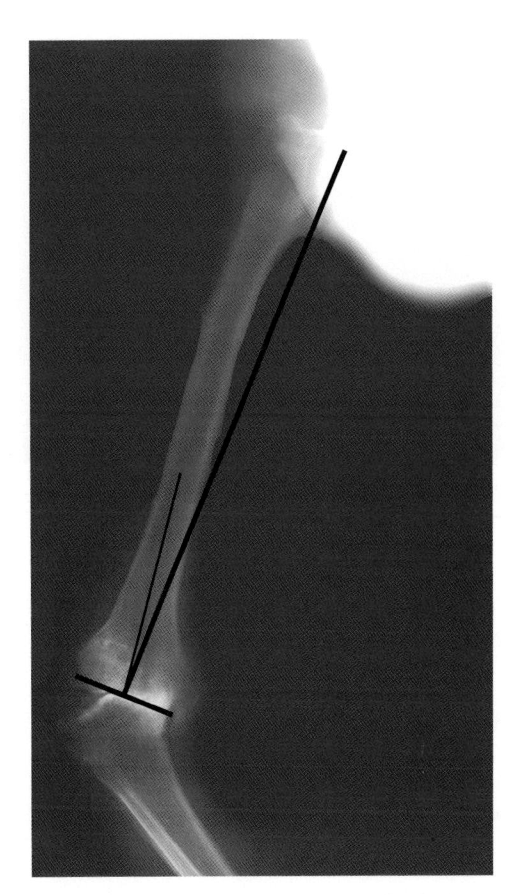

FIGURE 5–7. Drawing out the femoral resection for the purpose of establishing a neutral mechanical axis.

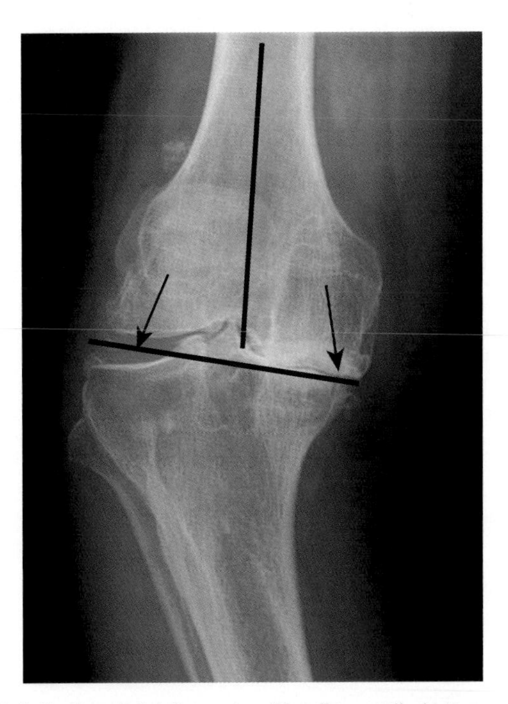

FIGURE 5–8. The distal femoral cutting jig usually bottoms out on eburnated bone medially and intact cartilage laterally.

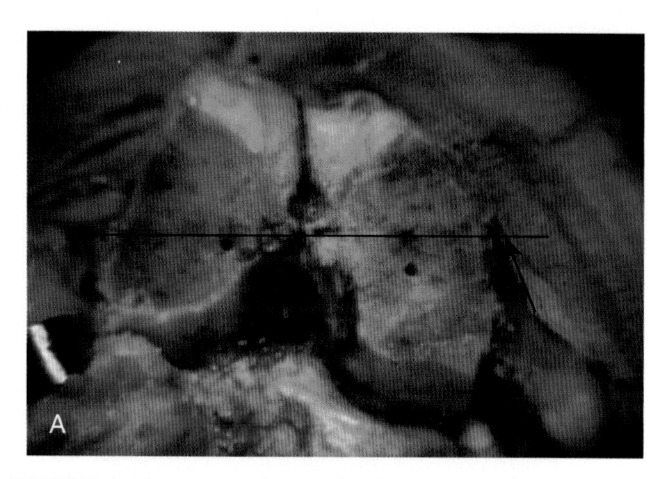

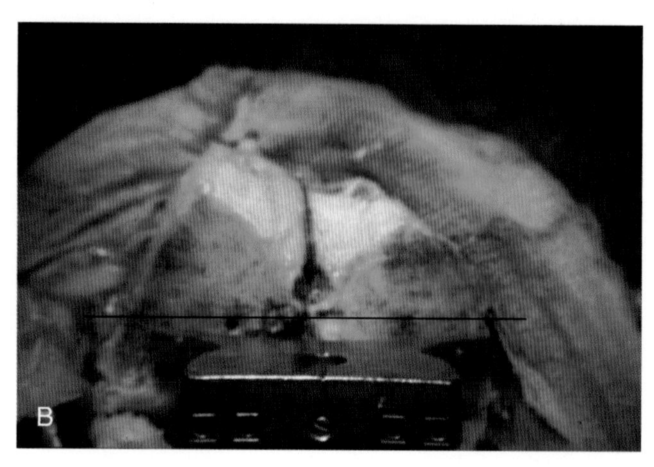

FIGURE 5–9. Severe varus knees often have "hyperplastic" medial condyles and need much more than 3 degrees of external rotation for flexion gap symmetry.

presence of a flexion contracture over 15 degrees, distal resection is increased (see Chapter 9).

FEMORAL COMPONENT ROTATION

Proper femoral component rotation is based on establishing a balanced, symmetric flexion gap to maximize flexion stability.

In the varus knee, this rotation must be performed after the knee is balanced in extension. Baseline parameters for proper femoral component rotation can be established by marking out the trans-sulcus angle (Whiteside line), the transepicondylar axis, and a line that is in 3 degrees of external rotation off the posterior femoral condyles (see Chapters 4, 7, and 15). The knee is then flexed 90 degrees, and the medial and lateral compartments are tensed with laminar spreaders. In severe varus knees, the Whiteside line and transepicondylar axes often yield flexion gap symmetry. Three degrees of external rotation off the posterior condyles is usually inadequate external rotation to provide symmetry. Most total knee systems have femoral sizing guides that can orient pinholes for the AP cutting jig in 3 degrees of external rotation. These pinholes will have to be adjusted to provide the proper increased external rotation to the femoral component. Patients with severe varus deformity often have "hyperplastic" medial femoral condyles that accentuate the need for increased external rotation (Fig. 5–9). When adjusting the pinholes for the AP cutting guide, the lateral pinhole is kept in its "anatomic" position. Increased external rotation is achieved by raising the medial pinhole until the two pinholes are parallel with the proposed tibial resection. Raising the medial hole serves to increase the flexion space on the medial side and relieve tightness in the medial compartment.

TIBIAL BONE STOCK DEFICIENCY

In severe varus deformity, the medial tibial plateau is always deficient. Excising bone down to the level of the medial deficiency may require an unacceptable amount of lateral resection. In this case some form of medial augmentation is necessary. The need for augmentation methods can be predicted preoperatively (see Chapter 12). The surgeon simply reconstructs the tibial joint line based on the normal lateral side. At the level of the lateral joint line, a line is drawn perpendicular to the long axis of the tibia (Fig. 5–10). The perpendicular distance from this line to the bottom of the medial deficiency is then measured. If the distance measured is 10 mm, no augmentation is necessary with an acceptable 10 mm lateral resection. If the distance measures 15 mm or more, some augmentation definitely is necessary. Deficiencies between 10 and 15 mm are addressed on a case-by-case basis.

Options for Restoration of Deficient Tibial Bone Stock

Restoration of tibial bone stock deficiency is addressed in detail in Chapter 12. Basically, the options are to use cement alone, cement with screw augmentation, bone graft, modular

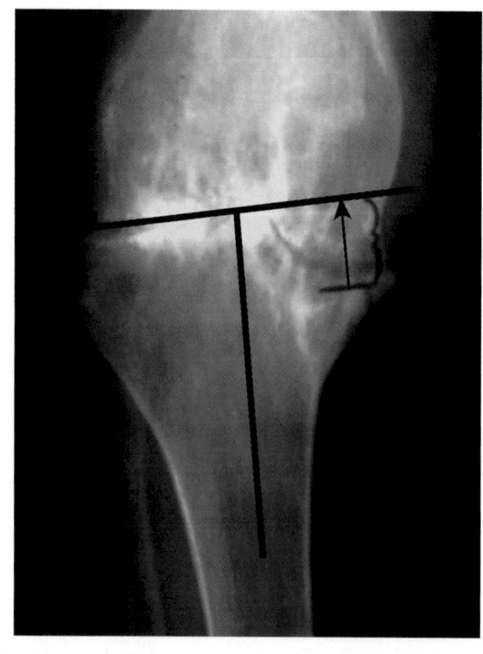

FIGURE 5–10. To predict the need for augmentation, measure the distance from the bottom of the defect to the reconstructed medial joint line.

metal wedges, or custom components. The optimal choice will vary with the extent of the deficiency, quality of the bone, and age of the patient.

RESIDUAL LATERAL LAXITY

In severe varus deformity, even after a significant medial release, there may still be some residual lateral laxity in extension. The question arises as to how much laxity is acceptable. In my experience, it is not a clinical problem if two criteria exist. The first is that the static alignment of the knee as determined by the angle of the femoral and tibial bone resections is no longer mechanically in varus alignment. If residual mechanical varus exists, the application of weight-bearing forces across the knee will promote the recurrence of varus and a progressive increase in the residual lateral laxity. This ultimately will lead to failure of the arthroplasty.

The second criterion is the observation that the lateral side does not gap open with the knee resting passively in the supine position. If it does, it means that the imbalance between the medial and lateral sides overwhelmingly favors the tight medial side and recurrent varus is likely.

If these two criteria are fulfilled, I have routinely seen dynamic stability restored to the knee via the iliotibial band. At the one-year follow-up, the residual lateral laxity can be documented when a varus stress is applied to the patient's knee when the patient is resting in the supine position. When the muscles are tensed via a straight-leg-raise maneuver, the laxity cannot be demonstrated.

Correcting Significant Residual Lateral Laxity

I must reemphasize that the mechanical axis of the knee as imparted by the angle of the bone resections from the femur and the tibia must not be in varus. There are then two options to diminish the residual lateral laxity. The first is to increase the amount of medial release and use a thicker insert to tighten the lateral side. The second is to tighten the lateral side by advancing the lateral collateral ligament.

A technique is described in the literature that advances the fibular head distally to diminish the residual lateral laxity. I have no experience with this technique.[2] My preference is the technique of medial release with a thicker insert (Fig. 5-11). One concern about this technique might be its effect on flexion gap stability if the flexion gap imbalance was not associated with the extension gap imbalance. Fortunately, the more pliable lateral structures can accommodate the thicker insert, and I have not yet seen problems with this technique.

Finally, if lateral laxity develops secondarily in a knee left in mechanical varus alignment, consideration might be given to correcting this malalignment using a custom angled tibial insert at the time of ligament rebalancing (Fig. 5–12).

POSTERIOR CRUCIATE LIGAMENT RETENTION IN SEVERE VARUS

It is widely thought that the posterior cruciate ligament (PCL) must be substituted in the face of severe varus deformity. This has not been my personal experience. I begin surgery on a severe varus knee attempting to preserve and balance but not substitute for the PCL unless an obvious need for this arises during the operation. I estimate that I am able to avoid a substituting technique in well over 90% of varus knees with angular deformity greater than 20 degrees. The PCL is almost always "intact" in these knees but certainly not "normal." It does not have to be normal. As long as the flexion gap is properly balanced and tensed, a stabilizing post does not appear to be necessary.

The PCL usually ends up being too tight after the medial side is released to balance the lax lateral side. PCL balancing

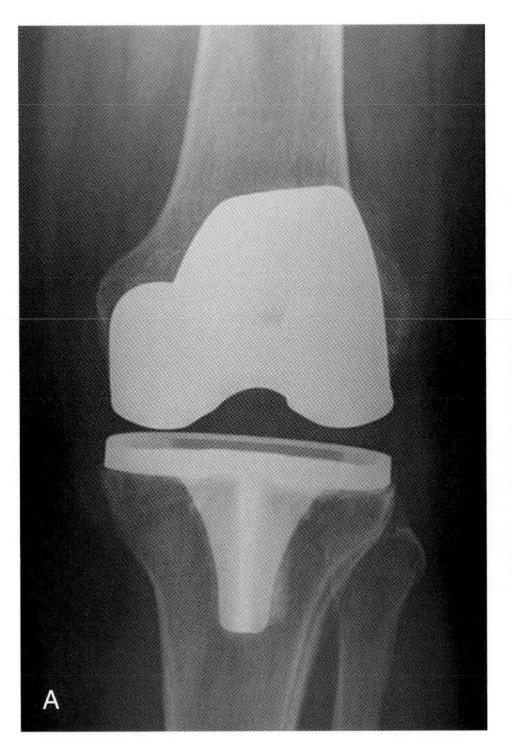

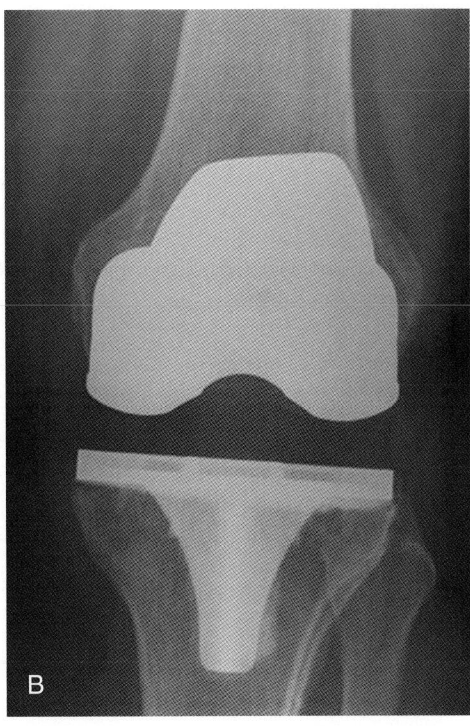

FIGURE 5–11. Residual lateral laxity can be treated with MCL release and thicker tibial insert.

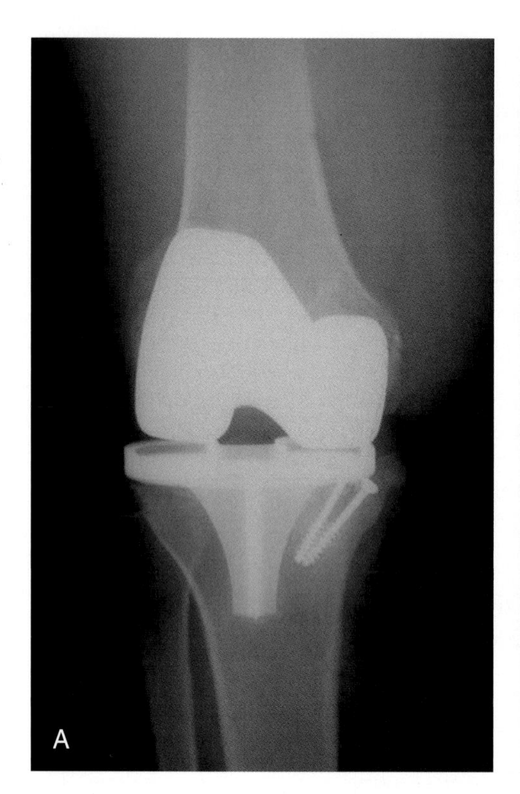

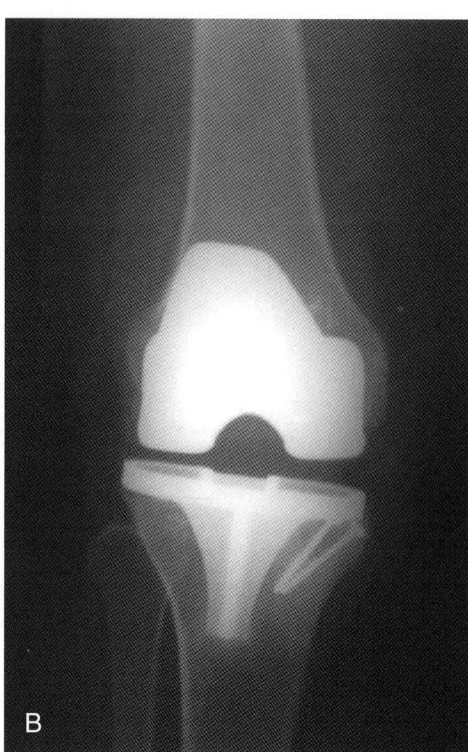

FIGURE 5–12. Use of a custom angled bearing to correct varus malalignment during an insert exchange.

and release are carried out using the POLO test, described in Chapter 2.[3]

INTERNAL TIBIAL TORSION IN SEVERE VARUS

Internal tibial torsion often is associated with severe varus deformity. It cannot be corrected without the use of rotationally constrained components or the combination of TKA plus a derotational osteotomy. It is usually best to accept this deformity and advise the patient that it will persist postoperatively.

SUMMARY

Severe varus deformity has no predilection for male or female patients. There usually is a history of bilateral varus alignment from childhood. The deformity gradually progresses over time. It may present at any time after age 50 years.

Tibial deformity is responsible for the varus angulation. The medial tibial plateau is deficient. The tibia is often partially dislocated laterally.

An initial MCL release should be performed during exposure by the removal of medial femoral and tibial osteophytes. The release is continued by dissecting the deep medial collateral ligament off the proximal medial tibia while gaining exposure.

An initial tibial bone resection should be performed. The tibial tray size is then determined, undersized, and shifted laterally. Uncapped medial tibial bone is then resected to gain more medial release. A formal medial collateral ligament subperiosteal release from the tibia is rarely necessary.

The flexion gap is balanced by proper femoral component rotation with the ligaments tensed. The PCL can be preserved or substituted. If preserved, it probably will need to be released to balance the knee.

Some residual lateral laxity may be acceptable if static alignment is mechanically in valgus. Medial tibial deficiency is augmented with cement, cement/screws, metal augments, or bone graft depending on the individual case. Preoperative internal tibial torsion may not be correctable without constrained articulations and should be accepted intraoperatively.

References

1. Dixon MC, Parsch D, Brown RR, Scott RD: The correction of severe varus deformity in total knee arthroplasty by tibial component downsizing and resection of uncapped proximal medial bone. J Arthroplasty 2004;19:19–22.
2. Teeny SM, Krackow KA, Hungerford DS, Jones M: Primary total knee arthroplasty in patients with severe varus deformity. Clin Orthop 1991;273:19–31.
3. Chmell MJ, Scott RD: Balancing the posterior cruciate ligament during cruciate-retaining total knee arthroplasty: description of the POLO test. J Orthop Tech 1996;4:12–15.

CHAPTER 6

Total Knee Arthroplasty in Severe Valgus Deformity

THE TYPICAL PATIENT

The typical patient with a severe valgus deformity is an elderly woman (Fig. 6–1). She usually is in her seventh or eighth decade and reports that she has had "knock-knees" her whole life. She also may give a history of patellofemoral problems through adolescence and young adulthood. These problems might be symptoms of chondromalacia or recurrent subluxation episodes. As the valgus deformity progresses, there is loss of lateral compartment joint space and gradual attenuation of the medial collateral ligament (MCL) (Fig. 6–2). A skyline view of the patella often shows patellofemoral involvement and possibly patellar dysplasia, with a very thin patella that is partially dislocated laterally, developing a concave shape to the lateral facet that mates with the convex shape of the lateral femoral condyle (Fig. 6–3). Patella alta often is present and can be appreciated on both the anteroposterior (AP) and lateral radiographs. Chondrocalcinosis is a frequent finding with calcification of the menisci or articular cartilage. A long film of the tibia will usually show a valgus bow. This valgus tibial deformity is problematic if the surgeon uses intramedullary tibial alignment devices (Fig. 6–4). The long film is necessary for template placement to show where to enter the tibia for the intramedullary device and may even show that its use is contraindicated.

The clinical diagnosis generally is osteoarthritis, although severe valgus can also be seen in rheumatoid patients. The osteoarthritic patient usually has a hypermobile knee and possibly hyperextension. The rheumatoid patient can share this clinical picture or may have a stiff knee and a flexion contracture (see Chapters 8 and 9).

CLINICAL FEATURES OF VALGUS VS. VARUS KNEES

Valgus knees have several clinical features distinct from varus knees. In my experience, patients with valgus deformity and lateral compartment disease often can tolerate significant structural damage better than those with varus knees of comparable severity. I have seen patients with 20-degree valgus deformities complain more about secondary trochanteric bursitis than about pain and disability from the knee itself. If a patient has "windblown" knees, the varus knee is almost always more symptomatic than the valgus knee and should be operated on first unless bilateral procedures are contemplated (see Chapter 13).

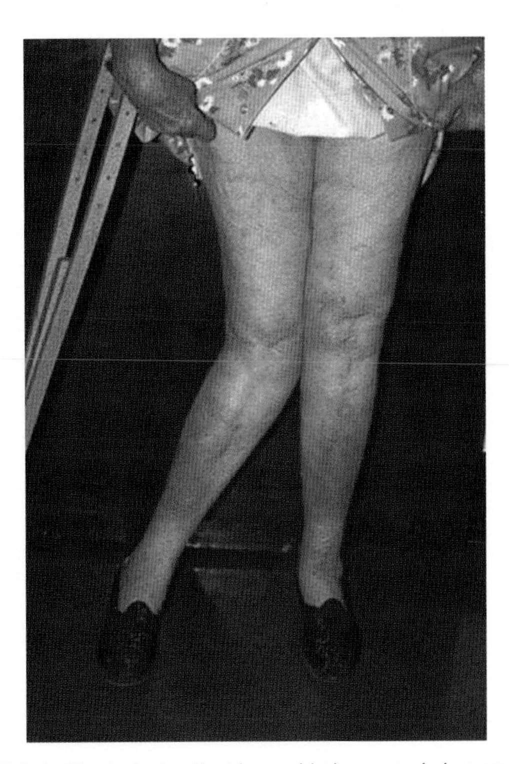

FIGURE 6–1. The typical patient is an elderly woman in her seventh or eighth decade.

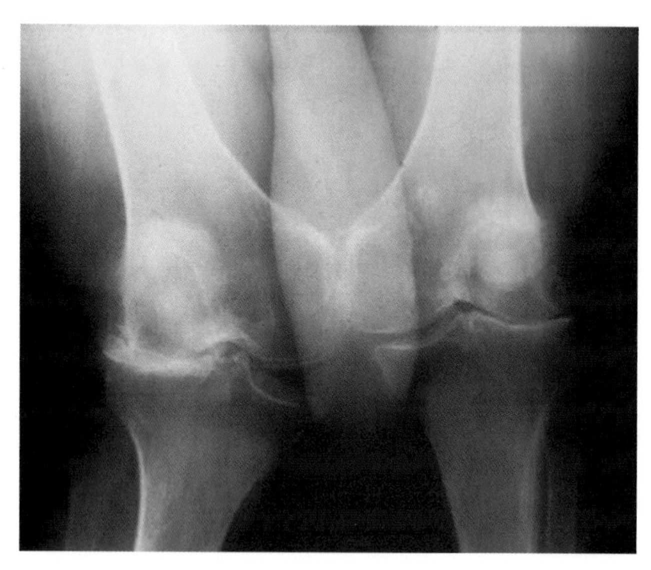

FIGURE 6–2. Note the loss of lateral joint space and attenuation of the MCL.

Another distinction between the valgus and the varus knee is the source of the deformity. In varus knees, the medial tibial plateau is deficient and the tibial joint line is in significant varus. The femoral joint line, however, still retains valgus between 5 and 9 degrees (see Chapter 5). In valgus knees, however, the valgus deformity comes from the femur. The tibial joint line is usually in neutral or even in the classic 2 to 3 degrees of varus, while the femoral joint line is in marked valgus (Fig. 6–5). This deformity is due to hypoplasia of the lateral femoral condyle, which is seen both distally and posteriorly (Fig. 6–6). Occasionally, there may also be a valgus metaphyseal bow. As the valgus progresses, the MCL becomes attenuated, allowing the deformity to increase, and at times the lateral femoral condyle erodes the lateral tibial plateau in its central portion (Fig. 6–7). The peripheral aspect of the lateral plateau remains intact so the resultant defect is a contained one. In the varus knee, the progressive erosion of the medial tibial plateau involves the periphery of the plateau so the defect is not contained and is more structurally significant.

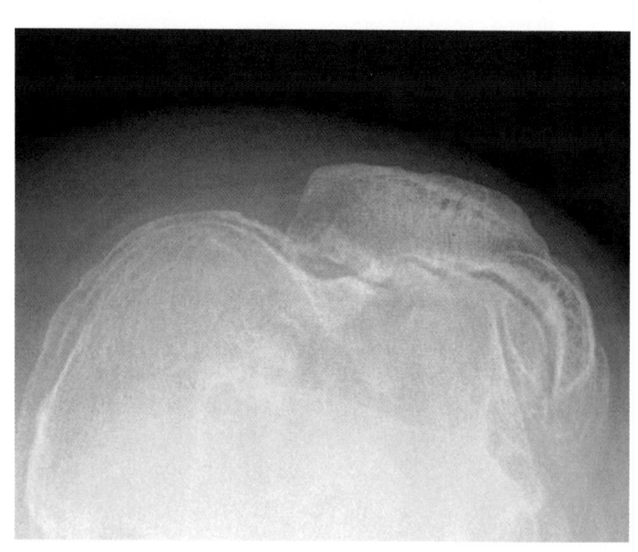

FIGURE 6–3. Patellofemoral involvement is common.

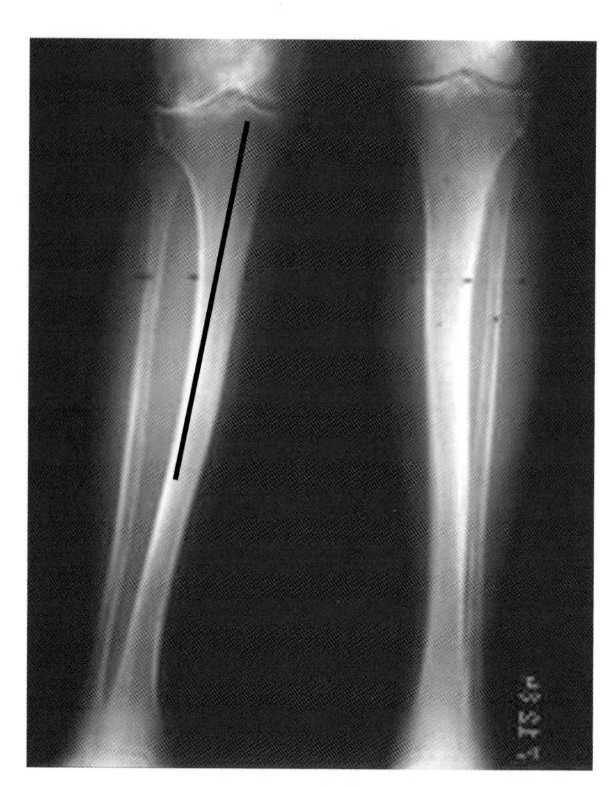

FIGURE 6–4. A valgus tibial bow makes the use of tibial intramedullary alignment devices problematic.

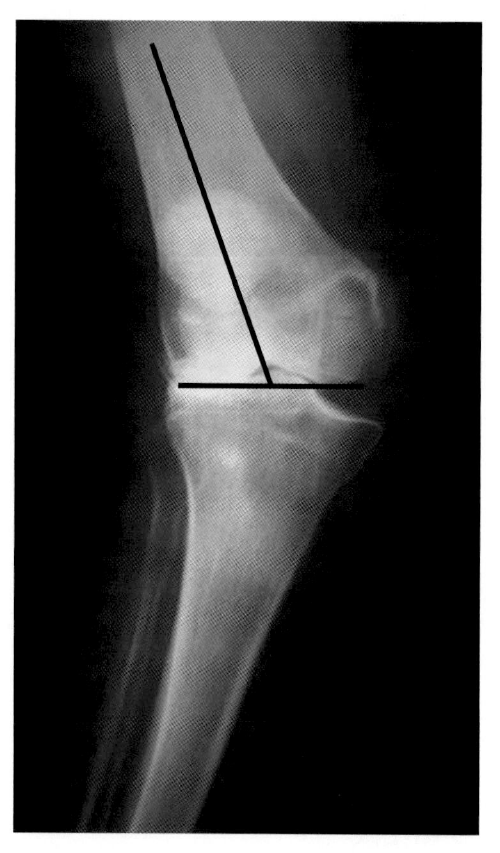

FIGURE 6–5. The valgus deformity comes from the femur rather than the tibia.

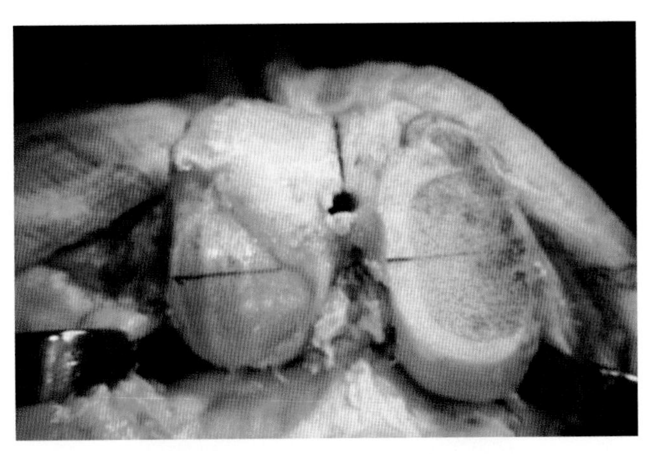

FIGURE 6–6. The lateral femoral condyle is hypoplastic both distally and posteriorly.

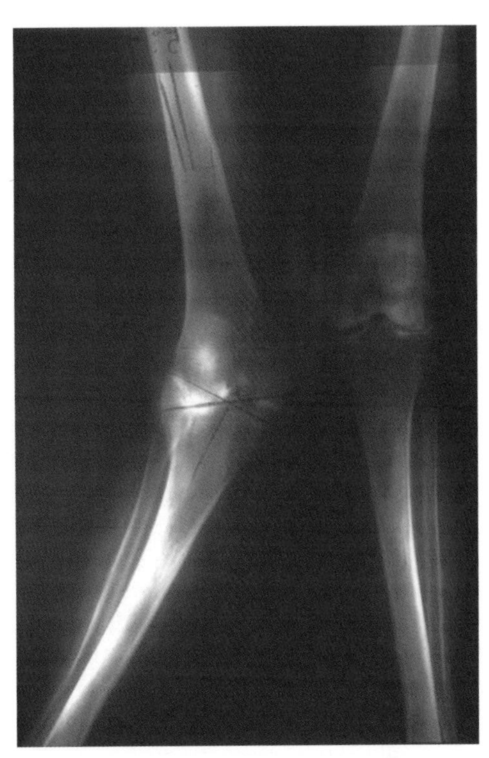

FIGURE 6–7. Sometimes the femoral condyle erodes into the central portion of the lateral tibial plateau.

Lateral Femoral Condyle Hypoplasia

As noted above, the typical severe valgus knee demonstrates hypoplasia of the lateral femoral condyle. This hypoplasia exists both distally and posteriorly. When performing the distal femoral resection in a valgus knee, the surgeon must resist the temptation to resect back to the level of this deficiency (Fig. 6–8). Instead, the deficient lateral side must be augmented. The consequence of excessive distal femoral resection in a valgus knee is twofold. First, the extension gap can end up being extremely large because of the extra distal medial resection coupled with a normal tibial plateau resection and an attenuated MCL. Second, the joint line is elevated, distorting the kinematics of the collateral ligaments and often

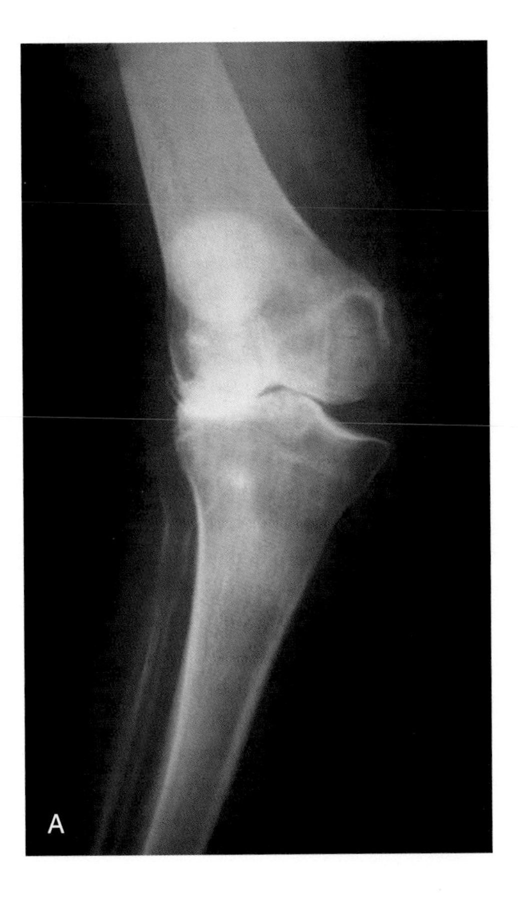

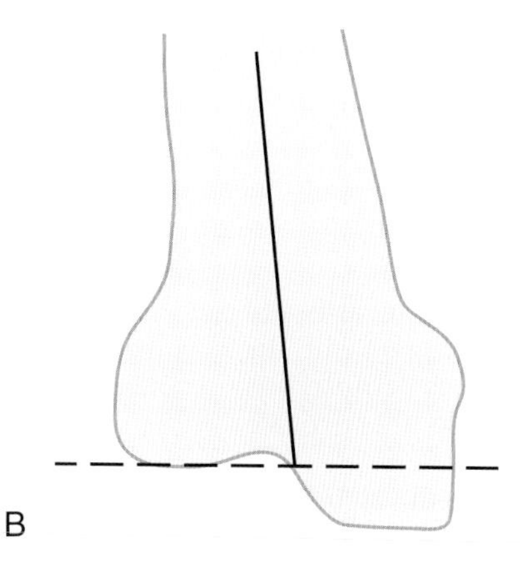

FIGURE 6–8. Avoid resecting back to the level of the condylar deficiency.

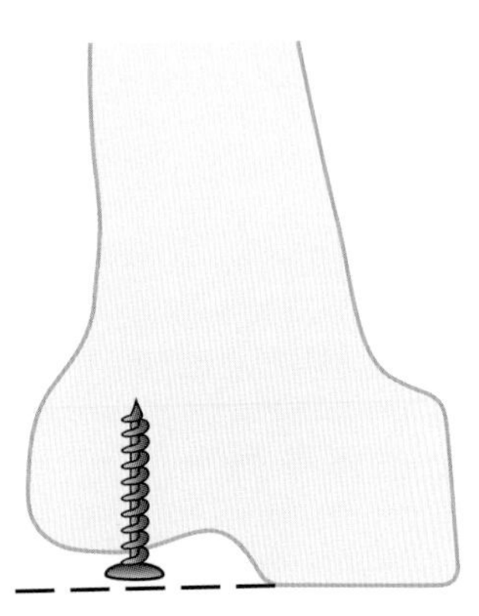

FIGURE 6–9. Resection should be based on the normal medial side with augmentation laterally using cement and screws, or wedges.

resulting in mid-flexion laxity. Both distal femoral and proximal tibial resections in a severe valgus knee should initially be conservative. It is not unusual for the distal lateral resection to be zero or even less. Augmentation methods (see Chapter 12) include cement alone, cement and screw augmentation, or metal wedge modular augments (Fig. 6–9).

Augmentation on the tibial side in severe valgus knees is occasionally necessary if the valgus is due to a depressed lateral plateau fracture or there is erosion of the femoral condyle into the central portion of the tibial plateau. It may also be necessary if the valgus is due to overcorrection following tibial osteotomy (see Chapter 10). Any central lateral plateau deficiency can be filled with cement with or without a supporting screw, depending on the discretion of the surgeon. Because the bone surface is greatly sclerotic, I do not recommend bone graft for these defects.

The wear pattern in the lateral compartment usually is posterior. The appropriate level of tibial resection generally is distal enough to eliminate this deficiency.

THE ANGLE OF DISTAL FEMORAL RESECTION

I prefer a 5-degree valgus angle resection for both varus and valgus knees. In severe valgus, it is tempting to cut the distal femur in as much as 7 degrees of valgus because it is then easier to balance the lax medial side. I do not advocate this for two reasons.

The first reason to choose 5 or less degrees of valgus is to attempt to overcorrect the deformity slightly so that the pathologically stretched and abnormal MCL and capsule are put under less tension during weightbearing. The less the overall valgus, the less tension on the medial side. Some surgeons even like to diminish the valgus angle to as little as 2 or 3 degrees. The result, however, is a need for more lateral release to balance the lax medial side.

A second reason to choose 5 or less degrees of valgus for distal resection is the fact that some of these knees have a distal metaphyseal valgus bow (Fig. 6–10). If the surgeon follows the center of the shaft from its midpoint to the joint line, it becomes apparent that the center shaft alignment exits medial to the true center of the intercondylar notch. Unless the surgeon enters the medullary canal at this medial position, the valgus angle chosen on the cutting jig will actually result in a few more degrees of valgus imparted to the resection (see Chapter 4).

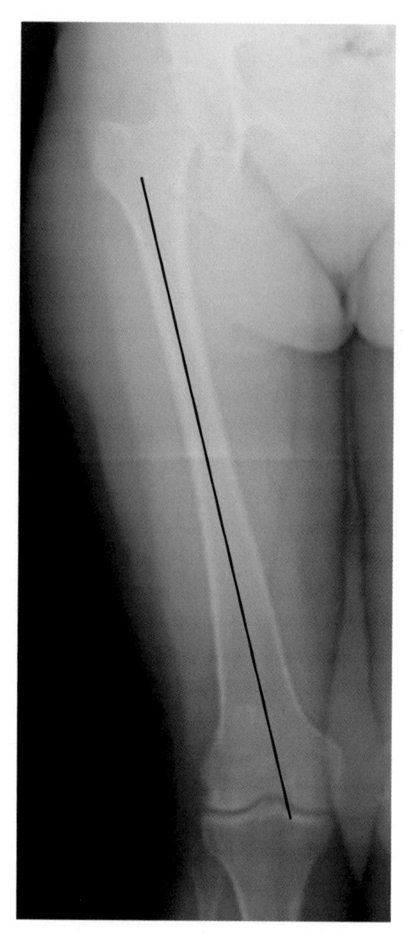

FIGURE 6–10. The entry point for a femoral intramedullary alignment rod must be displaced medially in the presence of a valgus metaphyseal bow.

BALANCING THE VALGUS KNEE IN FLEXION AND EXTENSION

Ligament balancing involves creating symmetric (rectangular) flexion and extension gaps. Unlike the varus knee, the valgus knee can be balanced in flexion independent of the balancing in extension. The flexion gap is balanced by proper rotational alignment of the femoral component (see Chapters 4, 7, and 15). In my experience, the lateral tissues in severe valgus knees are not extremely tight, nor are the medial tissues as lax in flexion as they are in extension (Fig. 6–11). After the conservative distal femoral resection is performed, the knee is flexed 90 degrees, and medial and lateral laminar spreaders are placed to tense the tissues. I still draw the Whiteside line and transepicondylar axis as reference points. Using the tensed flexion gap method, the femoral component is almost always externally rotated to establish symmetry. In extremely rare cases, the lateral collateral ligament (LCL) must be partially released from the femur to open up the lateral side of the flexion gap. This type of situation will always be present in the severe valgus knee that results from overcorrection of the tibial osteotomy (see Chapter 10). In these cases, I accept the fact that internal rotation of the

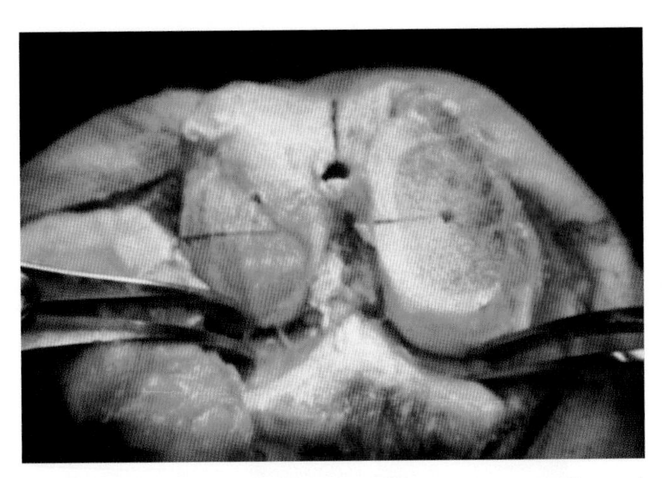

FIGURE 6–11. Medial laxity and lateral tightness are not usually a problem in flexion.

femoral component is necessary to establish symmetry, and I avoid release of the LCL to open up the lateral side in flexion. In my experience, this internal rotation of the femoral component (as much as 5 degrees in some cases) has not led to maltracking of the patella.

For the severe valgus knee in extension, the problem that needs to be resolved is pathologic medial laxity combined with pathologic lateral contracture. Medial laxity in extension can be resolved either by advancement of the medial structures or by lateral release of the tight structures or by a combination of both techniques. Healy and colleagues have published a technique of medial advancement that is attractive to me because the location of the femoral attachment of the MCL is not distorted.[1] The origin of the ligament is freed from the femur attached to a block of bone. This bone block with the ligament attached is then advanced to the metaphysis of the femur at the appropriate tension and secured with anchoring sutures that pass through and are tied over the lateral epicondyle (Fig. 6–12). I have no personal experience with this technique, but it would be my first choice should I elect to perform a medial advancement.

Obviously, I believe that medial lateral imbalance and extension can be resolved in almost all cases by performing a lateral release to balance the lax medial side. Through the years, I have developed a simple inverted cruciform release of the lateral structures that has worked for me even in extremes of deformity.[2] The advantages of the technique are its simplicity and effectiveness. The disadvantages of any lateral release are the resultant slight lengthening of the limb and a very small incidence of transient peroneal palsy.

Balancing the Extension Gap via a Lateral Release

The lateral release is performed after the bone resections are complete. The static alignment of the knee, of course, is determined by the bone cuts. The lateral release to balance the medial side provides stability to the knee in its corrected alignment. As noted above, the femoral and tibial resections should initially be conservative. After they are complete, the knee is brought into extension and the tibia is lined up beneath and against the femur. This placement will show the static alignment of the limb. Valgus stress is then applied to the knee, and I assess the width of the extension gap on the medial side (Fig. 6–13). It should be large enough to receive the thickness of a femoral and tibial component. For example, if the femoral component is 9 mm thick and the tibial component 8 mm thick, a minimum width of 17 mm is required. Owing to the stretched out MCL in a severe valgus knee, this minimum width is easily achieved.

Next, I apply varus stress to the knee and measure the lateral extension gap (Fig. 6–14). Most likely, it will be far less than the medial gap, confirming the need for lateral release to balance the knee.

Inverted Cruciform Release for Severe Valgus

This release starts similarly to the release recommended for patellar tracking (see Chapter 7). It is easier to perform the release without prosthetic components in place because the resultant laxity enhances exposure.

Prior to initiating the release, the lateral superior genicular vessels are isolated (Fig. 6–15). These will be preserved for their blood supply to the patella and overlying skin flap. A vertical release begins just below the vessels approximately one third of the way from the lateral edge of the femur to the edge of the patella. A vertical slit is made in the retinaculum until the subcutaneous fat is visualized (Fig. 6–16). One blade of a pair of scissors can then be placed into this slit and advanced distally to the level of the tibial bone resection (Fig. 6–17). A hemostat can be used to grasp the cut edge of the retinaculum at the level of the joint line or approximately 1 cm above the cut surface of the tibia. A slight varus stress is applied to the knee to put the cut edge on tension, and a horizontal cut is made posteriorly with a scalpel or scissors for approximately 2 cm. The anterior edge of the

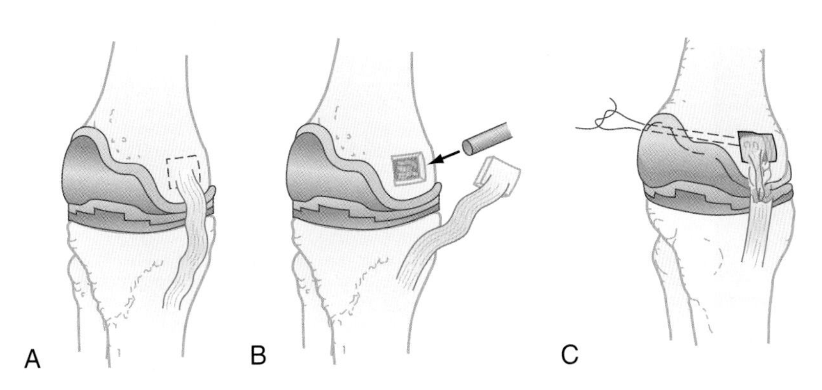

FIGURE 6–12. The MCL origin can be advanced by recession into the metaphyseal bone of the femur. (From Healy WL, Iorio R, Lemas DW: Medial reconstruction during total knee arthroplasty for severe valgus deformity. Clin Orthop Relat Res 1998;(356):161–169.)

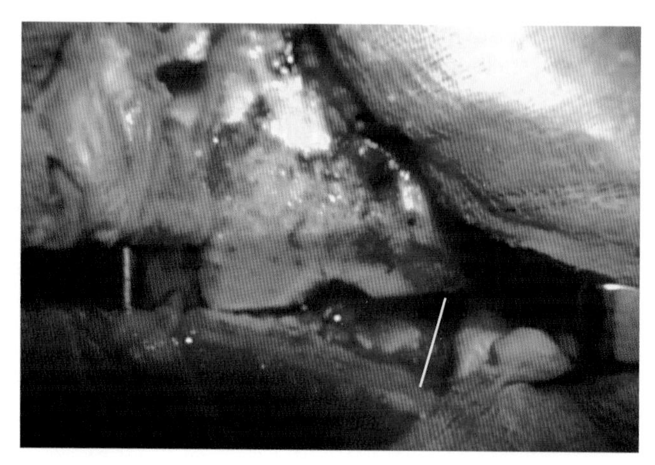

FIGURE 6–13. Valgus stress shows that the medial side opens sufficiently.

retinaculum is then grasped at the same level and a horizontal cut is made anteriorly toward the patellar tendon, again for approximately 2 cm (Fig. 6–18). The result is an inverted cruciform lateral retinacular release (Fig. 6–19). If a varus stress is applied, this release opens up in the shape of a four-pointed star.

This initial release may not yet be adequate. To ascertain adequacy, trial components are implanted using the thickness of insert on the tibial side that stabilizes the knee medially in extension (Fig. 6–20). The knee is then brought from flexion into extension. If the release is adequate, full extension is achieved. If it is inadequate, there is a lack of extension. As long as the surgeon has chosen the proper thickness to stabilize the medial side, the lack of extension does not signal the need for more distal femoral resection to increase the extension gap but rather signals the need for increasing the lateral release. This becomes apparent if the lateral soft tissues are palpated with the knee in the extended position. To propagate the release to the appropriate level, the knee is gently manipulated into extension. I often actually hear the soft tissue release occur as full extension is achieved. An obvious concern with this technique is the potential for peroneal nerve palsy. In using this technique in more than 50 consecutive cases, I have seen palsy detected once in the recovery room and it was resolved by loosening the operative dressing and flexing the knee by 45 degrees. This knee had preoperative valgus of 30 degrees. The palsy recurred each time the knee was fully extended over the next 24 hours and resolved each time when the knee was flexed. After 48 hours, the knee could be brought to full extension with no recurrence of palsy. A second patient had the onset of peroneal palsy 3 days following surgery. This palsy did not fully resolve until 6 months after surgery.

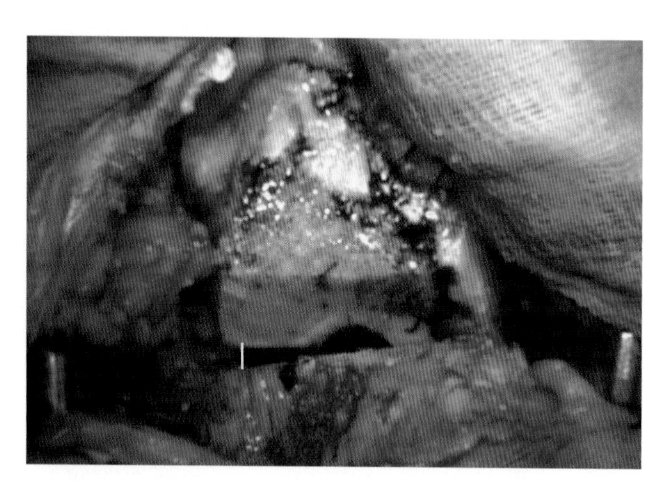

FIGURE 6–14. Varus stress shows that the lateral side is much tighter than the medial side.

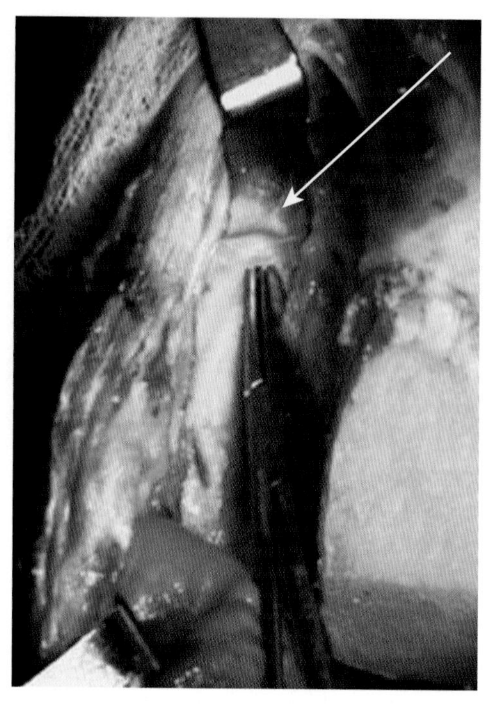

FIGURE 6–15. Isolation of the lateral superior genicular vessels.

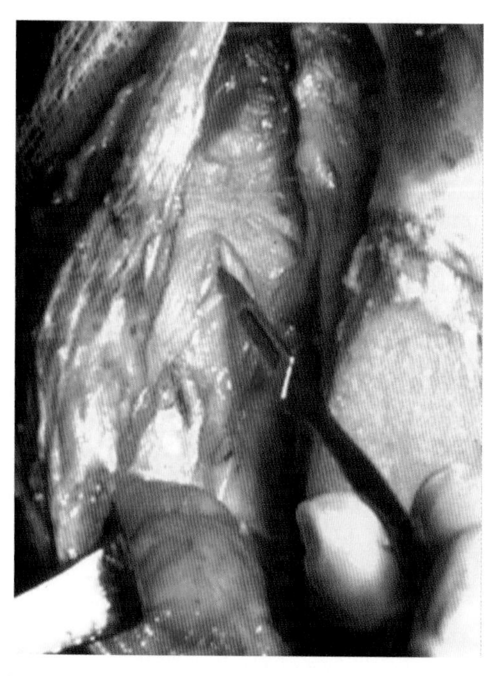

FIGURE 6–16. A vertical slit is made in the retinaculum.

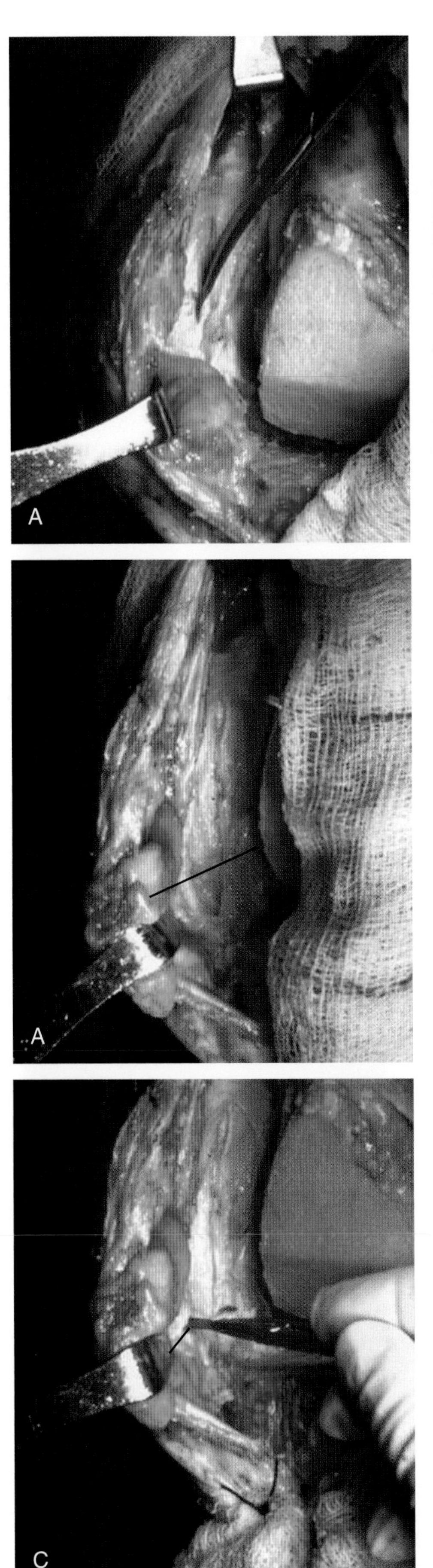

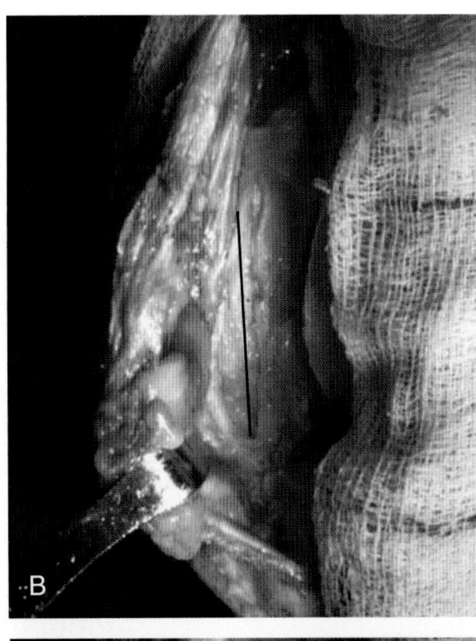

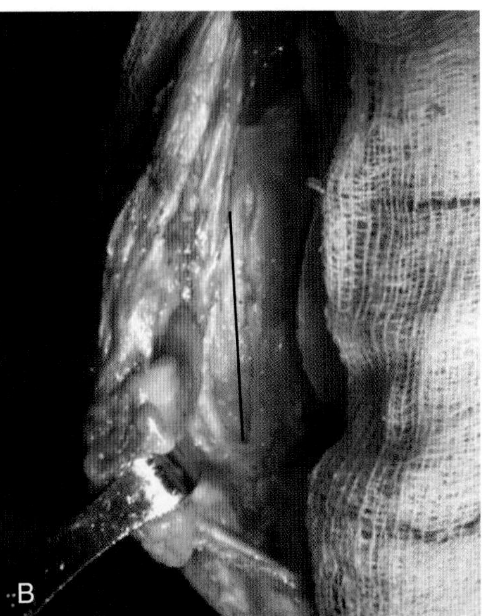

FIGURE 6–17. Vertical release from just below the vessels to the level of the tibial resection.

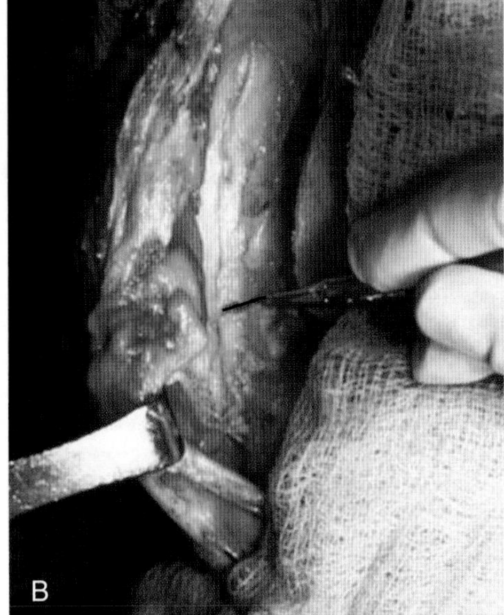

FIGURE 6–18. Horizontal release posteriorly and anteriorly at the level of the joint line.

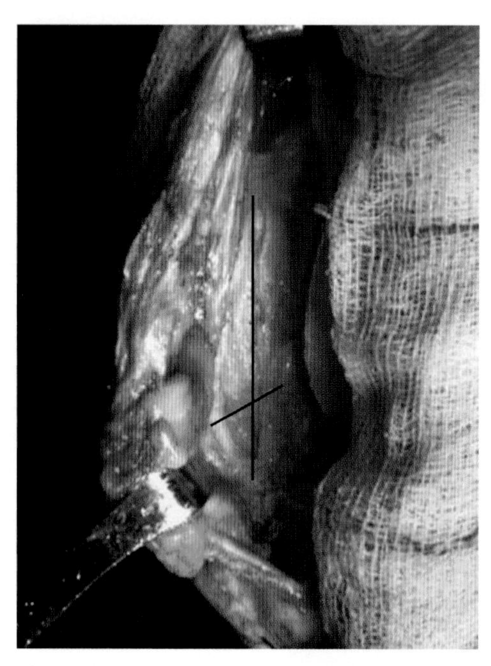

FIGURE 6–19. The result of the two retinacular incisions is an inverted cruciform release.

Lateral Collateral Ligament, Popliteal, and Biceps Tendon Release

It is now very rare for me to release the popliteus and LCLs from their femoral origins to correct a severe valgus deformity. I believe that the lateral retinaculum and capsule are all that need to be released for tightness in extension, while the LCL would be released mainly for tightness in flexion. Since lateral tightness in flexion is so rare, it is equally rare to need to perform this release.

Biceps release seems to be appropriate in the severe valgus knee with a combined flexion deformity. My preference is to never release the biceps tendon because I think that it protects the peroneal nerve from excessive longitudinal tension. I believe that flexion contractures must be resolved by other means (see Chapter 9).

POSTERIOR CRUCIATE LIGAMENT PRESERVATION VERSUS SUBSTITUTION

Either posterior cruciate ligament (PCL) retention or substitution is acceptable in the treatment of the severe valgus knee. I favor preservation of the PCL because of its medial stabilizing force (Fig. 6–21). However, if the medial side is pathologically lax and the lateral side is surgically released, the PCL will most likely be too tight and have to be released as well. The tightest fibers are usually those that are more lateral and anterior. The technique of PCL balancing is described in Chapter 2.

SUMMARY

Severe valgus usually is seen in the elderly female patient. It often is associated with patellofemoral disease, lateral femoral chondral hyperplasia, a valgus tibial bow, and medial laxity.

Excessive initial bone resection must be avoided. The flexion gap is balanced by appropriate femoral rotation with the ligaments tensed. The extension gap is balanced either by medial advancement or lateral release. I prefer a simple inverted cruciform release of the iliotibial band. This appears to be effective for all degrees of valgus. The LCL rarely needs to be released; when necessary, it is usually for tightness in flexion. In order to protect the peroneal nerve, the biceps should probably never be released.

The PCL can be preserved or substituted. A preserved PCL helps stabilize the medial side. A substituting technique removes the need for PCL balancing. Results of either technique can be gratifying and long lasting (Fig. 6–22).

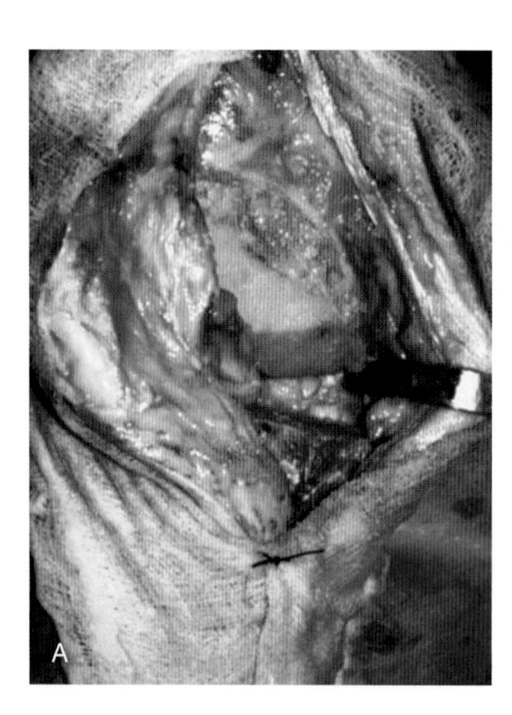

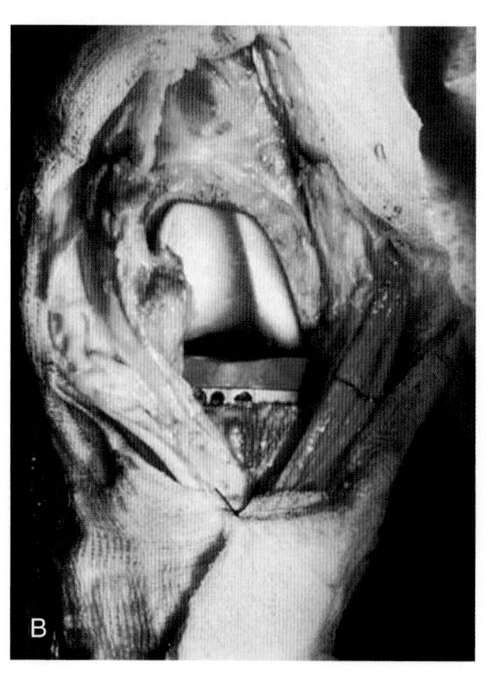

FIGURE 6–20. Trial components are tested to choose the thickness of insert that stabilizes the medial side.

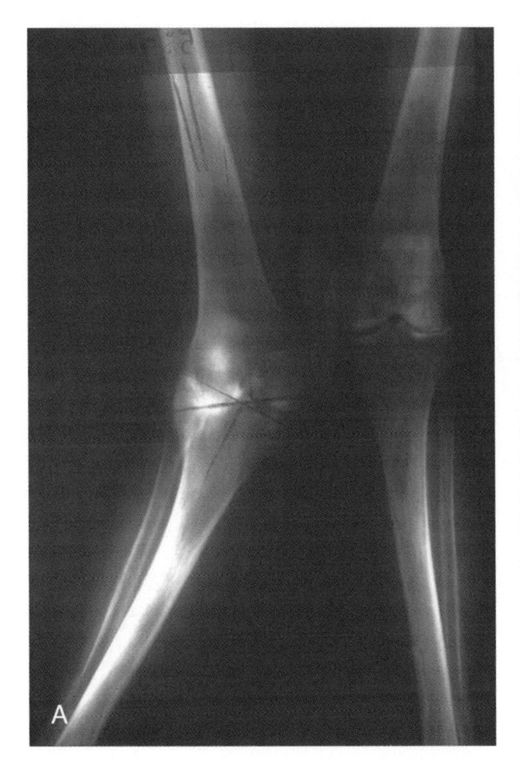

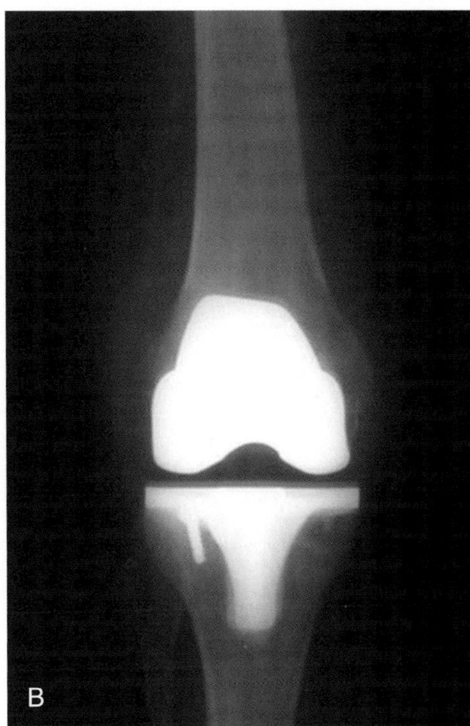

FIGURE 6–21. PCL retention in severe valgus is possible.

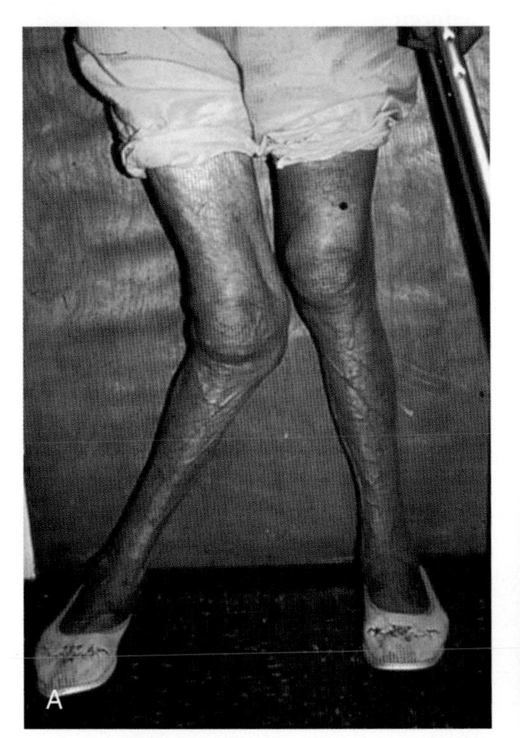

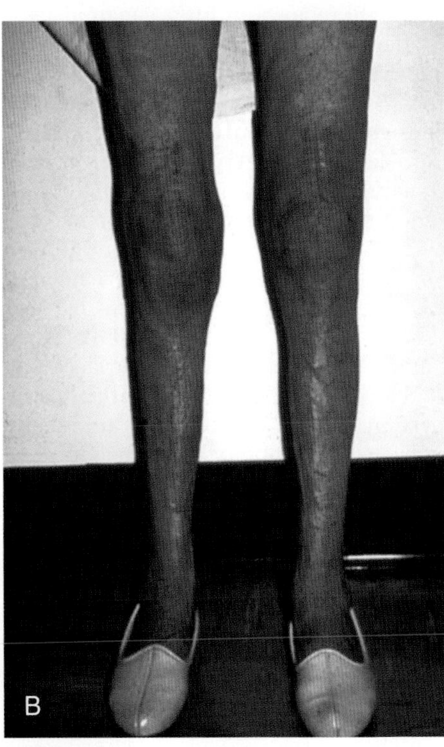

FIGURE 6–22. Preoperative (*A*) and postoperative (*B*) appearance following correction of a severe valgus deformity. (Courtesy of William H. Thomas, MD.)

References

1. Healy WL, Iorio R, Lemos DW: Medial reconstruction during total knee arthroplasty for severe valgus deformity. Clin Orthop 1998;356:161–169.
2. Politi J, Scott R: Balancing severe valgus deformity using a lateral cruciform retinacular release. J Arthroplasty 2004;19:553–557.

CHAPTER 7

Patellofemoral Complications Associated with Total Knee Arthroplasty

Patellofemoral complications are thought to account for as much as 50% of complications after total knee arthroplasty (TKA).[1] These statistics come from arthroplasties performed in the 1980s and early 1990s. With improvements in surgical technique and prosthetic design, the incidence is decreasing but is still significant. Problems include pain following an unresurfaced patella, maltracking, fracture, prosthetic loosening, osteonecrosis, and prosthetic wear.

THE UNRESURFACED PATELLA

One of the persistent controversies in TKA is whether the patella requires resurfacing. I have had more than 30 years of experience dealing with this question. In 1973, most prosthetic designs did not provide for even the possibility of patellar resurfacing of either trochlea or patella. In 1974, the first prosthesis in the form of the duopatellar design provided a femoral component with a trochlear flange and an optional polyethylene button for the patellar side of the patellofemoral joint.[2] At that time, 80% of our patients had rheumatoid arthritis. In 1974, we resurfaced only 5% of the patellae in both rheumatoid and osteoarthritic patients. Those patellae that were resurfaced were the ones having severe degenerative changes with exposed patellar bone at the time of arthrotomy. A 5-year review showed that 10% of the rheumatoid patients suffered secondary degeneration of the patella with cystic changes, pain, swelling, and sometimes the recurrence of rheumatoid synovitis (Fig. 7–1). By the end of the 1970s there was uniform agreement within our group to resurface the patella in all rheumatoid patients regardless of the operative findings.

Even in retrospect, we could not predict which rheumatoid patients would have problems and which would not. I don't mean to say that an unresurfaced patella in a rheumatoid patient will always encounter difficulty. I have some rheumatoid patients without a resurfaced patella who are still functioning well without patellofemoral symptoms more than 25 years after surgery.

Osteoarthritic patients fared better than rheumatoid patients (Fig. 7–2). Patients who did have secondary degeneration of the patella after TKA usually had a slight maltracking problem. The result would be areas of focal wear causing pain and possibly leading to progressive degeneration of the bone and progressive subluxation (Fig. 7–3). From this experience I developed certain selection criteria in the 1980s that led to selective patellar resurfacing in approximately 80% of osteoarthritic patients and left 20% of patellae unresurfaced. The indications for not resurfacing included noninflammatory osteoarthritis. That meant that patients with gout, pseudogout, or an inflamed synovium were resurfaced. In addition, the patients would have to have congruent

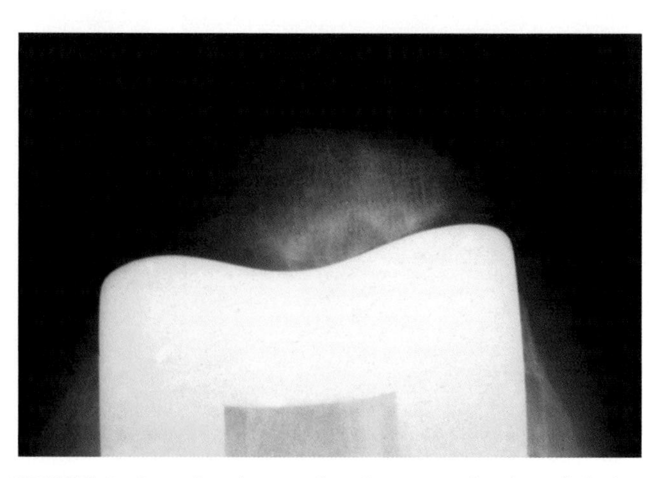

FIGURE 7–1. Secondary degeneration of an unresurfaced patella in rheumatoid arthritis.

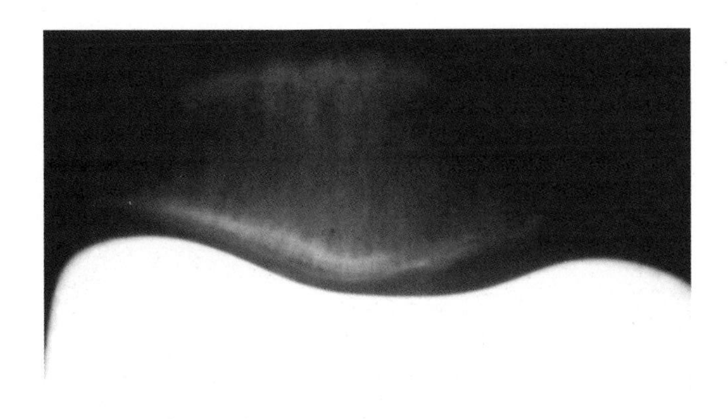

FIGURE 7–2. Twenty-year follow-up of an unresurfaced patella in osteoarthritis.

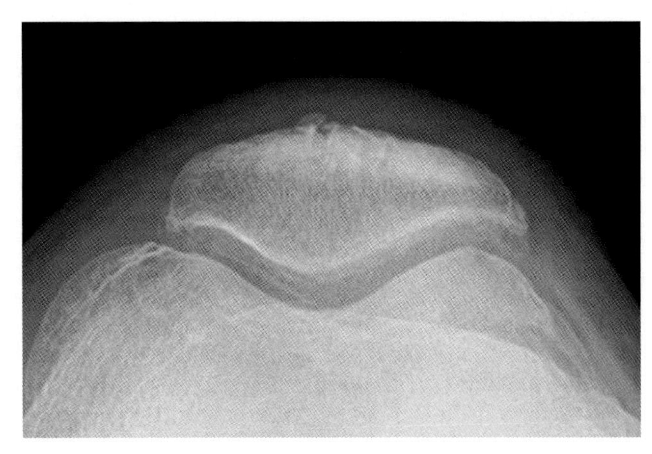

FIGURE 7–4. Preoperative skyline view of an ideal candidate for nonresurfacing.

tracking of the patella on the preoperative skyline with maintenance of a joint space. At surgery, there would be no areas of exposed eburnated bone. The unresurfaced patella would also have to track congruently with the trochlear flange of the prosthesis. Using these selection criteria, the 10-year survivorship of unresurfaced patellae was 97%.[3] On the other hand, resurfaced patellae from that era were experiencing a higher incidence of complications including accelerated wear of a metal-backed patella, potential wear and deformation of an all-polyethylene patella, patella stress fracture, and prosthetic loosening.

Second-decade evaluation of results showed that some patients with unresurfaced patellae could develop significant symptoms as late as 15 years after their arthroplasty and require secondary resurfacing. At the same time, improvements in prosthetic design and surgical technique were diminishing the complications seen with resurfacing. In addition, a patient with an unresurfaced patella might have pain that was attributed to the patellofemoral compartment but more likely did not originate from it. Unnecessary and unhelpful repeat surgery to resurface the patella could result. This situation prompted me to eliminate older patients and those with very low pain thresholds from the group that I might leave unresurfaced. For this reason, my personal incidence of not resurfacing the patella has diminished to less than 5% of cases. Today, if I do not resurface the patella it is after a careful preoperative discussion with the individual patient about the pros and cons of this decision. The advantages of not resurfacing are the conservation of patellar bone, avoiding resurfacing complications, easy salvage, and permitting high patellofemoral forces to be placed on this articulation without concern for prosthetic wear in active patients. The disadvantages are the possibility of incomplete pain relief and the fact that as comparative reoperation rates for resurfacing became known, they appeared to favor resurfacing in most patients. The ideal candidate for nonresurfacing is probably the young, heavy, active male patient (Fig. 7–4).

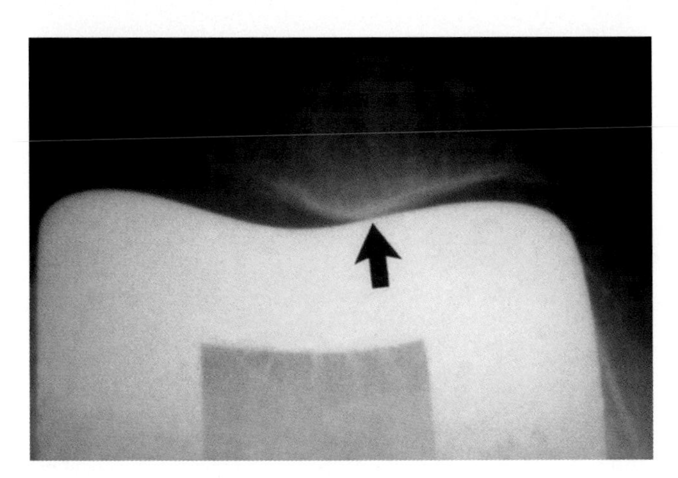

FIGURE 7–3. Subluxation of an unresurfaced patella with point contact and wear.

When considering not resurfacing the patella, always remember that the prosthetic geometry of the trochlear flange of the prosthesis utilized can make a difference. Obviously a flange that is not anatomic and flat will not tolerate an unresurfaced patella as easily as one that is anatomic in shape.

The reported results of nonresurfacing must be considered to be prosthesis-specific and not necessarily generic.

MALTRACKING OF THE PATELLA

Maltracking of the patella associated with TKA is usually the result of several factors converging in the same patient. Causes of maltracking include residual valgus limb alignment, valgus placement of the femoral component, patella alta, poor prosthetic geometry, internal rotation of the femoral or tibial component, excessive patellar thickness, asymmetric patellar preparation, failure to perform a lateral release when indicated, capsular dehiscence, and dynamic instability.

Residual Valgus Limb Alignment

Valgus limb alignment after total knee arthroplasty is usually the result of excessive valgus placement of the femoral component. I think this most often occurs when the surgeon places the intramedullary alignment device for the distal resection into a hole made at the center of the intercondylar notch (see Chapter 4). Preoperative templating will show that on most radiographs a line down the center of the shaft of the distal femur will exit several millimeters medial to the true anatomic center of the notch. If the entry hole is made lateral to the true exit point, the amount of valgus imparted to the distal cut will be up to several degrees greater than indicated by the instrument. The resultant increased valgus to the limb alignment increases the "Q-angle," encouraging lateral tracking of the patella.

Excessive Valgus Placement of the Femoral Component

Even if the surgeon counteracts valgus placement of the femoral component with some varus placement of the tibial component, correcting overall limb alignment, a valgus femoral component can compromise patellar tracking. The valgus placement shifts the most proximal portion of the trochlear flange medially so that the patella may not even be centered on the groove in full extension (Fig. 7–5).

Patella Alta

Patella alta can affect tracking in a similar manner. In this situation, the patella is positioned higher than the top of the prosthetic trochlear flange in full extension and may not be funneled properly into the groove of the trochlea. The predicament of patellar tracking is accentuated when the trochlear flange of the prosthesis is both narrow and shallow (Fig. 7–6).

Component Malrotation

Internal rotation of either the femoral or the tibial component can promote maltracking. On the femoral side this is caused by the fact that with internal rotation of the femoral component the trochlear groove is moved medially away

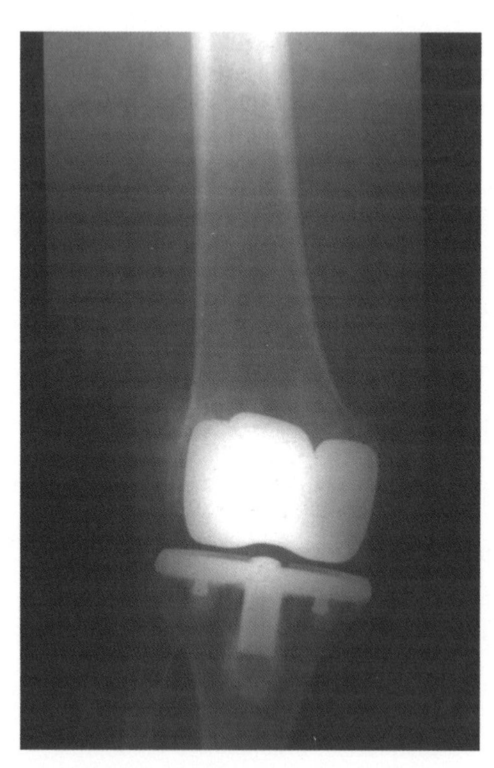

FIGURE 7–5. Excessive valgus placement of the femoral component, leading to patellar instability.

FIGURE 7–6. Narrow trochlear flange promoting patellar instability.

from the natural mediolateral position of the patella. I believe the effect of internal rotation of the femoral component on patellar maltracking may be overestimated. Depending on prosthetic geometry, it takes approximately 3 degrees of rotation of the femur to move the trochlear groove 1 mm. The amount of internal rotation, therefore, will determine its influence (Fig. 7–7).

The effect of rotation can be counteracted by undersizing the patellar component and shifting it medially as well as moving the femoral component as far laterally on the distal femur as possible so long as prosthetic overhang is not created.

Rotational Alignment of the Femoral Component

Although femoral component rotation does have an effect on patellar tracking, as stated above, I think that femoral component rotation by itself is not as significant as others believe. The major importance of femoral component rotation is to assist in the establishment of flexion gap symmetry. The technical details of determining femoral component rotation are discussed in Chapter 4.

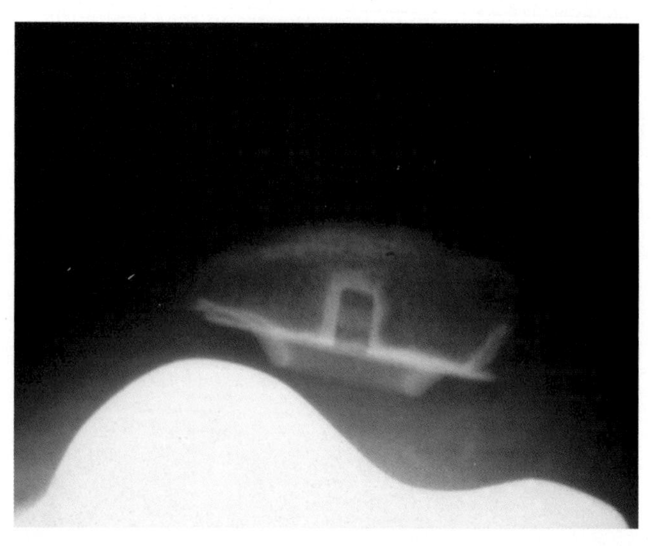

FIGURE 7–7. Marked internal rotation of the femoral component promoting patellar instability. The patella also has been asymmetrically prepared and is too thick.

Patellar Thickness

Excessive patellar thickness may also promote maltracking, mainly owing to its effect on overall shortening of the quadriceps excursion. For this reason, the surgeon should always measure the patient's patellar thickness prior to preparation of the bone. My colleagues and I have published a study showing that the average thickness of female patellae is between 22 and 24 mm whereas the average thickness of male patellae is between 24 and 26 mm.[4] In the case of a worn dysplastic patella, thickness can be restored to these values. The effect of thickness is more significant in preoperatively stiff knees than in very mobile knees.

Asymmetric Patellar Preparation

Asymmetric patellar preparation is another cause of maltracking. The most common fault is for the surgeon to not fully define the medial chondro-osseous junction by removing potential overlying soft tissue or synovium. The patellar cut is therefore shallow on the medial side but complete on the lateral side (see Fig. 7–7). This immediately imparts a tilt to the prosthetic component, promoting maltracking.

Need for Lateral Release

Prior to wound closure after TKA implantation, patellar tracking should be evaluated to assess the potential need for lateral release. The incidence of lateral release in the past was quite high in some series. I recall some surgeons reporting that their lateral release rate was 100%.

For most surgeons the lateral release rate was around 30% until the last 5 years when prosthetic geometry was improved and implantation techniques also improved by eliminating the technical errors mentioned above. Most experienced surgeons will report a lateral release rate less than 5% for varus knees. It is usually higher for valgus knees because they are often associated with patella alta and preoperative subluxation. I make a distinction between a lateral release required to correct a valgus deformity and a lateral release required to balance the patella. The release for valgus is distal to the lateral superior genicular vessels, whereas the release for the patella has to extend proximal to these vessels (see Chapters 4 and 6).

"Rule of No Thumb" Test

The classic intraoperative test for patellar tracking is referred to as the "rule of no thumb."[5] In this test, first suggested by F. Ewald, the patella is returned to the trochlear groove in extension with the capsule unclosed. The knee is then passively flexed, and whether or not the patella tracks congruently without capsular closure is assessed. If it does and the medial facet of the patellar component contacts the medial aspect of the trochlear groove, no lateral release need be considered. If the patella dislocates or tilts, lateral release may be necessary. The test should be repeated with one suture closing the capsule at the level of the superior pole. If tracking then becomes congruent without excessive tension on the suture, no release is necessary. If tilting still persists, some surgeons like to assess tracking with the tourniquet deflated so that any binding effect on the quadriceps can be eliminated from the test. A tight posterior cruciate ligament (PCL) can also impart apparent patellar tilt as the femoral component is drawn posteriorly while the tibia (with its tubercle) moves anteriorly.

Dynamic Patellar Instability

Dynamic instability is another form of patellar subluxation that must be considered. In this clinical situation, intraoperative testing for patellar tracking shows no evidence of subluxation. Postoperatively, however, the patella is partially dislocated laterally with full active extension and proceeds to shift medially into the trochlear groove on initiation of flexion. This may not cause a functional disability to the patient but is a rather disconcerting clinical finding that could, in fact, lead to accelerated patellar wear. This syndrome is most likely to occur in patients who have significant preoperative swelling that has stretched out the medial structures. Although the "rule of no thumb" test shows congruent tracking passively, the stretched out medial capsule combined with normal postoperative swelling allows dynamic lateral subluxation in full active extension. Sometimes the symptoms disappear as the postoperative effusion resolves. If the syndrome persists, resolution requires reoperation with advancement of the medial capsule.

Testing for Dynamic Instability

It is possible to test for and prevent this syndrome. The surgeon should be aware of the possibility when operating on patients with large, chronic, preoperative effusions. At the initiation of closure, two or three sutures are placed in the capsule at the level of the superior pole of the patella. With the knee in extension, medial capsular laxity is assessed by attempts to manually dislocate the patella laterally. If this is possible, the sutures are removed and a medial advancement is performed so that subluxation in extension is not possible.

VASCULAR SUPPLY TO THE PATELLA

It is important to maintain the integrity of the blood supply to the patella. The major sources are the medial and lateral superior and inferior genicular vessels. The medial genicular vessels are obviously interrupted during a standard medial arthrotomy. This emphasizes the importance of preserving lateral sources of blood supply if possible. The lateral inferior genicular artery is almost always sacrificed as a normal part of exposure for TKA (see Chapter 4). The vessel lies just lateral to the rim of the lateral meniscus. After the meniscectomy is completed, the surgeon should search for the open lumen of the artery and vein in the posterior aspect of the lateral compartment and coagulate these vessels to minimize postoperative bleeding (see Fig. 4–7).

The lateral superior genicular artery is the more important of the two lateral vessels and can be preserved even if a lateral release is required for valgus or patellar tracking (see Chapter 6). The vessels can be found in the lateral gutter at the level of the superior pole of the patella and in the fatty tissue just beneath the synovial layer. They form the base of a hypotenuse triangle with the angle of the triangle the curtain of the vastus lateralis muscle fibers and the height

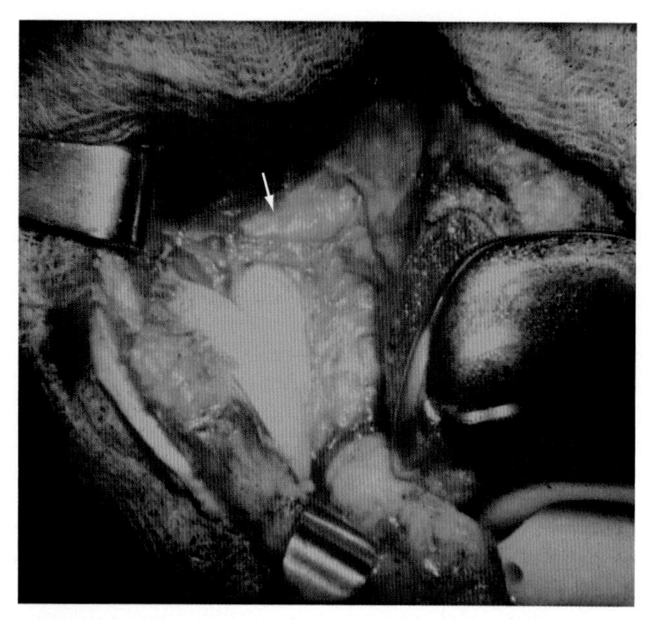

FIGURE 7–8. The lateral superior genicular vessels exposed in the lateral gutter of the knee.

of the triangle the lateral cortex of the femur (Fig. 7–8). A lateral release for valgus begins distal to these vessels. When a lateral release is necessary for patellar tracking, it can be performed beneath the vessels, preserving them. The vertical part of the release distal to the vessels facilitates tracking in extension (Fig. 7–9). The part that is proximal to the vessels facilitates tracking in flexion and is directed at a 45-degree angle to the vertical release making it perpendicular to the fibers of the vastus lateralis.

Although sacrifice of the lateral superior genicular vessels does not necessarily lead to an avascular complication of the patella or the skin flap, postoperative bone scan studies demonstrate that this is a possibility.[6] If full-blown osteonecrosis were to occur in patellar bone, the potential for stress fracture or component loosening would be increased.

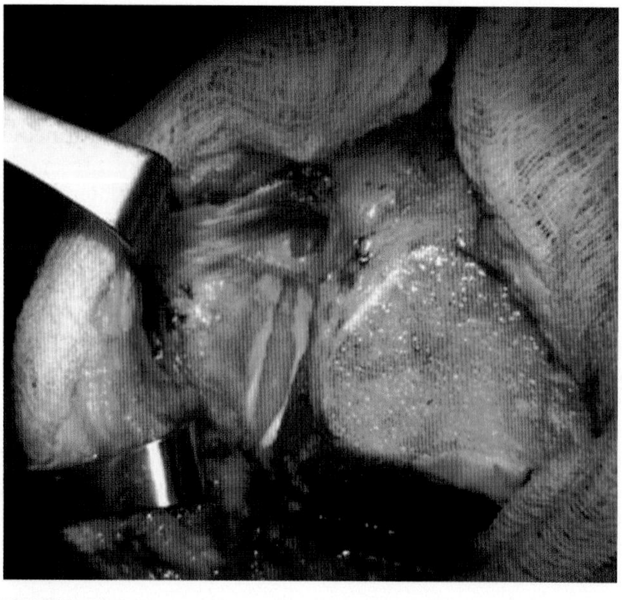

FIGURE 7–9. A lateral release with preservation of the superior genicular vessels.

PATELLA FRACTURE

Patella fractures can be the result of direct trauma, osteonecrosis, or high stresses across the patellar component fixation holes (Fig. 7–10).[7] In addition, small, usually insignificant, avulsion fractures can be seen at the superior or inferior pole of the patella (Fig. 7–11). Most fractures, regardless of the cause, do not need surgical treatment unless the extensor mechanism is disrupted or the patellar component is no longer fixed in a major fragment of the patella.

Initial treatment involves immobilization of the knee in a removable brace for several weeks allowing gentle passive flexion to 90 degrees once each day to maintain range of motion. Isometric quadriceps exercises are started immediately. Immobilization is gradually discontinued after 4 weeks and active extension initiated. If the patellar component has lost its fixation, surgery is necessary to remove it and repair any quadriceps disruption. All major fragments of patellar bone are initially preserved to try to maintain as much of the quadriceps mechanism integrity as possible. At times, a secondary complete patellectomy may be necessary, followed by "tubing" of the quadriceps mechanism to reinforce and thicken it (Fig. 7–12).

The incidence of stress fracture of the patella appears to be related to the fixation method. Large central fixation lugs have a higher incidence of stress fracture than smaller lugs whether central or peripheral.

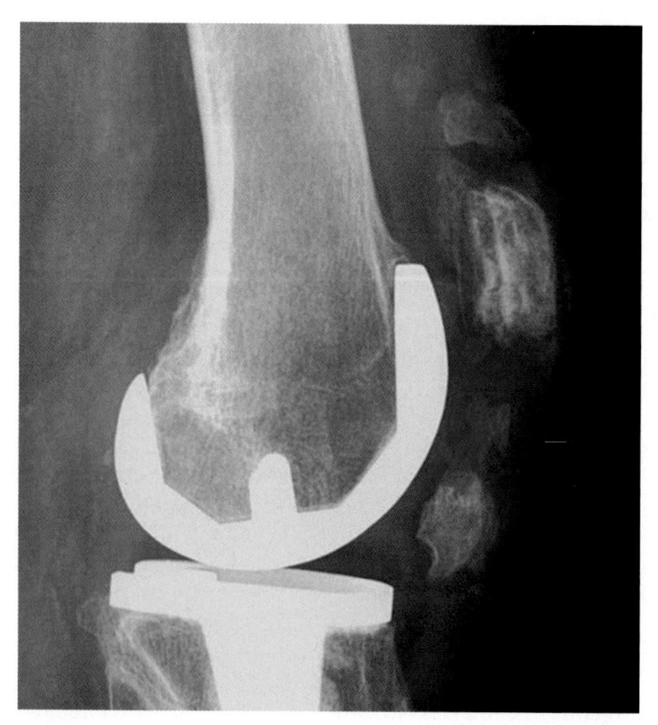

FIGURE 7–10. Stress fracture through the inferior pole of the patella.

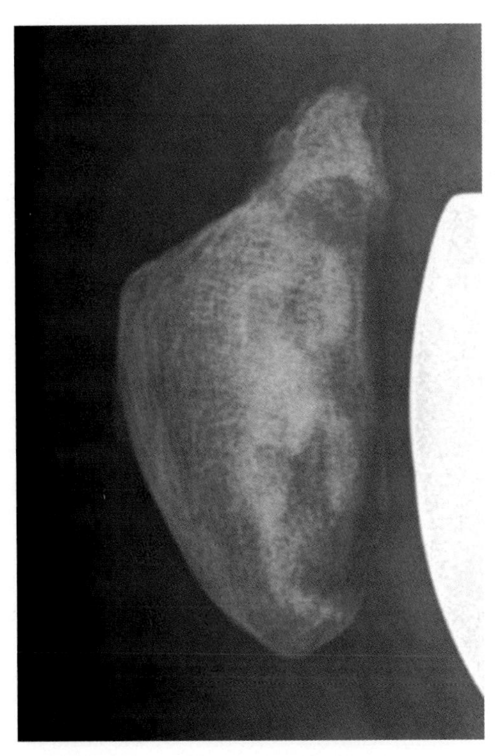

FIGURE 7–11. Small avulsion fractures at the superior pole of the patella are usually transiently symptomatic.

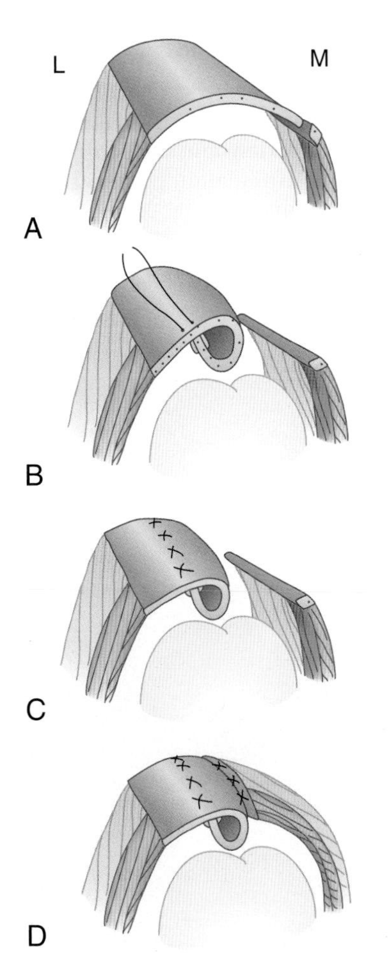

FIGURE 7–12. A method of "tubing" of the quadriceps to thicken and define the quadriceps mechanism.

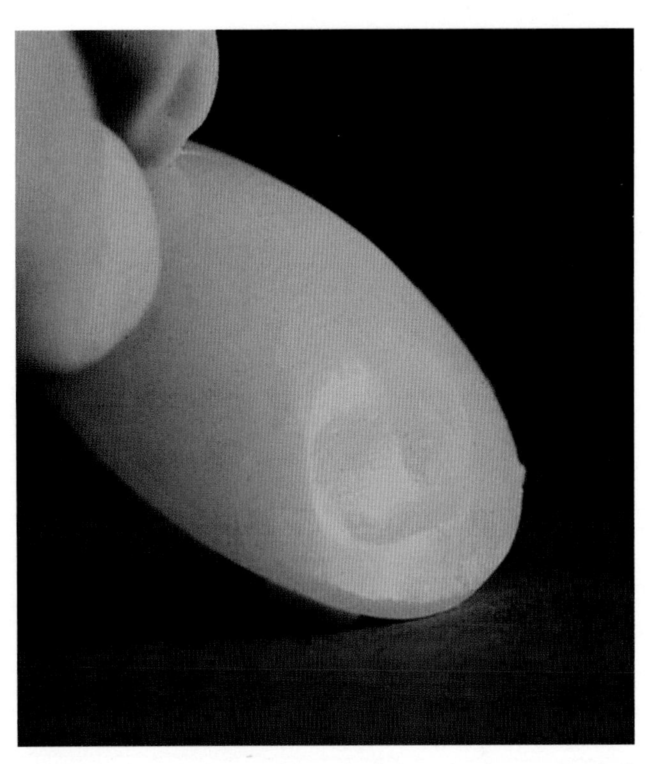

FIGURE 7–13. Deformation of the polyethylene due to poor prosthetic geometry.

PATELLAR LOOSENING

Patellar loosening also appears to be related to the fixation method. While large central lugs have a higher incidence of stress fracture, small central lugs have a higher incidence of loosening. Prosthetic components with three peripheral lugs appear to have the lowest overall incidence of both stress fracture and loosening and are the preferred method of patellar fixation.

Loosening can also be associated with osteonecrosis and with progressive deformation of the polyethylene owing to asymmetric wear forces transmitted to the surface of the patella as a result of poor prosthetic geometry (Fig. 7–13).

PROSTHETIC WEAR

Wear and defamation of an all-polyethylene patellar component, as described above, may lead to loss of fixation and patellar loosening, but isolated wear of an all-polyethylene component usually is not a situation that leads to reoperation. It is wear of metal-backed patellar components that is of concern. These components were introduced in the early 1980s at the time when tibial components began to become metal-backed. Metal backing theoretically has two advantages. One is the possibility of better distribution of forces across the fixation interface, as was shown for metal-backed tibial components. The other is the possibility of cementless fixation with bone ingrowth into a porous backing. Unfortunately, metal-backing a patella requires thinning the overlying polyethylene to the point where high stresses often lead to breakdown of the surface with exposure of the metal backing to the trochlea and resultant metal synovitis and

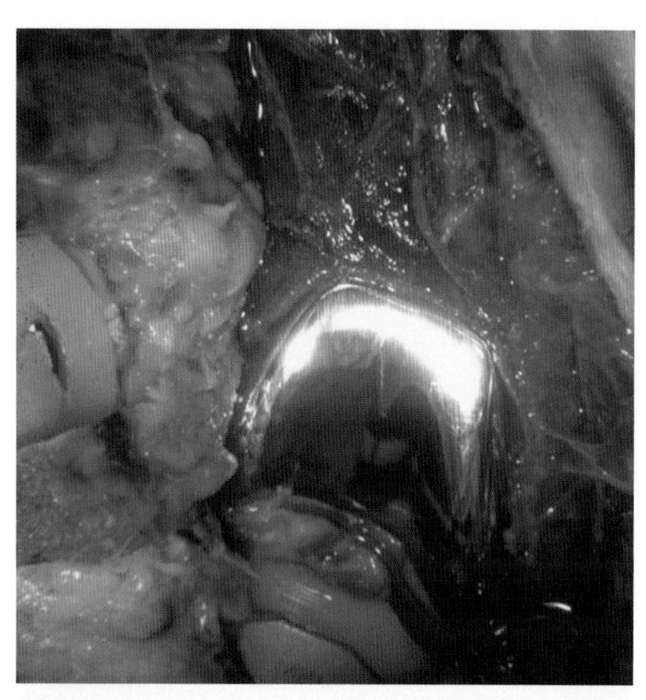

FIGURE 7–14. A worn, metal-backed patellar component with resultant metal synovitis.

urgent need for revision (Fig. 7–14). At the same time, the introduction of cemented, three-pegged all-polyethylene components provided a cemented method of fixation with high initial success and few late complications.

The mobile-bearing metal-backed patellar component is the only design that so far has enjoyed high success despite the metal backing. This is most likely due to the high conformity and low stresses permitted with a mobile-bearing articulation.

Attempts to minimize wear of all-polyethylene components have grown out of a better understanding of the kinematics of this articulation. The earliest designs from the mid-1970s provided a dome-shaped patella, which may have articulated congruently with the trochlear groove in extension but additionally allowed high stresses and point contact in flexion when the patellar component came down onto the femoral condyles (Fig. 7–15). This, of course, is where the highest forces are seen across the patellofemoral joint when a person arises from a chair or goes up stairs. The forces can be as high as five times body weight. Retrievals showed that the patella began to wear or "cold-flow" into a shape that had peripheral concavities articulating with the convexity of the condyles in flexion (see Fig. 7–13). In the early 1980s, the shape of the patellar component evolved into a so-called sombrero shape to allow for increased contact between metal and plastic in high flexion (Fig. 7–16). Alternatively, other designs kept the concave shape of the trochlear groove partway onto the femoral condyles (Fig. 7–17). This allows a dome-shaped patella to have high contact and good congruency in flexion as well as extension. In addition, the round-on-round shape of the articulation permits patellar tilt to occur without the possibility of edge-loading (Fig. 7–18). Total knee systems today provide various designs that allow the surgeon to choose either type of articulation.

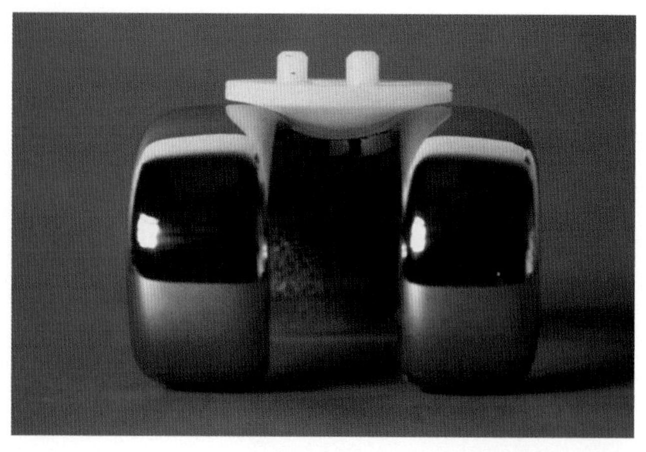

FIGURE 7–16. The sombrero-shaped patella provides more metal-to-plastic contact in flexion.

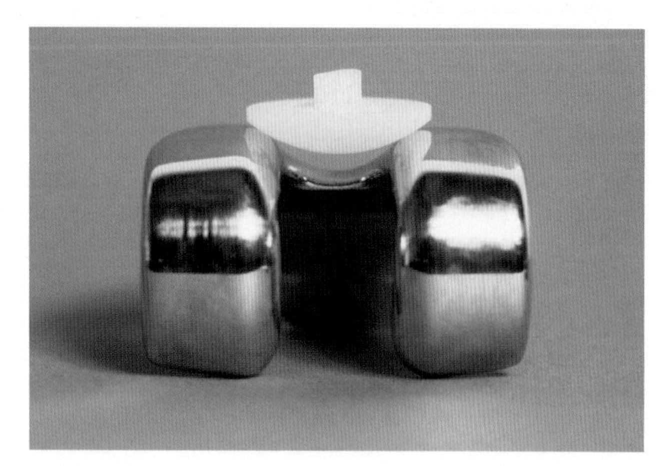

FIGURE 7–15. Point contact between the dome-shaped patella and femoral condyles occurs in high flexion in old condylar designs.

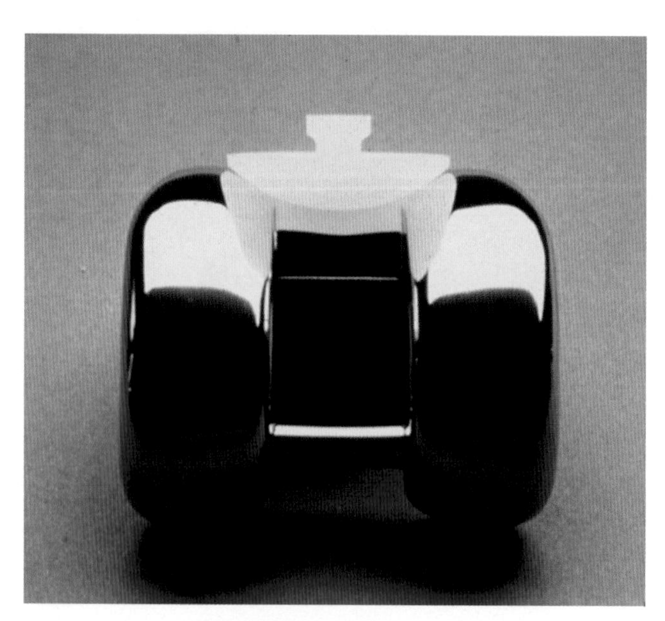

FIGURE 7–17. An alternative articulation that prolongs the trochlear groove onto the femoral condyles.

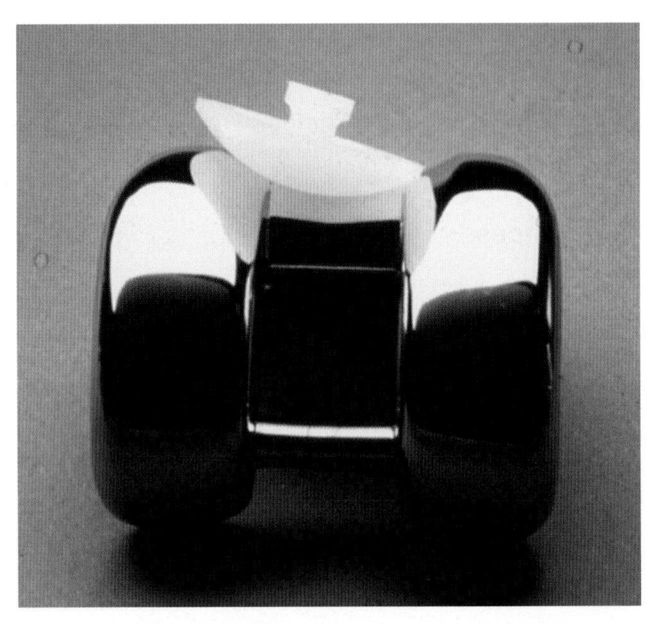

FIGURE 7–18. This articulation allows patellar tilt to occur while maintaining good metal-to-plastic congruency.

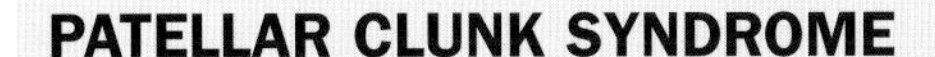

PATELLAR CLUNK SYNDROME

The patellar clunk syndrome occurs when scar tissue builds up at the superior pole of the patella and becomes trapped in the intercondylar housing of a posterior stabilized femoral component. For this reason, the clunk syndrome is not seen in PCL-retaining designs. Instead of a clunk, the patient may experience palpable and audible crepitus that is due to the presence of this scar tissue.

The clunk syndrome can be minimized if the design of a posterior stabilized femoral component has a smooth transition from the trochlea to the intercondylar housing. It can be further minimized by surgical removal of all residual synovium from the quadriceps tendon just above the superior pole of the patella (see Chapter 4). This surgical maneuver also appears to minimize or eliminate the potential for crepitus in a cruciate-retaining design.

PREPARING THE DYSPLASTIC PATELLA

Some patients have a dysplastic patellofemoral articulation associated with patella alta and lateral subluxation or even dislocation. On the skyline radiograph, the patella is thin and the lateral facet articulates with the convexity of the lateral trochlear and femoral condyle rather than in the trochlear groove (Fig. 7–19). In these cases, the basic principles of patellar preparation still guide the surgical technique.

The maximum thickness of this type of dysplastic patella may be as little as 15 mm. This does not mean that the patella after resurfacing must retain this thickness. If the patient is female, the patellar composite can be between 22 and 24 mm thick after resurfacing; if male, the patellar composite can be between 24 and 26 mm.

In dysplastic cases, I find it very helpful to draw the planned resection on the preoperative skyline radiograph (Fig. 7–20).

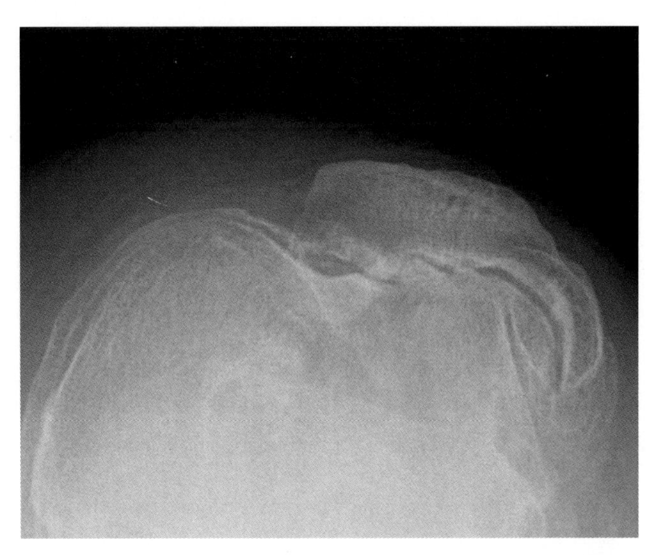

FIGURE 7–19. Dysplastic patella with a thin, concave, lateral facet.

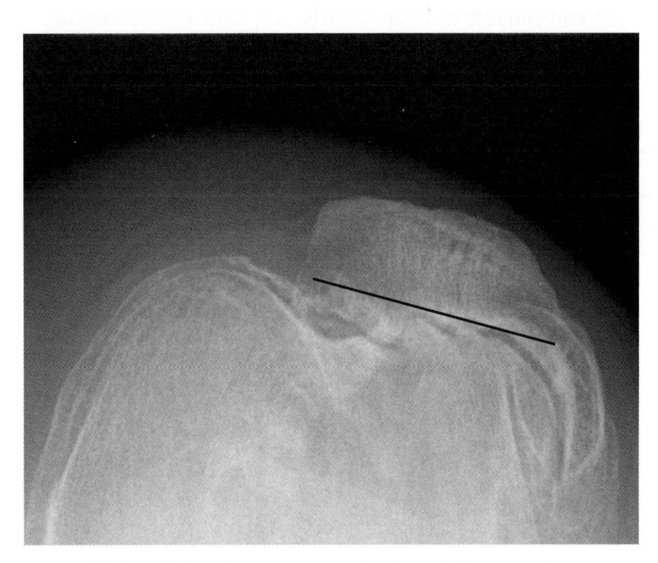

FIGURE 7–20. Preoperative planning of the resection.

The medial half of the patella is left between 12 and 13 mm thick, and the lateral resection often just entails removal and flattening of the rim of the lateral convexity. The two medial pegs of a three-pegged patella are fixed in the medial half of the patella, where the bone stock is acceptable. The single lateral peg enhances fixation via a shallow lateral peg hole. Bone cement can fill the thin deficient convex side of the patella (Fig. 7–21).

SUMMARY

Patellofemoral problems following TKA have been said to account for as much as 50% of complications requiring reoperation. These problems include wear of an unresurfaced patella, maltracking, patella fracture, prosthetic loosening, osteonecrosis, and prosthetic wear. With improvements in prosthetic design and surgical technique, these complications are becoming less frequent. The

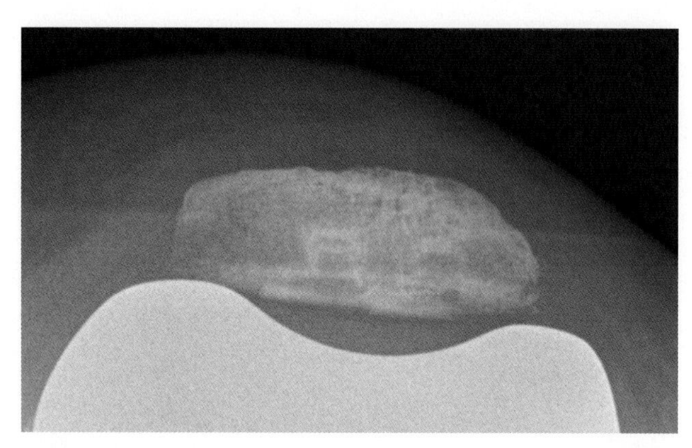

FIGURE 7–21. Postoperative radiograph after resurfacing the dysplastic patella.

main controversy that persists is whether or not to resurface the patella during TKA.

As complications from resurfacing continue to diminish, I am in favor of resurfacing patellae in all patients with rheumatoid and inflammatory arthritis as well as all elderly patients regardless of the operative findings. I reserve non-resurfacing for approximately 5% of my patients who are young, heavy, active osteoarthritics who concur with this decision after a preoperative discussion of its rationale.

References

1. Brick GW, Scott RD: The patellofemoral component of total knee arthroplasty. Clin Orthop 1988;231:163–178.
2. Scott RD: Duopatellar total knee replacement: the Brigham experience. Orthop Clin North Am 1982;13:89–102.
3. Kim BS, Reitman RD, Schai PA, Scott RD: Selective patellar non-resurfacing in total knee arthroplasty. Clin Orthop 1999;367:81–88.
4. Chmell MJ, McManus J, Scott RD: Thickness of the patella in men and women with osteoarthritis. Knee 1996;2(4):239–241.
5. Scott RD: Prosthetic replacement of the patellofemoral joint. Orthop Clin North Am 1979;10:129–137.
6. Wetzner SM, Bezreh JS, Scott RD, et al: Bone scanning in the assessment of patellar viability following knee replacement. Clin Orthop 1985;199:215–219.
7. Scott RD, Turoff N, Ewald FC: Stress fracture of the patella following duopatellar total knee arthroplasty with patellar resurfacing. Clin Orthop 1982;170:147–151.

CHAPTER 8

Stiffness Before and After Total Knee Arthroplasty

Among the goals of total knee arthroplasty (TKA) are relief of pain and restoration of function. Adequate range of motion is necessary for return to certain activities. For example, to walk normally on level ground, a person needs 70 degrees of knee flexion. Ninety degrees is necessary to ascend most stairs (depending on the height of the rise), while 100 degrees is needed to descend stairs and clear the trailing leg. One hundred five degrees is required to arise from a regular chair without using arm support. It is essential, therefore, for patients to achieve maximal potential motion.

Multiple causes for stiffness after TKA are possible. They are related to the patient's diagnosis, preoperative range of motion, prosthetic geometry utilized, surgical technique, intraoperative range of motion after capsular closure, postoperative rehabilitation, and wound healing factors.

The diagnoses most often associated with stiffness include juvenile rheumatoid arthritis, rheumatoid arthritis in some adults, psoriatic arthritis, and posttraumatic arthritis (especially if there have been multiple surgical procedures). Other patient factors include the patient's pain threshold, the presence of patella baja, ipsilateral hip involvement, heterotopic ossification, and overzealous physical therapy.

Ipsilateral arthritic involvement of the hip sometimes is overlooked as a cause of preoperative knee pain. It is not unusual for a patient to consult me for treatment of a painful knee after TKA when, in fact, the pain is referred from the hip. These painful knees often have diminished range of motion. It is difficult to rehabilitate a knee after TKA when it is below a stiff, painful hip. This is one reason to replace the hip before the knee in a patient with ipsilateral hip and knee involvement (see Chapter 11). When a TKA patient is evaluated postoperatively for pain and stiffness resulting from ipsilateral hip arthritis, a common clinical finding is that the patient's affected leg lies in external rotation in the supine position. (This might also occur, of course, if the patient has a knee flexion contracture).

A radiograph of the pelvis is essential to avoid missing an arthritic hip preoperatively prior to replacement of the ipsilateral knee. For preoperative planning, I always obtain a long standing film of the patient that includes hips, knees, and ankles. This allows me to screen for hip pathology as well as any anatomic deformity of the femur. I also ask a simple screening question during the preoperative workup. I ask patients if they have any difficulty whatsoever reaching their feet to cut toenails or tie shoes. If these activities of daily living are normal, significant hip pathology is unlikely. If the patient reports a disability with these functions, hip pathology must be eliminated.

EXPOSING THE STIFF KNEE

Exposure of the ankylosed knee can be difficult. Extreme care must be taken to avoid excessive stress on the patellar tendon insertion that might lead to patellar tendon avulsion. The two most common methods to facilitate exposure are a proximal release or a tibial tubercle osteotomy. I prefer the proximal release to avoid the potential morbidity of tubercle osteotomy, which includes wound healing difficulties, problems with union of the osteotomy, and the potential for stress fracture at the osteotomy site. The classic proximal release is the so-called "quadriceps snip" initially described by Insall.[1] I perform a modification of the snip in which the medial arthrotomy is taken to the top of the quadriceps tendon on the medial side and then brought distally along the lateral side of the tendon in an inverted V configuration (Fig. 8–1).[2] I prefer this release because it is easy to close and seal the joint to prevent leakage of the hematoma.

This procedure also can be extended to a formal V-Y quadricepsplasty to lengthen the quadriceps mechanism when appropriate. The proximal quadriceps release effectively takes tension off the patellar tendon and allows the patella

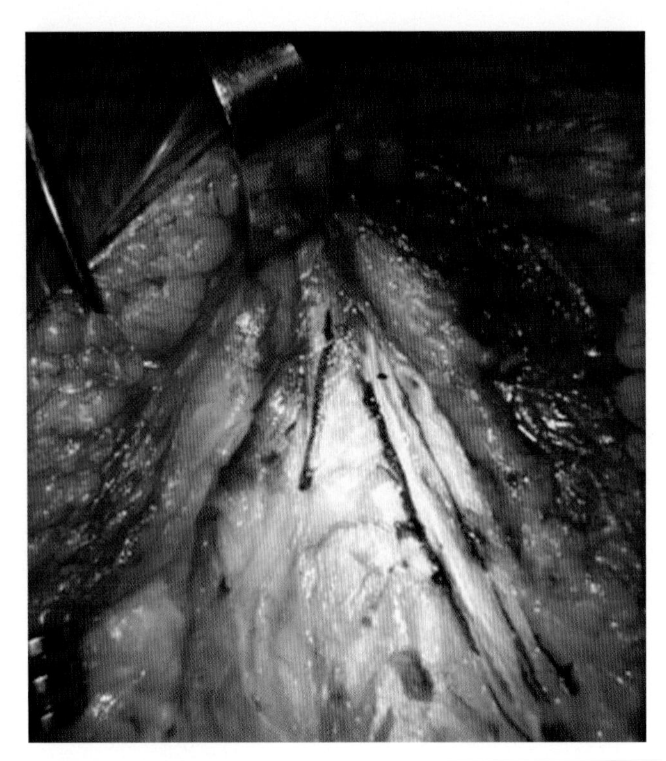

FIGURE 8–1. An inverted V incision in the quadriceps tendon facilitates eversion of the patella.

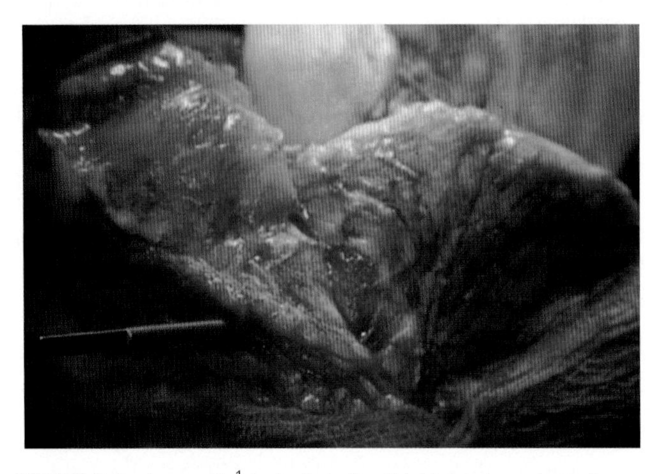

FIGURE 8–2. A smooth $\frac{1}{8}$-inch pin in the tibial tubercle protects the patellar tendon from avulsing.

to be turned rather like the page of a book. The surgeon then has access to lateral parapatellar scar tissue and the lateral retinaculum to perform a preliminary lateral release to further facilitate eversion and exposure. Despite these measures, I think it is advisable to place a smooth, $\frac{1}{8}$-inch pin into the tibial tubercle to further prevent the patellar tendon from avulsing or peeling off its insertion (Fig. 8–2).

EXPOSING THE ANKYLOSED KNEE IN EXTENSION

When the knee is ankylosed in extension (the knee has limited potential to flex), I recommend the following sequence of maneuvers. An inverted V or quadriceps snip is performed upon initial exposure. Flexion of the knee is achieved by gentle manipulation. If the anterior cruciate ligament (ACL) is present, it is surgically released. In certain knees (in postseptic or juvenile rheumatoid arthritis), a joint line osteotomy using a saw or osteotomes may be required. A prophylactic tubercle pin is placed. During preparation of the femur, maximal trochlear resection is performed short of notching the anterior cortex. During preparation of the patella, maximal patellar resection is performed, leaving a remnant of as little as 10 mm in thickness. These two measures enhance flexion by increasing the quadriceps excursion. At the same time, the surgeon should avoid overstuffing the joint with too large a femoral component and too thick a patellar composite.

At the time of closure, flexion against gravity is measured with the capsule closed anatomically. If this range is deemed to be inadequate for the specific patient, consideration can be given to extending the inverted V quadriceps incision to a formal V-Y quadriceps lengthening (Fig. 8–3).[2] The disadvantage of V-Y quadriceps lengthening is the resultant extensor lag, which will depend on the amount of lengthening. The quadriceps usually will recover to an acceptable amount, but the patient may have to be braced during ambulation until active extension is –15 degrees or better.

EXPOSING THE ANKYLOSED KNEE IN FLEXION

I recommend the following measures in exposing the knee that will not straighten owing to a severe flexion contracture. A quadriceps snip or inverted V proximal quadriceps release is indicated. For most primary knees, I start with femoral resection. For the knee with a severe flexion contracture, a conservative tibia-first resection is a reasonable way to help mobilize the knee. When the tibial resection is performed, it is advisable to apply no posterior slope to the cut. This is because every degree of posterior slope is a degree of flexion imparted to the prosthetic components.

In most primary knees, I preserve the posterior cruciate ligament (PCL) (see Chapter 2). One of my indications for PCL resection and substitution is the knee with a severe flexion contracture. PCL resection facilitates release of the posterior capsule, whereas substitution helps correct those knees with posterior subluxation of the tibia in association with a contracture (Fig. 8–4).

Whether the PCL is preserved or substituted, it is important to remove all posterior femoral and tibial osteophytes, which tent up the posterior capsule. Further posterior capsule release can be achieved by using an elevator or osteotome to strip the capsule from the femur and tibia. Distal femoral resection is increased by 2 mm for every 10 to 15 degrees of contracture up to a limit of 12 to 14 mm. Resection greater than this amount can compromise the integrity of the collateral ligaments. Stabilization with a Total Condylar III type of prosthesis must sometimes be considered for persistent flexion gap laxity.

At the time of capsular closure, the medial capsule is advanced distally on the lateral capsule to minimize the extensor lag that would be created by use of an anatomic capsular closure (Fig. 8–5) (see Chapter 9).

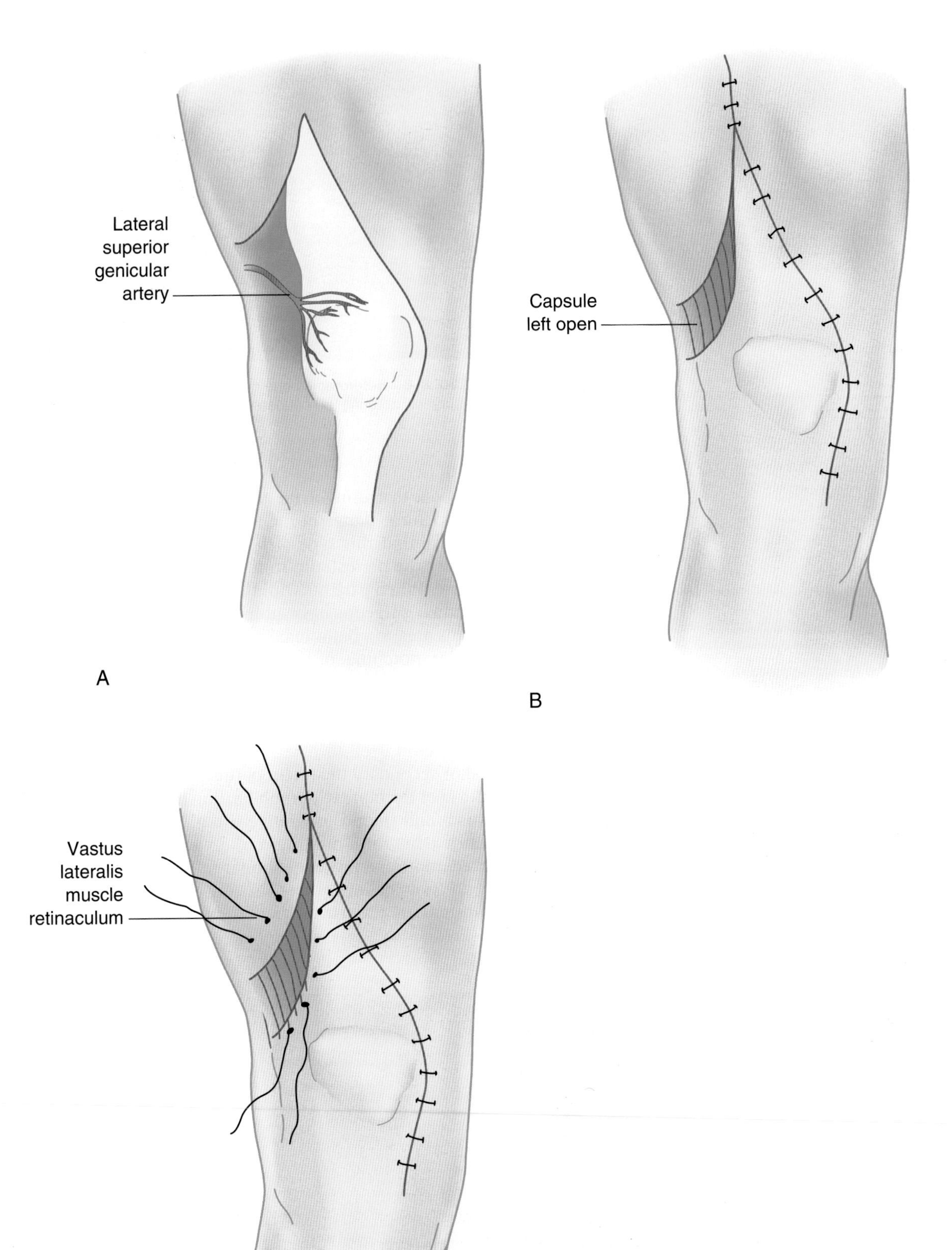

FIGURE 8–3. *A*, An inverted V quadriceps incision can be extended to permit a V-Y quadriceps lengthening. *B*, The lateral capsule must be left open to allow the advancement. *C*, The joint is sealed by advancing the retinaculum of the vastus lateralis muscle. (*A–C* from Scott RD, Siliski JM: The use of a modified V-Y quadricepsplasty during total knee replacement to gain exposure and improve flexion in the ankylosed knee. Orthopedics 1986;8:45–48.)

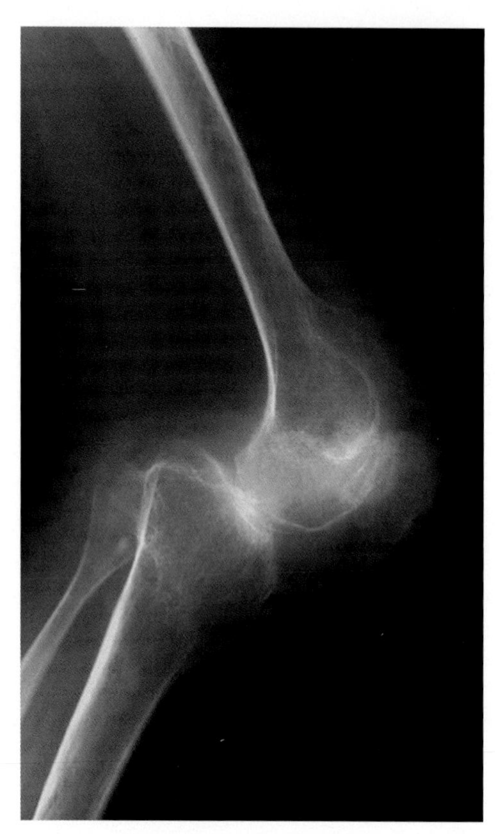

FIGURE 8–4. A severe flexion contracture with posterior tibial subluxation requires PCL substitution.

HETEROTOPIC BONE FORMATION

Heterotopic bone formation in TKA can often be seen in small amounts in the quadriceps mechanism. It is rarely the cause of symptoms or significant stiffness.

There are times, however, when heterotopic bone formation can limit range of motion. This is usually in association with bone that forms on the anterior shaft of the femur just above the trochlear flange of the femoral component (Fig. 8–6). I theorize that this type of bone formation results from disturbing the periosteum in this area during the surgical procedure. When patients with this finding have been referred to me, their surgeons have admitted to incising the periosteum in this area to obtain maximum exposure and prevent inadvertent notching of the anterior cortex. Some have also admitted to the use of subperiosteal extramedullary alignment devices. I think it is important to preserve the subsynovial fat overlying the periosteum in this area and never to incise the periosteum itself.

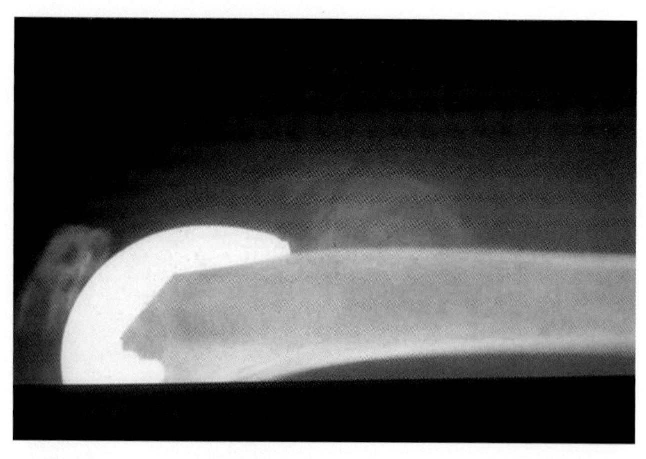

FIGURE 8–6. Heterotopic bone can restrict flexion, possibly caused by the surgeon violating the periosteum of the anterior cortex of the femur.

For secondary treatment of this problem, I recommend removal of the bone with mobilization of the quadriceps mechanism and the postoperative use of indomethacin 25 mg 3 times a day for a minimum of 6 weeks. Some surgeons use irradiation in a protocol similar to that used in the hip, but I do not believe there is any published literature to substantiate the use of irradiation in the knee.

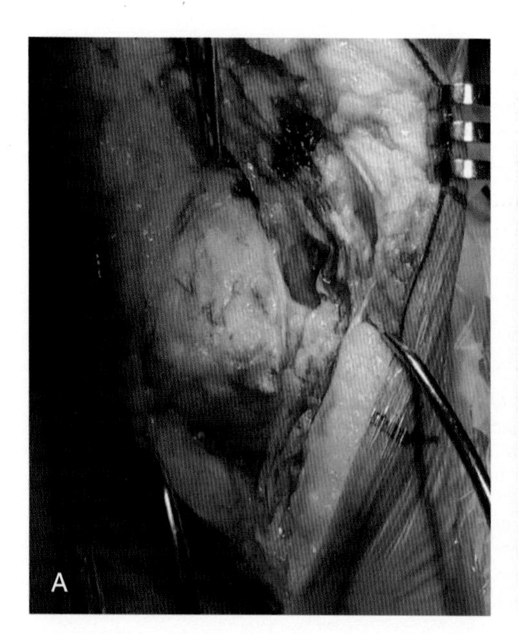

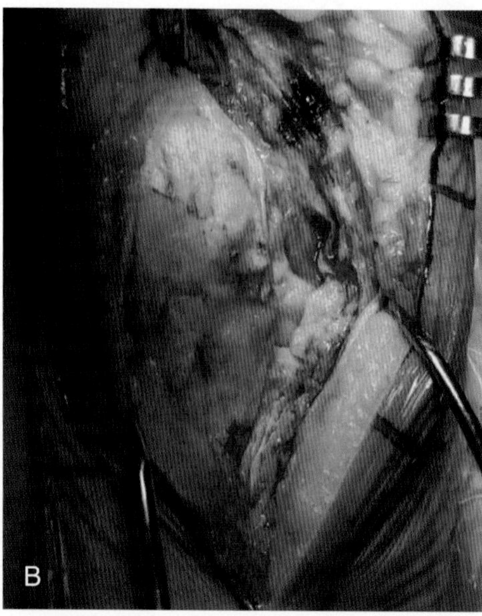

FIGURE 8–5. After correction of a severe flexion contracture, advancement of the medial capsule distally on the lateral capsule will minimize an extensor lag.

OVERZEALOUS PHYSICAL THERAPY

Whereas properly executed physical therapy facilitates recovery from TKA, overzealous therapy can be counterproductive. It can result in excessive pain and swelling that limits flexibility and creates apprehension in the patient. In this event, therapy should be postponed or limited to that which maintains progress without inflaming the soft tissues.

MANIPULATION OF THE KNEE

When patients fail to achieve satisfactory range of motion after TKA, manipulation under anesthesia is considered. Over the past 20 years, the incidence of performing knee manipulation after TKA has decreased significantly.

In the 1970s, postoperative knee manipulation was performed in up to 20% of patients. Some postoperative protocols immobilized the knee for 1 to 2 weeks after which knee manipulation frequently was necessary. In those times, patients also remained in hospital for up to 2 weeks and were not discharged home until at least 90 degrees of flexion was achieved. We now know that most patients, given time, can achieve their potential range of motion without the need for formal manipulation. My own incidence of knee manipulation today is approximately 1%. The need for potential manipulation is assessed by recording the patient's intraoperative flexion against gravity with the knee capsule closed at the end of the procedure (Fig. 8–7). The patient's progress toward achieving this potential is then monitored. For example, if a patient's flexion against gravity after replacing an ankylosed knee is 45 degrees and this is achieved within the first postoperative month, the patient is congratulated and no manipulation is indicated. On the other hand, if the patient's flexion against gravity at the end of the knee arthroplasty is 120 degrees and progress stops at 70 degrees of flexion, the patient is a candidate for manipulation.

Most surgeons are taught to correlate the patient's potential motion with the preoperative motion. This statistic bears up when the average of a group of patients' preoperative flexion is compared with the average of their postoperative flexion. In reality, patients with 70 degrees of preoperative flexion, for example, may improve to 90 degrees, whereas patients with 140 degrees may regress to 120 degrees. This allows the averages of the preoperative and postoperative groups to remain similar.

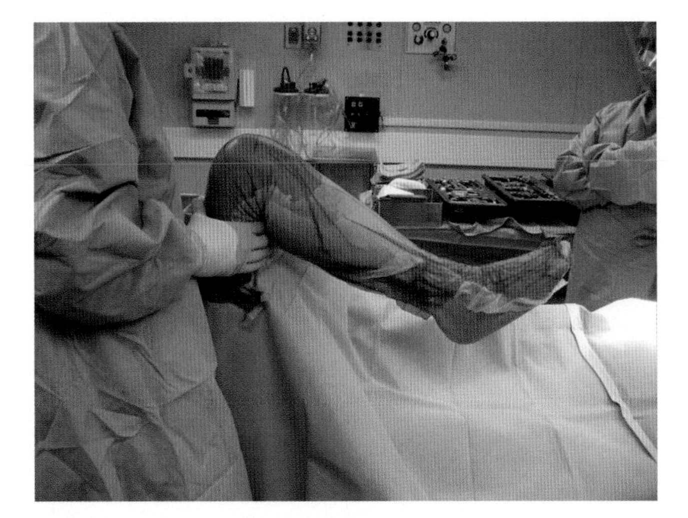

FIGURE 8–7. Flexion against gravity with the capsule closed is the best predictor of ultimate postoperative knee flexion.

The best indicator of an individual patient's potential is the intraoperative flexion against gravity with the capsule closed at the end of the procedure.[3] This is a measure of quadriceps excursion influenced by multiple preoperative factors as well as intraoperative technical factors such as sizing of the femur, prosthetic geometry, and patellar thickness.

Timing of Knee Manipulation

In the rare case in which knee manipulation may be indicated, it should be delayed until 4 weeks or more after surgery. This delay allows monitoring of the patient's progress to determine whether adequate range of motion evolves with time and physical therapy. If, for example, a patient leaves the hospital with 70 degrees of flexion, I ask the patient or therapist to call in the degree of flexion at weekly intervals. If progress ceases or regresses after several weeks, knee manipulation is scheduled. If there is gradual improvement, progress is monitored until it reaches a plateau and patient function and satisfaction are assessed. Although the surgeon may be disappointed, some patients find, for example, that 85 degrees of flexion is satisfactory. For others, this degree would be unacceptable.

Technique of Knee Manipulation

Patients are admitted directly to the operating room on the day of manipulation. Aspirin is used for anticoagulation. Ideally, the manipulation is done under spinal or epidural anesthesia. With the patient in the supine position, the hip is flexed 90 degrees and the patient's passive flexion against gravity is measured. When pain has been limiting flexion, gravity itself may satisfactorily manipulate the knee. Usually, however, some gentle force must be applied. The posterior aspect of the knee is cradled in both hands while the patient's ankle is placed in the axilla of the manipulating surgeon. When the surgeon leans forward and backward, gentle manipulation is applied through the anterior aspect of the ankle. I do not favor sudden, violent manipulation of the knee because of the potential to cause fracture. Sometimes adhesions can be heard or felt to give way, and other times the scar yields in much the same way as taffy is pulled. Successful manipulation can take seconds or may involve 5 to 10 minutes of gentle, persistent rocking forces.

When the manipulation is complete, a measurement of flexion against gravity is taken and recorded.

Following manipulation, the patient is placed immediately in a continuous passive motion (CPM) machine with the dial set at the maximum flexion achieved at manipulation. Ice is applied to the knee.

When the spinal or epidural effect wears off, oral medications are utilized and the patient is urged to ride a stationary bicycle prior to discharge. Faithful use of a stationary bicycle at home assures that adequate range of motion will not be lost. The patient is encouraged to ride the bicycle for 10 to 15 minutes twice a day and slowly lower the seat until maximum motion has been achieved and maintained.

Manipulating into Extension

At times, patients who achieved full extension at surgery will regress and develop a flexion contracture. The contracture usually improves with continued physical therapy and resolution of postoperative swelling. Permanent flexion contractures of 10 degrees or less do not appear to be symptomatic or disabling. Flexion contractures greater than 15 degrees cause gait abnormalities and fatigue on prolonged standing and walking. Manipulation to regain extension is performed similarly to that used to gain flexion. With the patient in the supine position under spinal or epidural anesthesia and the hip extended, the ankle is supported by one hand of the surgeon while the suprapatellar area is compressed with the other. Gentle, persistent extension force may have to be applied for as long as 5 or 10 minutes. Any improvement in extension is held by the application of a well-padded cylinder or long leg cast. The patient sleeps in the cast overnight. The process is repeated daily until progress ceases or full passive extension is achieved. The final cast is bivalved and lined the next morning for use as a resting splint upon discharge. The process is repeated daily until satisfactory passive extension is achieved or progress ceases. Dynamic extension splints such as the Dyna-Splint are sometimes helpful at resolving flexion contractures or maintaining those that have been corrected.

SUMMARY

The causes of preoperative and postoperative stiffness are multifactorial. The problem of postoperative stiffness often can be anticipated preoperatively. It can be resolved or minimized by certain intraoperative and postoperative measures regarding surgical technique, prosthetic design, and rehabilitation.

References

1. Garvin KL, Scuderi G, Insall JN: Evolution of the quadriceps snip. Clin Orthop 1995;321:131–137.
2. Scott RD, Siliski JM: The use of a modified V-Y quadricepsplasty during total knee replacement to gain exposure and improve flexion in the ankylosed knee. Orthopedics 1986;8:45–48.
3. Lee DC, Kim DH, Scott RD, Suthers K: Intraoperative flexion against gravity as an indication of ultimate range of motion in individual cases after total knee arthroplasty. J Arthroplasty 1998;13:500-503.

CHAPTER 9

Flexion Contracture Associated with Total Knee Arthroplasty

A fixed flexion contracture can result from several disease processes, including osteoarthritis, rheumatoid arthritis, and posttraumatic arthritis. There often is a common pathway that starts with pain and leads to decreased motion and posterior capsular scarring. The scarring promoted by the inflammatory component of rheumatoid arthritis also plays a role. In arthrosis resulting from osteoarthritis or trauma, osteophytes play a significant role. Osteophytes develop posteriorly and in the intercondylar area (Fig. 9–1). The intercondylar osteophytes form a mechanical block to extension and they also alter cruciate kinematics. Osteophytes often overgrow the entire intercondylar notch, obscuring the posterior cruciate ligament (PCL), in knees where there is advanced arthritis and an absent anterior cruciate ligament.

Posterior osteophytes can impede flexion because of impingement and scarring. They limit extension by scarring and by tenting up the posterior capsule. When a flexion contracture becomes chronic and long-standing, secondary hamstring contracture can occur.

The goals of total knee arthroplasty (TKA) are to provide adequate pain relief along with a knee that is stable and has a functional range of motion. The amount of knee flexion necessary for various activities of daily living is discussed in Chapter 11. How much knee extension is necessary for a good functional result remains controversial. In a gait analysis study, Perry and colleagues reported in 1975 that −15 degrees of extension was necessary for a good functional result.[1] In my experience, a permanent flexion contracture of 15 degrees after TKA may or may not be dysfunctional for the patient. On the other hand, I have yet to see a patient with a 10-degree flexion contracture complain of disability. In other words, −10 degrees of extension is acceptable, −10 to −15 degrees is borderline, and −15 or more is not acceptable.

Another controversy exists about how much of a preoperative flexion contracture has to be corrected at the time of surgery. An article often quoted is that of Tanzer and Miller from 1989.[2] They reported a small series of 35 TKAs with preoperative flexion contractures of less than 30 degrees. Only five of the knees in the series had flexion contractures greater than 20 degrees. The authors noted that the flexion

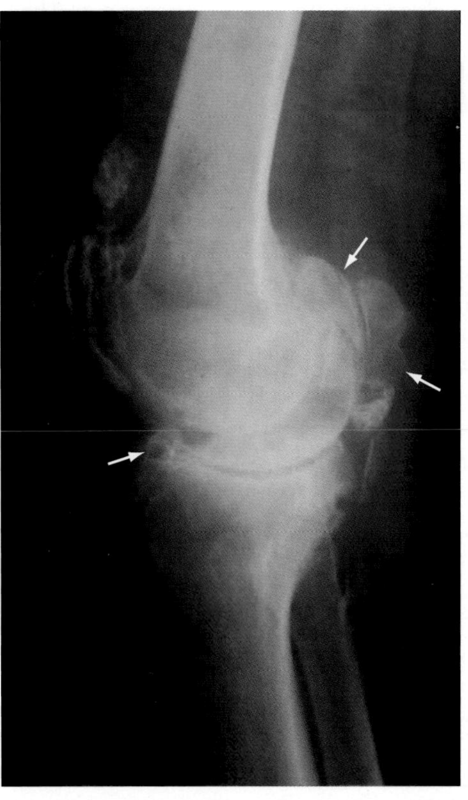

FIGURE 9–1. Posterior osteophytes and intercondylar osteophytes play a major role in flexion contractures associated with osteoarthritis.

contractures tended to improve after surgery and complete correction intraoperatively was not necessary. To an extent, I am in agreement with this, as discussed below. I feel it is very important not to overcorrect for flexion contractures and end up with a knee with hyperextension. In short, I would rather have a knee with a 5-degree contracture rather than one with 5 degrees of hyperextension. Similarly, I would rather have a knee with 10 or 15 degrees of a flexion contracture rather than 10 or 15 degrees of hyperextension.

TREATMENT OPTIONS

Treatment options for flexion contractures can be sorted into three categories: preoperative, intraoperative, and postoperative measures. Postoperative measures are discussed under "Ancillary Measures."

Preoperative Measures

Preoperative measures such as manipulation and serial casting or dynamic splinting are usually amenable only to patients with inflammatory arthritis without osteophyte formation (which can cause a bony block to extension). This type of treatment is especially appropriate for the adult or juvenile rheumatoid patient with bilateral hip and knee flexion contractures about to undergo hip and knee replacement surgery. In this situation, the hip arthroplasty is almost always performed first (see Chapter 11). While the patient is under anesthesia for the hip surgery, the knee is gently manipulated (stretched) for 3 to 5 minutes. Maximal extension is recorded, and a longleg cast is applied at approximately 5 degrees less than the maximal extension. The cast must be well padded to avoid undue skin pressure. The following day, the cast is bivalved and lined as a resting cast. Ideally, the anesthetic utilized is an epidural, which can be left in place for several days, permitting daily manipulations with a new cast until progress ceases. In rheumatoid patients, I have seen preoperative flexion contractures of 90 degrees almost entirely corrected prior to attempting TKA (Fig. 9–2). Obviously, this method is preferable to excessive bone resection to achieve an adequate extension gap. Because these patients are always osteopenic, care must be taken to avoid forceful manipulation and the possibility of a fracture (usually supracondylar). As noted above, this preoperative manipulation method is not appropriate for the osteoarthritic patient with a bony block to extension.

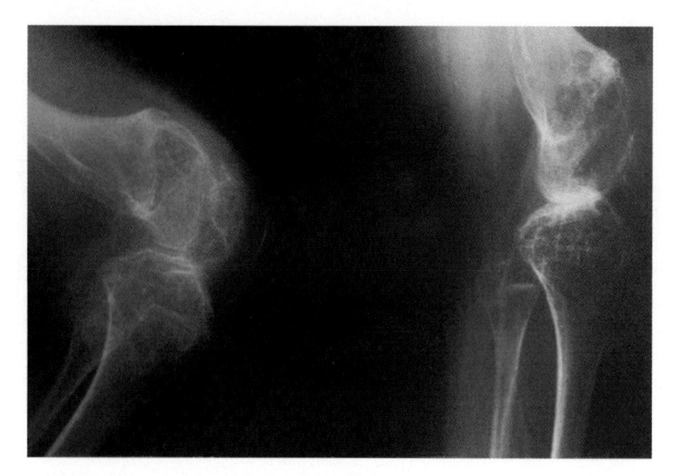

FIGURE 9–2. Correction of a 90-degree flexion contracture by serial casting technique.

Intraoperative Measures

Various intraoperative measures can be utilized to correct a flexion contracture. It may be difficult to expose this knee, and the measures I recommend are covered in Chapter 8. The treatment options include removal of osteophytes both anteriorly and posteriorly. The posterior capsule can be stripped from both femur and tibia. Additional distal femoral resection is necessary for severe contractures. Occasionally, extra proximal tibial resection will be appropriate in the presence of patella baja. The amount of posterior tibial slope applied to the tibial resection should be zero rather than the usual 3 to 5 degrees. Finally, PCL substitution is helpful to facilitate release of posterior structures and to correct posterior tibial subluxation, which either preexists in severe contractures or occurs as extension is achieved (Fig. 9–3).

Osteophyte Removal

Anterior osteophytes in the intercondylar notch can build up and limit extension because of impingement. They will be removed with routine bone resection, allowing room for adequate extension to occur. Posterior osteophytes are more common in varus knees than valgus knees and more prevalent medially than laterally. The posterior capsule often

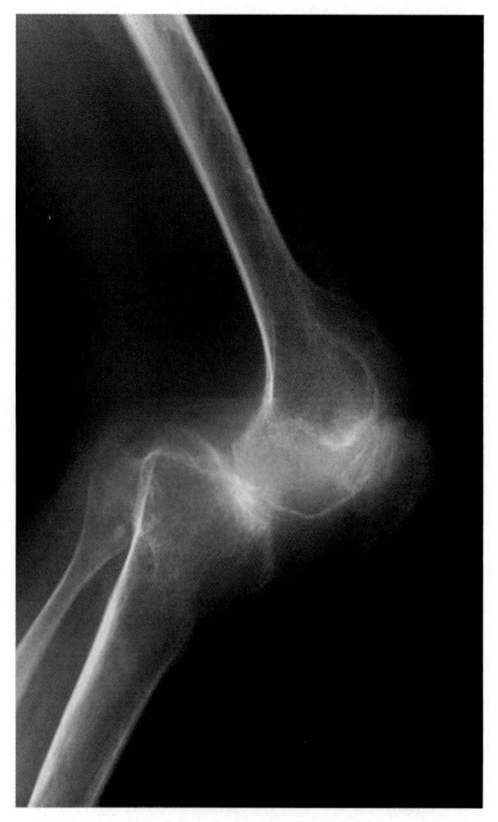

FIGURE 9–3. This severe flexion contracture with posterior tibial subluxation requires PCL substitution.

contracts around the osteophytes, and their removal releases the posterior capsule enough in many cases to gain full extension with routine amounts of distal femoral bone resection when preoperative contractures are 15 degrees or less. The posterior osteophytes are best accessed and cleared after preliminary femoral and tibial preparation.

The trial femoral component is inserted without a trial tibial component. The knee is flexed and held upward with a bone hook. A curved $\frac{3}{8}$-inch osteotome is passed sequentially tangent to the metallic posterior condyles so that it removes any uncapped femoral bone and frees up the posterior osteophytes. The same maneuver is an efficient way to strip some of the posterior capsule from its femoral attachment. After the contour of the femoral component has been outlined on the posterior condylar bone, the trial femur is removed and the uncapped femur and remaining osteophytes are resected (Fig. 9–4). An osteotome can also be used to strip the posterior capsule from the back of the tibia. I rarely do this maneuver, however, and gain most of the capsular stripping from the femoral side.

Additional Distal Femoral Resection

The initial amount of distal femoral resection should be based on the thickness of the femoral component to be implanted. If the component is 9 mm thick, for example, an anatomic resection would consist of 9 mm including cartilage. If the amount resected is based on bone, a conservative initial distal femoral resection should be 7 mm, allowing for 2 mm of cartilage. It is important not to perform too much initial distal femoral resection in a PCL-retaining knee. This could lead to a flexion-extension gap mismatch that is difficult to fix. For example, too much distal femoral resection will lead to a knee that is tighter in flexion than in extension. To repair this, the surgeon will have to perform a PCL release, apply more posterior slope to the tibial resection, or consider downsizing the femoral component to increase the posterior condylar resection and increase the flexion gap without affecting the extension gap. A final solution would be to cement the femoral component proud of the distal cuts. These four solutions can be effective but will not need to be considered if the surgeon prepares the knee initially so that, if anything, the extension gap is tighter than the flexion gap. The solution to this mismatch is simple: the surgeon revisits the distal femoral cut to increase the extension gap without affecting the flexion gap. The chamfer cuts will also have to be redone, but the entire maneuver will take only a few minutes. For this reason, I use the method of increasing the distal femoral resection for flexion contracture only in knees with initial flexion contractures greater than 15 degrees when the patient is under anesthesia. I increase the distal femoral resection by 2 mm for every extra 15 degrees of flexion contracture. For example, if a knee has 0 to 15 degrees of flexion contracture, the distal resection for a 9 mm femoral component is 7 mm of bone. For a flexion contracture between 15 and 30 degrees, the distal resection is 9 mm of bone. Between 30 and 45 degrees of flexion contracture, the distal resection is 11, and over 45 degrees it may go as high as 13 mm. I would never increase the distal resection more than this amount because the level of the origin of the collateral ligaments is soon approached and the resultant elevation of the joint line significantly disturbs the kinematics of the knee. This elevation of the joint line will usually require PCL substitution and even Total Condylar III constraint if significant joint line elevation leads to flexion instability.

Algorithm Based on Personal Experience

Through the years I have developed an algorithm for the treatment of severe flexion contracture based on a large experience with patients who had bilateral, severe flexion contractures that rendered them nonambulatory. Most of these patients had rheumatoid arthritis.[3] Many also had hip involvement. I found that the patient with inflammatory arthritis could be treated somewhat differently from the patient with osteoarthritis.

In my experience, preoperative flexion contracture under anesthesia is the best guide for determining treatment. The intraoperative correction gained is the best guide for determining the final result except for the patient with inflammatory disease and a preoperative contracture greater than 40 degrees under anesthesia.[4] In these specific patients, I

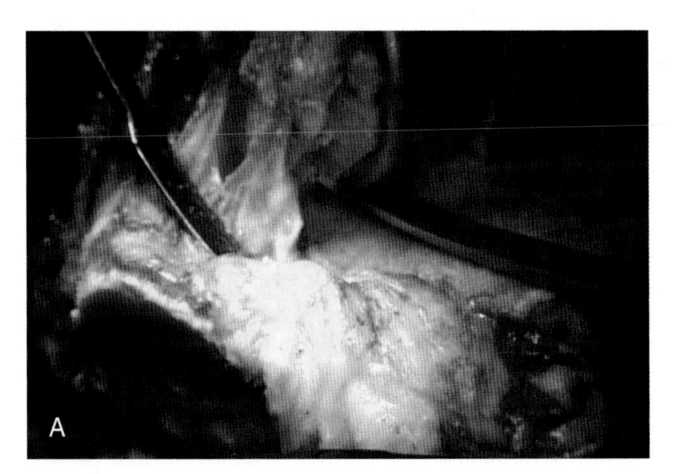

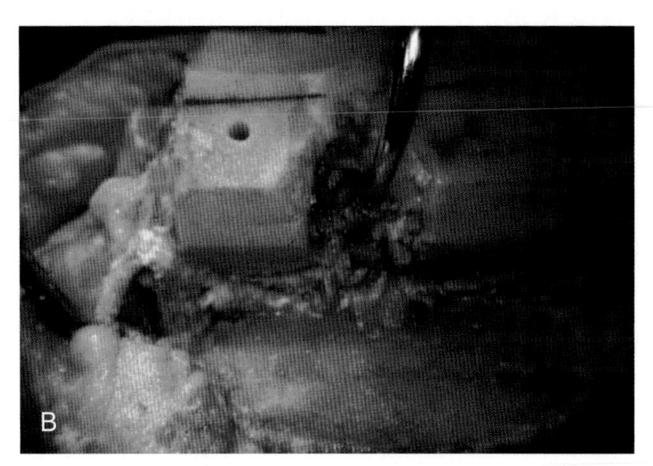

FIGURE 9–4. After the posterior prosthetic femoral condyles are outlined with an osteotome, retained osteophytes and uncapped posterior condylar bone are removed.

follow a "rule of one third." This rule states that the intraoperative correction needs to be only to within one third of the flexion contracture noted prior to surgery under anesthesia. The residual one third will resolve satisfactorily with postoperative physical therapy, sometimes supplemented by serial casting or the use of a dynamic splint. For example, if the patient's preoperative contracture is 45 degrees, the correction need only be to 15 degrees intraoperatively. If the contracture is 60 degrees, the correction need only be to 20 degrees. The worst flexion contracture I have seen was of 110 degrees. The intraoperative correction was to –40 degrees. Epidural anesthesia was left in place, and after three serial casts applied daily, the contracture was corrected to zero. No hamstring tendon releases have been necessary, although this may be required in selected patients. This rule of one third does not apply in the presence of a flexion deformity resulting from a fracture or osteotomy.

Summary of Treatment Guidelines

For flexion contractures of less than 15 degrees, a normal distal femoral resection (7 mm of bone for a 9-mm prosthesis) is performed. All anterior and posterior osteophytes are removed, and the posterior capsule is stripped from the femur if necessary.

For flexion contractures from 15 to 45 degrees, the distal femoral resection is increased by 2 mm for every 15 degrees of correction needed. So, for a 9-mm thick femoral component, a contracture from 15 to 30 degrees has 9 mm of distal resection. One from 30 to 45 degrees has 11 mm of resection. If there is greater than 45 degrees of contracture, the resection is 13 mm. Resection much greater than 13 mm is to be avoided because, depending on the size of the patient, the PCL and medial collateral ligament (MCL) origins are not much more proximal.

For flexion contractures between 45 and 60 degrees, preoperative manipulation and casting should be considered, and a PCL-substituting technique should always be used. For flexion contractures greater than 60 degrees, preoperative manipulation and casting again are appropriate, and Total Condylar III stability must often be utilized to resolve flexion gap laxity.

OTHER IMPORTANT CONSIDERATIONS REGARDING FLEXION CONTRACTURES

Contractures Due to Bony Deformity

For flexion contractures secondary to a healed fracture or osteotomy, corrective osteotomy may be indicated depending on the amount of bony deformity. This could be performed as a separate procedure or in conjunction with the TKA with the use of a long-stemmed component to fix the osteotomy.[5]

Bilateral Contractures

In the patient with severe bilateral flexion contractures, both replacement operations should be done simultaneously or within a few weeks of one another. Otherwise, there is a significant risk of the corrected knee regressing to the level of the flexion contracture of the uncorrected knee.

Patella Baja

Flexion contractures associated with patella baja are a significant challenge. If the surgeon attempts to gain extension by increasing the distal femoral resection, the patella baja will be worsened. All the other corrective measures, therefore, must be maximized, including osteophyte removal and posterior capsular stripping and manipulation. The surgeon also should consider lowering the joint line by increasing the normal amount of tibial resection to increase the extension gap. The increased tibial resection, of course, will loosen the flexion gap also. For that reason, the surgeon should consider using an anterior-down femoral sizing technique and try to slightly oversize the femoral component in the anteroposterior dimension. If this is done, the increased tibial resection has less influence on loosening the flexion gap (Fig. 9–5).

Posterior Slope

In severe flexion contractures, the surgeon should consider applying no posterior slope to the tibial resection. Every degree of posterior slope for any given amount of tibial resection will inhibit the correction of the flexion contracture. For example, given the same amount of tibial resection posteriorly, a tibial cut with 0 degrees of posterior slope will allow 10 more degrees of extension than one with 10 degrees of posterior slope.

Capsular Closure

The capsular closure should be modified following correction of a severe preoperative flexion contracture. If the capsule is closed anatomically, an extensor lag is likely to persist in a patient with a long-standing contracture. The reason becomes apparent when noting the laxity that will exist in the patellar tendon when the knee is in full extension with an anatomic repair. The extensor lag is minimized by advancement of the medial capsule distally on the lateral capsule. The best way to determine the amount of advancement is to place the knee at rest in full extension and grasp the lateral capsule at the level of the superior pole of the patella and pull it proximally to eliminate the distal laxity. The medial capsule is then sutured directly across to the advanced lateral side (see Fig. 8-5). In some knees, this maneuver might limit motion on the other side of the arc by decreasing quadriceps excursion. This effect can be assessed merely by flexing the knee against gravity after the capsular closure. Usually, the amount of decrease in flexion is not enough to obviate the positive effect of the advancement.

Ancillary Measures

Finally, ancillary measures can be taken in the perioperative period to minimize the chance of a postoperative flexion contracture.

The patient should avoid lying supine with a pillow under the knee for any length of time. Any pillow or roll should be under the ankle. If necessary, a trochanteric roll should be utilized to prevent the knee from rolling into external rotation.

A knee immobilizer is helpful at night. It often provides comfort to patients in the first week or so after surgery and prevents them from sleeping with the knee in a flexed position.

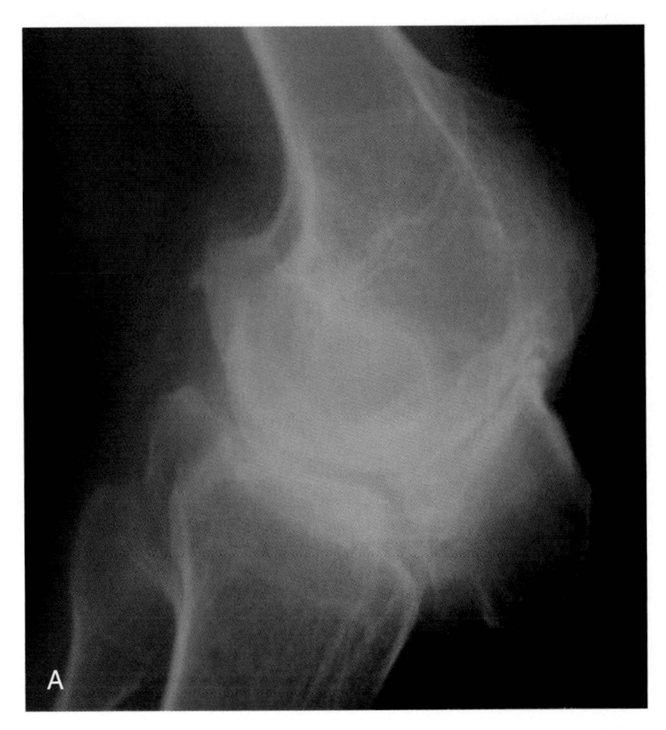

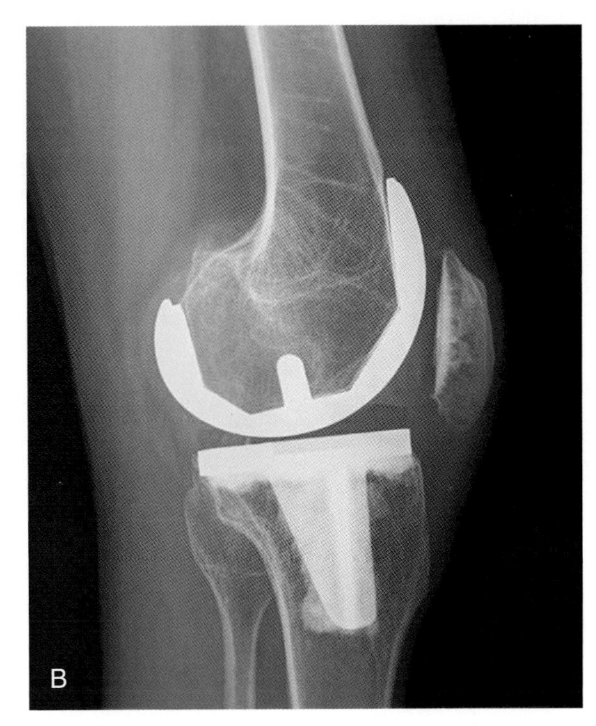

FIGURE 9–5. Resolution of a flexion contracture associated with patella baja.

Too much time on a continuous passive motion (CPM) machine should be avoided. Although the CPM may facilitate flexion, its overuse may promote a flexion contracture. In patients who develop a flexion contracture following surgery and do not respond to normal measures, a dynamic splint can be used to correct the flexion contracture and maintain extension over several weeks.

SUMMARY

Many factors play a role in causing a flexion contracture in association with TKA. The pathways that lead to the flexion contracture may differ in rheumatoid arthritis and osteoarthritis. Soft tissue contracture and inflammation play a major role in rheumatoid arthritis, whereas osteophytes play the most significant role in osteoarthritis. The final goal of correction is to achieve and maintain a contracture of less than 15 degrees. Contractures between 10 and 15 degrees may still be symptomatic, and those of 10 degrees or less rarely cause difficulties.

Perioperative and intraoperative treatment measures can alleviate flexion contractures. Intraoperative correction determines the final result in most cases except in inflammatory cases where the preoperative contracture is greater than 40 degrees. In these cases, the preoperative contracture under anesthesia need only be corrected to within one third of its initial amount and the remainder usually resolves with postoperative physical therapy and serial casting or splinting.

References

1. Perry J, Antonelli D, Ford W: Analysis of knee joint forces during flexed knee stance. J Bone Joint Surg 1975;57:961–967.
2. Tanzer M, Miller J: The natural history of flexion contracture in total knee arthroplasty: a prospective study. Clin Orthop 1989;248:129–134.
3. Chmell MJ, Scott RD: Surgical management of juvenile rheumatoid arthritis. In Kelley WM, Harris ED, Ruddy S, Sledge CB (eds): Textbook of Rheumatology, 5th ed. Philadelphia, WB Saunders, 1996, pp 1773–1781.
4. Slater J, Fox J, Vidolin JP, et al: Severe flexion contracture of the arthritic knee: results and treatment guidelines. Orthop Trans 1994;17:963–964.
5. Scott RD, Schai PA: Tibial osteotomy coincident with long stem total knee arthroplasty. Am J Knee Surg 2000;13:127–131.

CHAPTER 10

Total Knee Arthroplasty After Osteotomy

Conversion of osteotomy to total knee arthroplasty can be extremely difficult for a number of reasons. These include the presence of prior incisions, with operative exposure, the presence of retained hardware, joint line angle distortion, malunion, nonunion, patella baja, offset tibial shafts, and relative deficiency of the lateral tibial plateau (Fig. 10–1).

PRIOR INCISIONS

Incisions made prior to a standard total knee arthroplasty exposure must be respected. Unlike the hip, the knee does not tolerate multiple parallel or crisscrossing incisions. The vascular supply and lymphatic drainage are dominant on the medial side, resulting in a lateral flap being most vulnerable. Vulnerability may be increased when a lateral retinacular release has been performed for valgus patellar tracking with compromise of the lateral superior genicular vessels. The most vulnerable knee is one with a long lateral parapatellar incision when the surgeon plans a parallel median parapatellar incision for a medial arthrotomy (see Chapter 15). Unfortunately, this type of incision has been used frequently in the past for osteotomy by some surgeons. When there is a long lateral incision, it must be utilized and extended and a medial flap raised in order to perform a standard medial arthrotomy. If the osteotomy is in marked valgus and the surgeon is familiar with the lateral approach, a lateral incision and lateral arthrotomy can be performed. Most experienced osteotomy surgeons now use midline incisions or short oblique incisions that can either be utilized easily later for total knee arthroplasty or ignored.

An oblique lateral incision (Coventry method) from the fibular head to the tibial tubercle, for example, can be ignored. If the surgeon is contemplating making a new medial incision parallel to an old lateral incision, the "delayed technique" or "sham incision" can be considered (see Chapter 15).

OPERATIVE EXPOSURE

Because postosteotomy patients sometimes lose mobility and have scarring about the osteotomy site, exposure can be difficult. Exposure also is compromised by the presence of patella baja. For this reason, a proximal quadriceps release

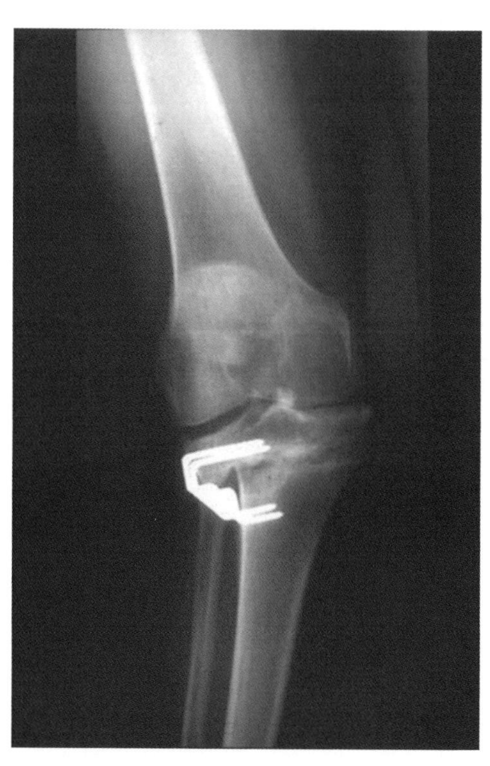

FIGURE 10–1. A failed tibial osteotomy with a nonunion, malalignment, a valgus joint line, and retained hardware.

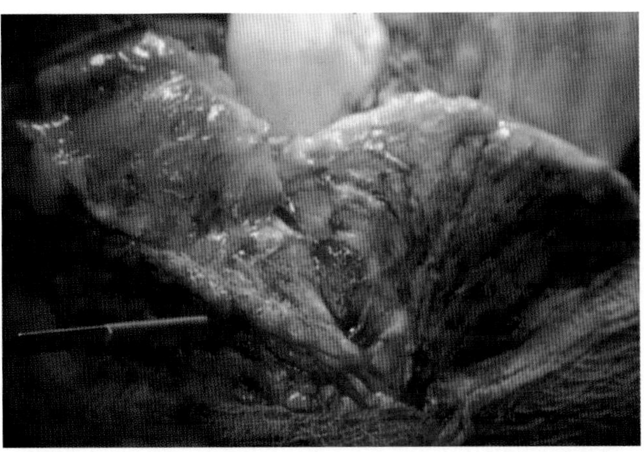

FIGURE 10–2. A smooth $\frac{1}{8}$-inch pin protects the patellar tendon from avulsing.

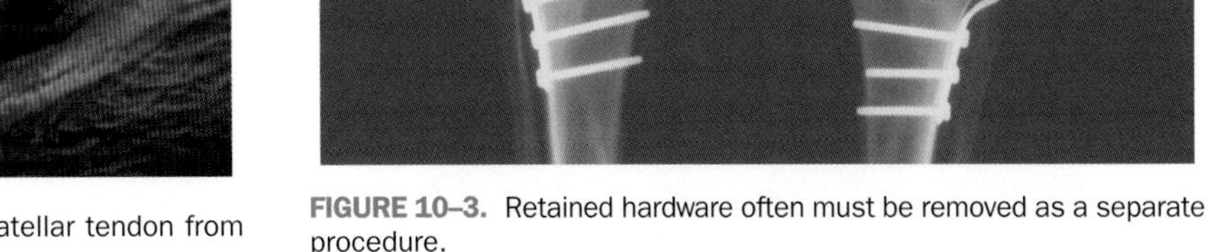

FIGURE 10–3. Retained hardware often must be removed as a separate procedure.

usually is appropriate to protect the patellar tendon (see Chapter 8). A smooth $\frac{1}{8}$-inch pin placed in the tibial tubercle further protects the patellar tendon from avulsion (Fig. 10–2). Dissection in this area can be compromised by the healing of the osteotomy, and the surgeon must proceed with care.

PATELLA BAJA

Patella baja often follows osteotomy. The surgeon can employ several techniques to resolve this situation (see Chapter 9). These include attempts to lower the joint line by decreasing the distal femoral resection and increasing the proximal tibial resection. When this is done, the anteroposterior cam of the femoral component should be moved posteriorly to prevent flexion gap laxity caused by lowering the joint line (see Fig. 9–5).

The patellar thickness should be minimized and the patellar tendon freed from scar about the tubercle and proximal bone. Sometimes the inferior portion of the polyethylene of the patellar component and the anterior portion of the polyethylene of the tibial component have to be relieved with a rongeur or similar tool to prevent impingement of the patellar plastic on the tibial plastic. At the time of closure, the medial capsule is advanced distally on the lateral capsule to allow the patella to be pulled as proximal as possible (see Fig. 8–5).

RETAINED HARDWARE

The presence of previously placed hardware about the knee following osteotomy can present problems owing to the need to remove the hardware and to the prior incisions utilized to implant it (Fig. 10–3). Some hardware can be retained if it does not cause symptoms and is not located where it would impede placement of the components (Fig. 10–4). If hardware does have to be removed, the decision has to be made about whether to remove it as a separate procedure or at the time of arthroplasty. Screws and staples usually can be removed at arthroplasty. Plates that have to be removed through a large separate incision are probably best removed 4 to 6 weeks prior to the arthroplasty, giving the separate incision time to heal. If there is concern about chronic low-grade sepsis at an osteotomy site or a hardware site, cultures can be obtained at the time of hardware removal.

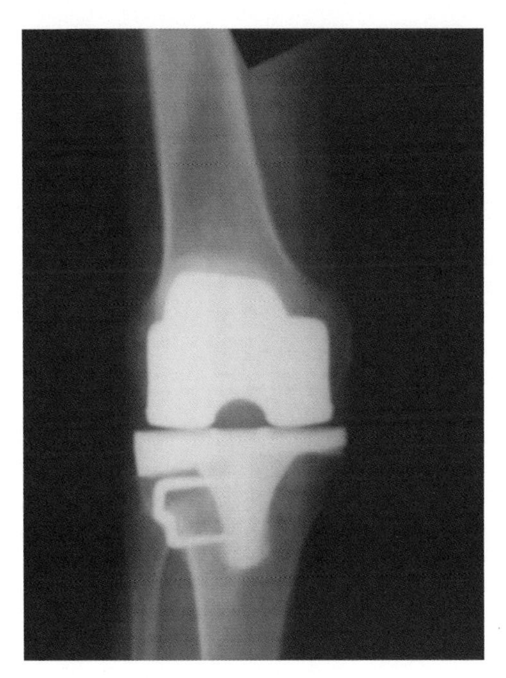

FIGURE 10–4. Asymptomatic staples can be retained if they do not interfere with stem replacement.

UP-SLOPED JOINT LINE

Joint line distortion after osteotomy can be in two planes. Abnormality in the varus-valgus plane is discussed below. In the flexion-extension plane, the most common distortion is a conversion of the normal down-slope of the tibia in the sagittal view to an up-slope of varying degree (Fig. 10–5). The up-sloped joint line demands a tibial resection at 90 degrees to the long axis of the tibia in the sagittal view. Down-sloping the cut must be avoided because of the abnormal amount of bone that would need to be resected from the posterior aspect of the tibia and the resultant distortion of knee kinematics. It is often difficult to preserve and balance

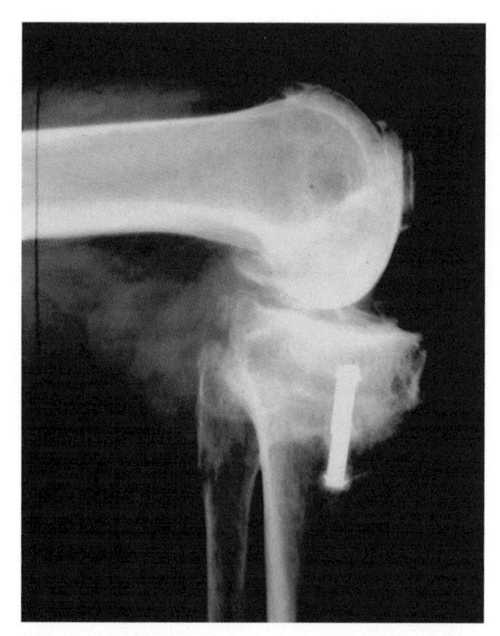

FIGURE 10–5. An up-sloped joint line calls for little or no posterior tibial slope to the tibial resection.

the posterior cruciate ligament in the presence of an up-sloped joint line.

NONUNION

When an osteotomy fails as a result of nonunion, the conversion to total knee arthroplasty must involve addressing the nonunion. I have had consistent success using a technique that prepares the tibia in a standard fashion but utilizes a long-stemmed tibial component to internally fix the nonunion (Fig. 10–6). The fibrous tissue of the nonunion is accessed from the intramedullary hole for the stem and circumferentially curetted. This area is then grafted with bone obtained from the standard resections from the femur, patella, and tibia.

The long stem of the tibial component is either cemented or press fit depending on the anatomy of the patient and the bone quality of the tibial diaphysis. Postoperative rehabilitation of these patients can usually proceed in a routine manner.

MALUNION

When malunion of the tibia is present following osteotomy, it can be in the form of excessive varus, valgus, flexion, and extension. Significant deformities in the flexion-extension plane are rare. Most do not have an impact on the patient's ability to achieve satisfactory flexion and extension and knee stability. For example, in the presence of a marked anterior bow of the tibia that imparts flexion to the overall alignment of the leg, full functional extension can be achieved by allowing hyperextension at the joint surfaces. This becomes a problem only when the prosthetic components themselves do not allow their surfaces to hyperextend (such as in some posterior stabilized designs). Conversely, if the tibial bow is in extension, clinical hyperextension can be avoided by tightening the extension gap.

If the malunion is in the varus or valgus plane, a decision has to be made about whether the secondary deformity can be corrected through the joint with ligament release or whether corrective osteotomy is necessary. For elderly patients, correction through the joint is usually appropriate (Fig. 10–7). A semiconstrained prosthesis, such as a Total Condylar III, may be required. In younger patients, an osteotomy is more appropriate. This can be done as a two-stage procedure or as a one-stage procedure fixing the reosteotomy with a long-stemmed tibial component. If a two-stage procedure is selected, the patient may be rewarded with enough improvement by the realignment procedure that the total knee arthroplasty can be postponed for a number of years. One-stage procedures require significant preoperative planning of the osteotomy in two planes.[1] As for nonunions, the osteotomy can be fixed with a cemented or a press-fit long-stemmed tibial component, depending on bone quality (Fig. 10–8).

CONSEQUENCES OF OVERCORRECTION OF A VARUS TIBIAL OSTEOTOMY

An osteotomy that has failed and healed in excessive valgus can be one of the most difficult total knee arthroplasty conversions. This is a result of three factors. The first is a valgus joint line in a knee that had a varus joint line prior to osteotomy. This situation distorts the kinematics of the collateral ligaments and posterior cruciate ligament when the static alignment is corrected. The second is the lateral plateau deficiency created by the valgus joint line (Fig. 10–9*A*).

The third is the effect on the rotational alignment of the femur articulating in flexion on a valgus joint line. The surgeon is forced to internally rotate the femoral component to reestablish flexion gap symmetry (Fig. 10–9*B*). The use of standard measures for femoral component rotation such as the Whiteside line, the transepicondylar access, or 3 degrees of external rotation off the posterior condyles will cause further distortion of the flexion gap by further external rotation of the femur. The flexion gap would be impossible to balance unless the surgeon performed a large, possibly complete, release of the lateral collateral ligament. More effective and easier to perform is internal rotation of the femoral component with the flexion gap tensed until symmetry is achieved. This maneuver is contrary to classic teaching for femoral component rotation and raises concern about compromise of patellar tracking. Although it obviously makes tracking more difficult, my experience shows that the internal rotation is not catastrophic. The lateral retinaculum is released anyway for correction of the valgus deformity in extension, and this facilitates patellar tracking. Consider also that for every 3 degrees of rotation of the femoral component, the trochlear groove moves only about a millimeter medially or laterally depending on whether the rotation is internal or external. This effect can be counteracted by undersizing the patellar component and placing it somewhat medial on the cut surface of the patella. One or two millimeters of medial shift can easily be achieved by this method. In addition, the surgeon can move the femoral component laterally on the end of the femur, thereby moving the trochlear

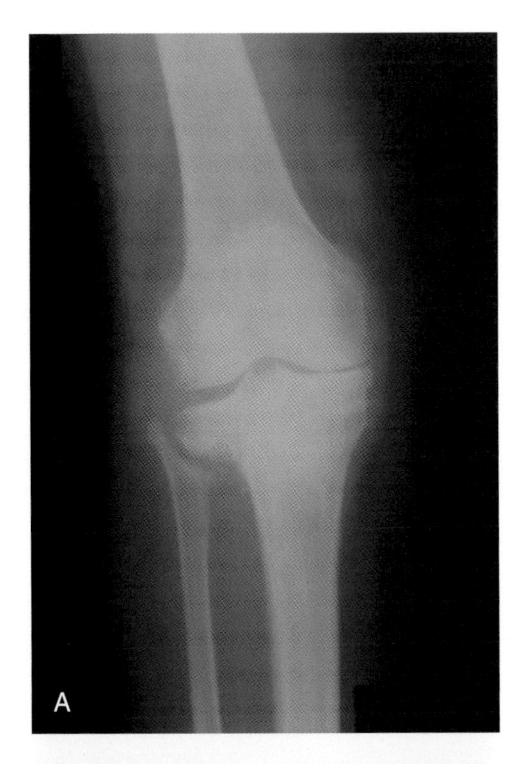

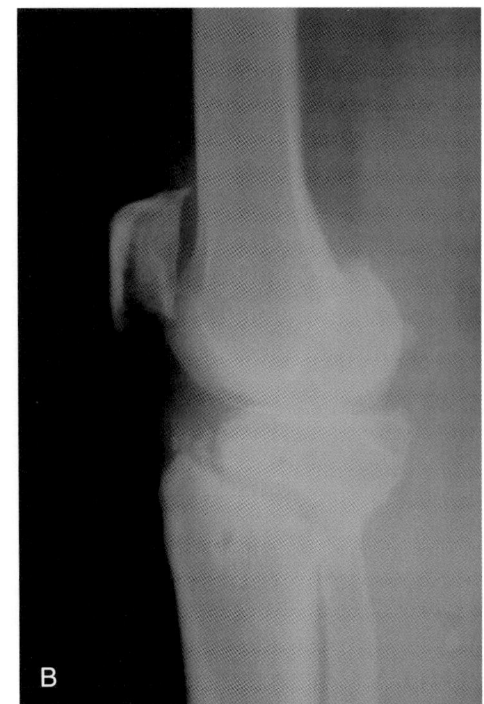

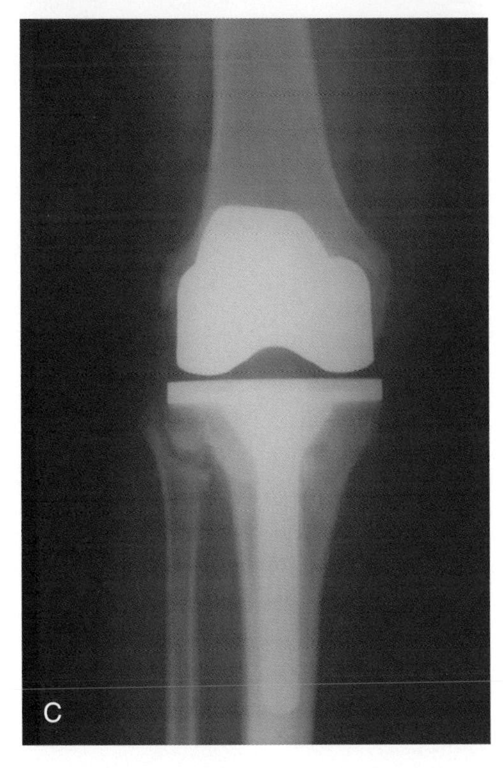

FIGURE 10–6. *A*, A failed osteotomy with a nonunion in malalignment. *B*, The lateral radiograph shows marked posterior displacement of the proximal fragment. *C*, The postoperative radiograph shows good restoration of alignment.

groove laterally along with it. Again, one or two millimeters of lateral shift is easily achieved. It is most important to proceed with internal rotation of the femoral component and establish a knee that is stable in flexion and avoid lateral collateral ligament releases.

Lateral plateau deficiency can be resolved in one of several ways. Minor deficiencies can be treated by slightly lowering the tibial resection until the cut is below the level of the deficiency. This method is reasonable as long as a significant amount of medial bone stock is not sacrificed. I limit the amount of medial resection to no more than 4 mm (Fig. 10–10).

A second option is to undersize the tibia by one size and shift the component medially away from the periphery of the lateral plateau. This will preserve medial bone stock and decrease the need for a lateral augmentation method.

Lateral augmentation can be accomplished by bone graft, screw/cement augmentation, or metallic wedge augmentation.

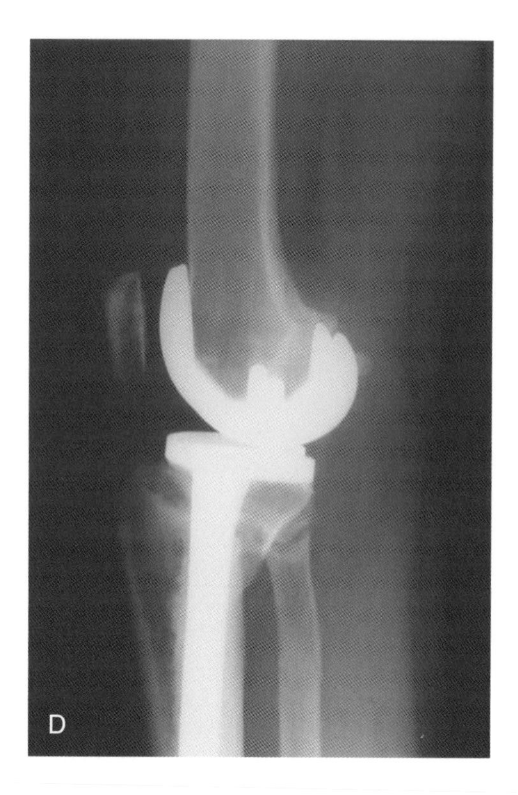

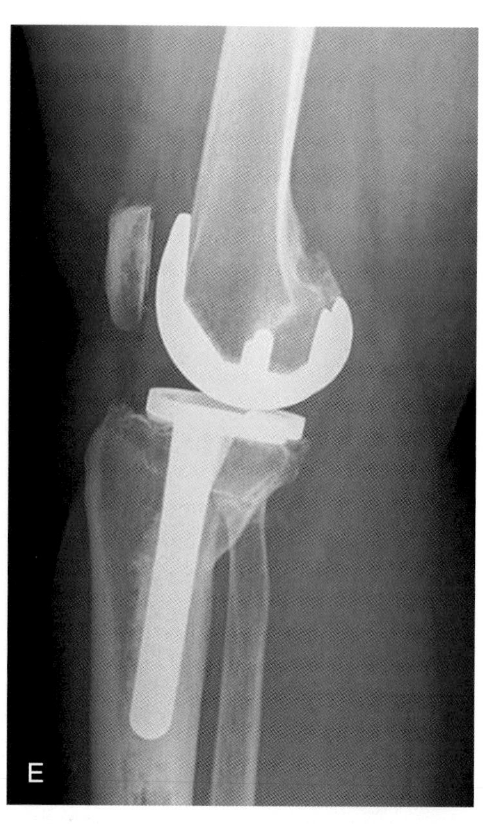

FIGURE 10–6 (cont'd). *D*, The nonunion has been grafted and immobilized with a cemented long-stemmed tibial component. *E*, Four years later, the osteotomy has fully healed and remodeled.

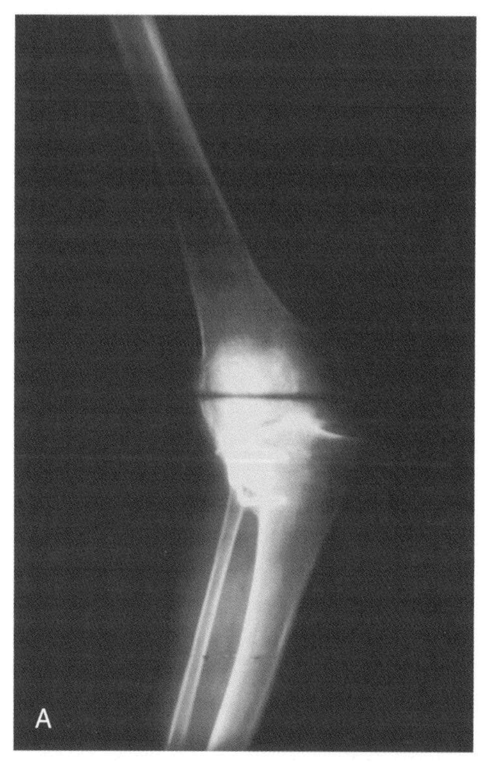

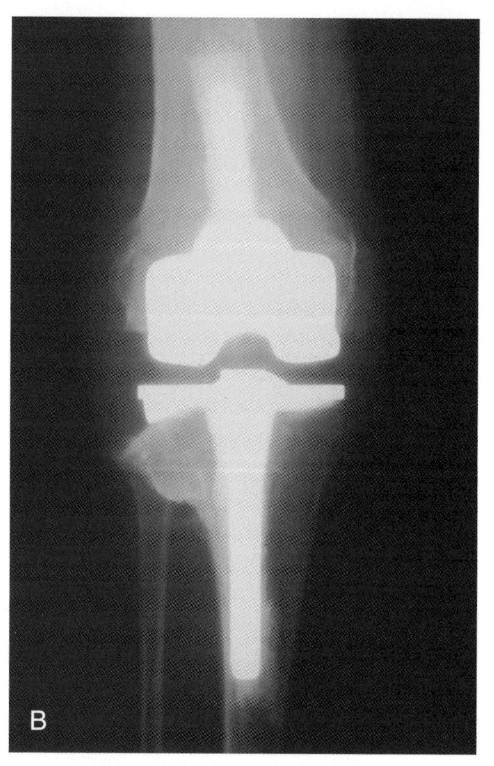

FIGURE 10–7. *A*, Malunion of an osteotomy in an elderly patient with a severe secondary valgus deformity. *B*, Alignment has been corrected by the knee arthroplasty with a large lateral release, lateral wedge augmentation, and stabilized components.

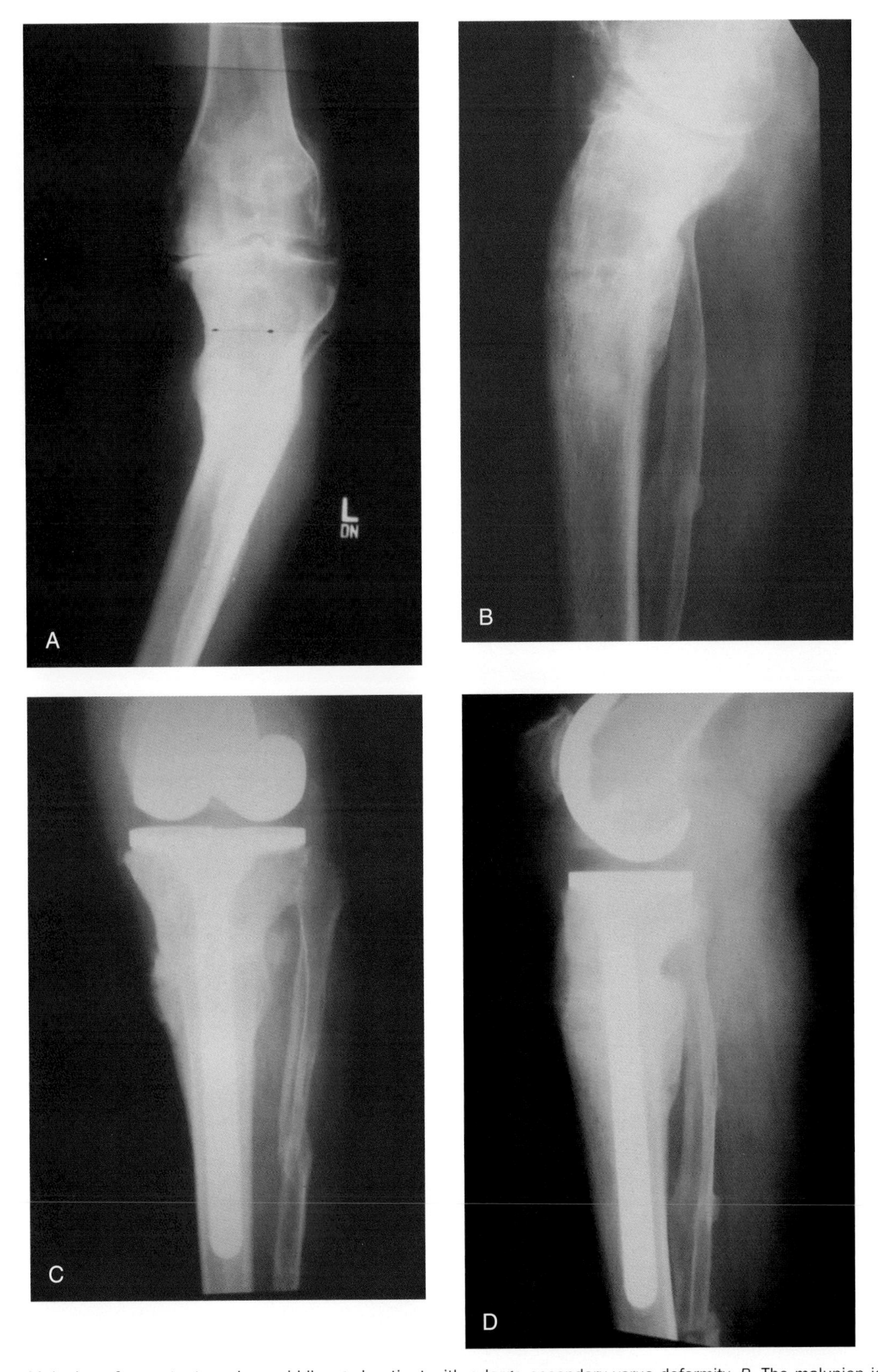

FIGURE 10–8. *A*, Malunion of an osteotomy in a middle-aged patient with a large secondary varus deformity. *B*, The malunion is in two planes. *C*, The malunion was corrected with an osteotomy and long-stemmed tibial component during the total knee arthroplasty. *D*, The deformity was also corrected in the sagittal plane.

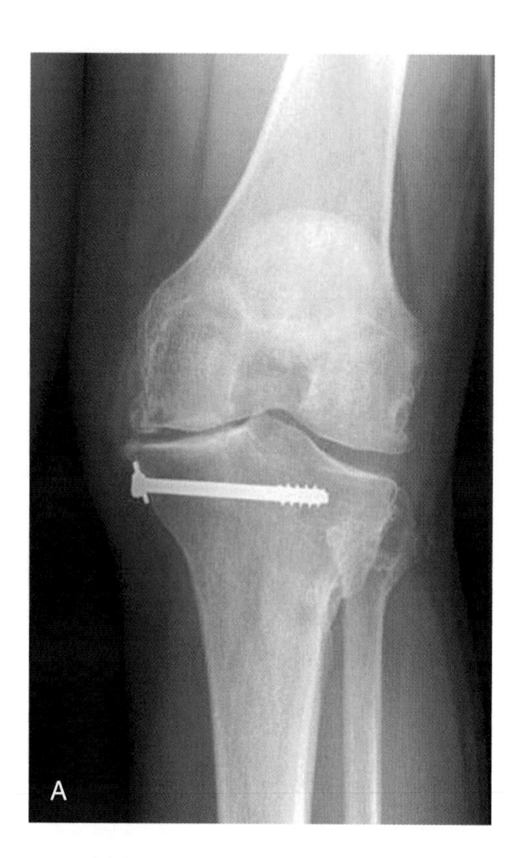

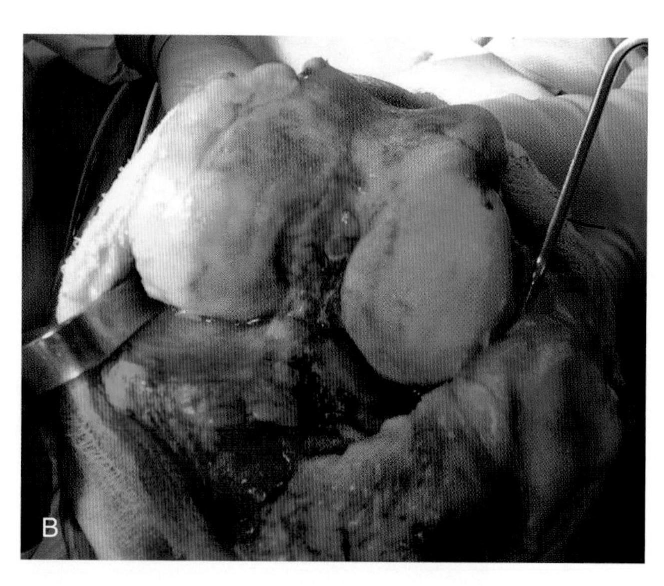

FIGURE 10–9. *A*, A failed osteotomy with a valgus tibial joint line. *B*, Intraoperative view showing the femur externally rotated on the valgus joint line. The femoral component will have to be internally rotated to restore flexion gap symmetry with a 90-degree tibial resection.

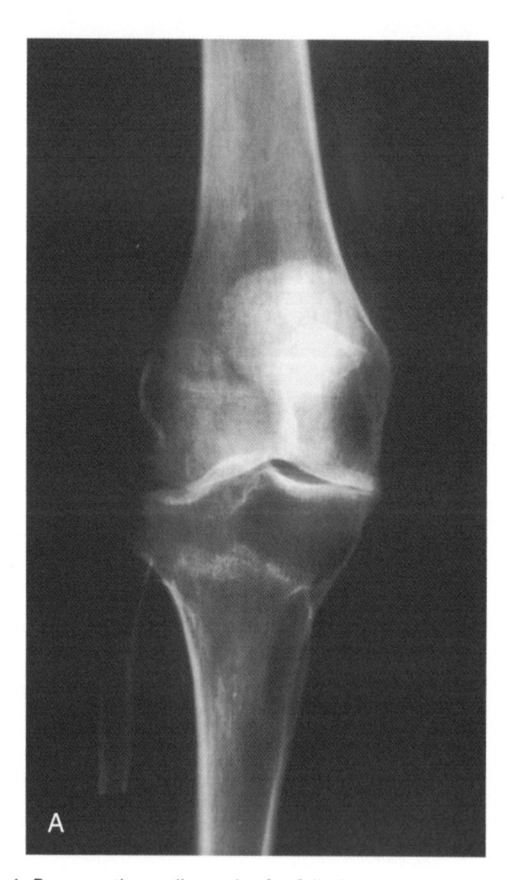

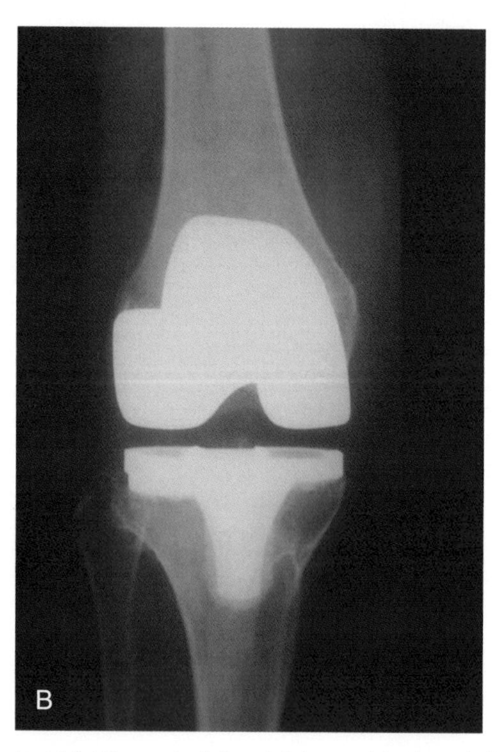

FIGURE 10–10. *A*, Preoperative radiograph of a failed osteotomy with a valgus joint line and relative deficiency of the lateral tibial plateau. *B*, At surgery the tibial component was undersized and shifted medially to minimize the lateral deficiency.

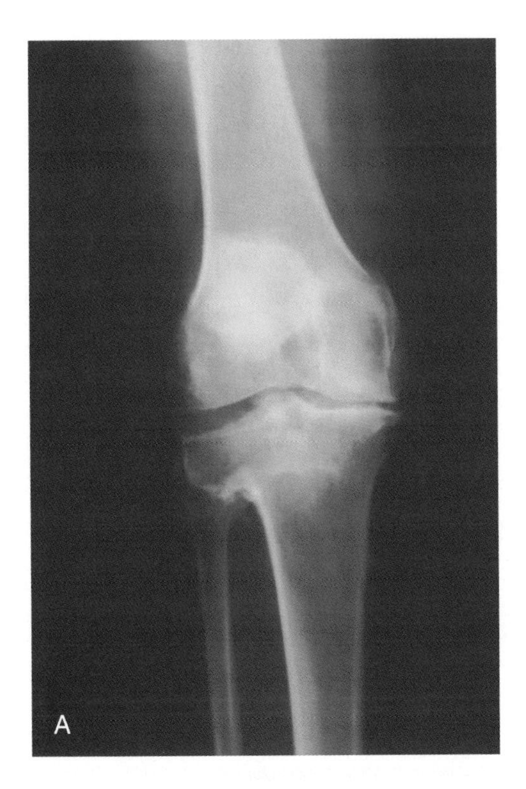

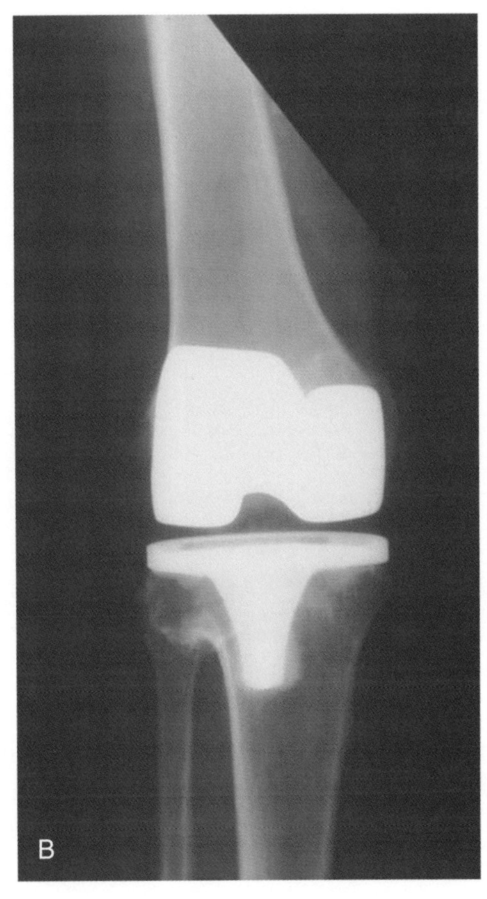

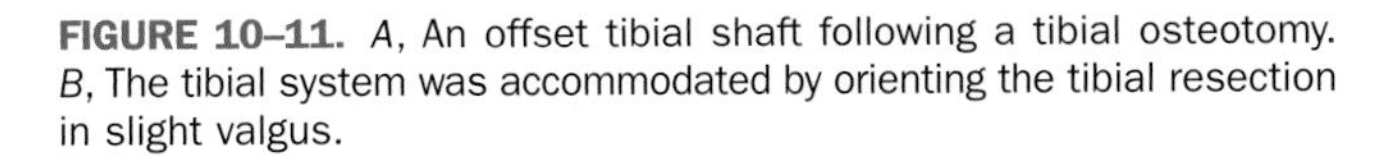

FIGURE 10–11. *A*, An offset tibial shaft following a tibial osteotomy. *B*, The tibial system was accommodated by orienting the tibial resection in slight valgus.

I use bone graft mainly for contained defects. The problem with bone grafts for large peripheral defects is that the interface between the graft and the tibia is not one that would promote healing unless more lateral bone is sacrificed below a sclerotic surface. Screw augmentation is attractive for posterior quadrant defects again, as an alternative to removing more bone for a suitable base for graft or metal wedge. Modular metal wedges are best used for large defects associated with severe overcorrection (see Fig. 10–7).

OFFSET TIBIAL SHAFTS

After a closing-wedge tibial osteotomy, offset shafts frequently are created. These tibias must be templated preoperatively when conventional stemmed components are being contemplated.

For a conventional stem to be accommodated, the component must sometimes be shifted medially and undersized. Alternatively, the tibial resection can be made in a few degrees of valgus counteracted by a femoral resection in 2 or 3 degrees of valgus rather than 5 or 6 degrees (Fig. 10–11). Another alternative is a tibial component with an offset stem, provided by most total knee systems (Fig. 10–12).

UNICOMPARTMENTAL REPLACEMENT AFTER FAILED TIBIAL OSTEOTOMY

At times, the surgeon must decide whether unicompartmental arthroplasty is an appropriate way to salvage a failed high tibial osteotomy (HTO). If the patient otherwise fulfills the selection criteria for unicompartmental knee arthroplasty (UKA; see Chapter 17), this is a reasonable consideration. It is problematic, however, if the osteotomy has failed in valgus in the presence of persistent unicompartmental disease on the medial side (Fig. 10–13). The valgus angulation, of course, would not be corrected by the arthroplasty, and in fact it is usually accentuated. UKA after HTO, therefore, is possible only when the HTO has failed into recurrent varus.

SUMMARY

Total knee arthroplasty (TKA) after a failed HTO can be a difficult technical procedure owing to multiple factors. These include the presence of prior unusable incisions, exposure difficulties, and retained hardware. The tibial joint line often is distorted by an abnormal up-slope rather than down-slope and a valgus angulation. Malunions and nonunions can occur. Malunion into valgus creates the

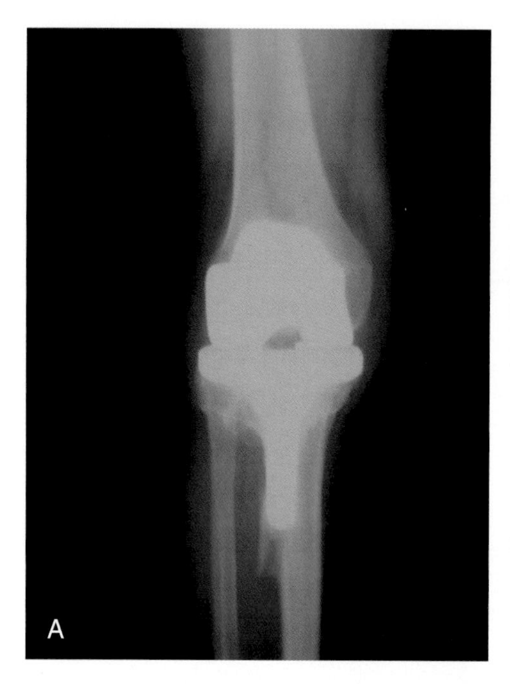

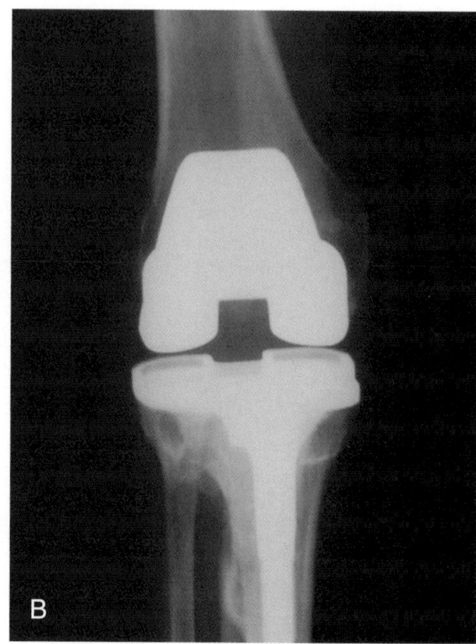

FIGURE 10–12. *A*, In this case, the offset tibial shaft failed to accommodate a standard stem. *B*, The knee was salvaged by use of an offset tibial stem.

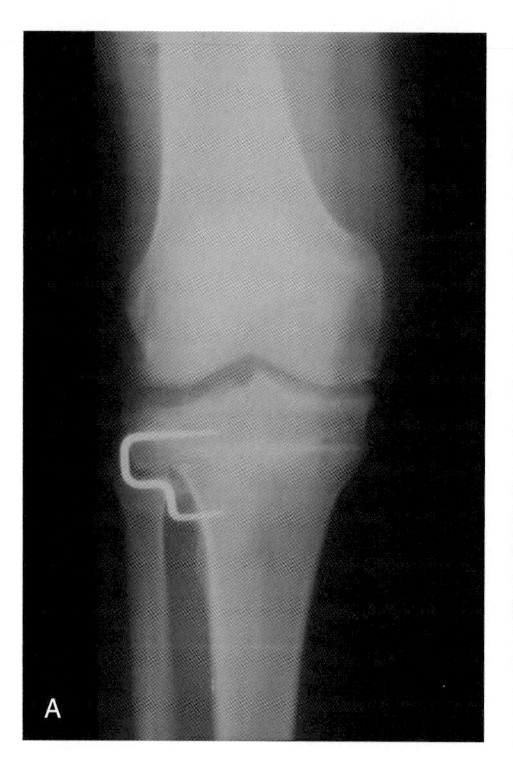

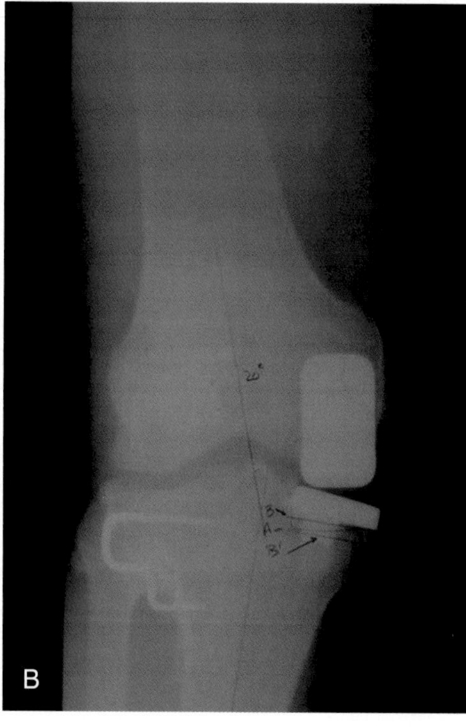

FIGURE 10–13. *A*, A failed osteotomy in valgus anatomic alignment. *B*, Unicompartmental replacement was unsuccessful.

valgus joint line and relative lateral plateau deficiency. Patella baja often is associated with osteotomy and can add to the risks of exposure and with limiting the postoperative range of motion. Finally, after a closing-wedge osteotomy, offset tibial shafts are frequent. The surgeon must be prepared for the availability of offset tibial stems depending on the results of preoperative templating.

Reference

1. Scott RD, Schai PA: Tibial osteotomy coincident with long stem total knee arthroplasty. Am J Knee Surg 2000;13:127–131.

CHAPTER 11

Total Knee Arthroplasty in Rheumatoid Arthritis

Total knee arthroplasty (TKA) in patients with rheumatoid arthritis has unique features different from those encountered in patients with osteoarthritis. Through the years, I have taken care of a large number of rheumatoid patients requiring TKA, both adults and juveniles. When I started practice in 1975 at the Robert Breck Brigham Hospital, 85% of patients undergoing TKA had rheumatoid arthritis. Since that time, this percentage has reversed itself to the point where only 5% of my patients have rheumatoid disease. There are a number of reasons for this change. The percentage of patients with rheumatoid arthritis was high in the mid-1970s because TKA was new and many potential candidates were withheld from the surgeon's care until the success of the procedure was established. Once the backlog of patients had been operated on, the percentage of rheumatoid arthritis patients decreased. Another factor was the training of residents and fellows who stayed in our geographic area. They had developed their own expertise with this procedure, and fewer rheumatoid patients were referred into our center. A third important reason for the decrease is the marked improvement in the medical treatment of rheumatoid arthritis. Fewer patients now progress to the stage of permanent structural damage requiring arthroplasty.

IPSILATERAL HIP INVOLVEMENT

Ipsilateral hip involvement is more frequent in rheumatoid arthritis than in osteoarthritis. The hip should always be thoroughly evaluated prior to TKA, and with few exceptions, the hip should be replaced prior to the knee surgery. I can think of at least six reasons for this. The first is that it is best to resolve any knee pain that is referred from the hip first. At times, the knee arthroplasty can even be delayed owing to the pain relief gained by replacing the hip. In cases in which it is critical to resolve the source of the knee pain, the hip joint should be injected with bupivacaine under fluoroscopic control (Fig. 11–1). The patient can then report on the extent of pain relief gained. If the pain relief is considerable, both patient and surgeon are more comfortable with the decision to proceed with the hip first.

The second reason is especially important in the juvenile rheumatoid patient. Since the hip surgery is relatively easy and painless for the patient (compared with the knee surgery), the surgeon gains the patient's confidence. On the contrary, if the knee is operated on first, the pain and difficult rehabilitation that the patient endures without a significant gain in function discourages the patient who still has pain and lack of function.

A third related reason is the fact that a person can exercise a hip above a painful arthritic knee, whereas it is difficult to exercise a knee below a painful, stiff, arthritic hip. I believe that a stationary bicycle is extremely helpful during rehabilitation of knee arthroplasty but is not important to rehabilitation of a hip replacement. The use of a bicycle is not possible when the hip above is painful and stiff.

The fourth reason is to resolve the tension of muscles that cross both the hip and knee joint, especially the hamstrings. If, for example, both hip and knee have flexion contractures and the knee is operated on first, resolving that contracture, a subsequent hip replacement that lengthens the hip can retighten the hamstring muscle.

The fifth reason also is related to preoperative knee contractures. At the time of hip arthroplasty, a contracted knee can be manipulated and casted to improve passive extension prior to the knee replacement. If epidural anesthesia is utilized, it can be maintained for several days and serial casts can be applied (see Chapter 9 and Fig. 9–2).

Sixth and finally, it makes sense to avoid twisting and torquing a well-balanced TKA while dislocating and exposing a stiff hip for replacement.

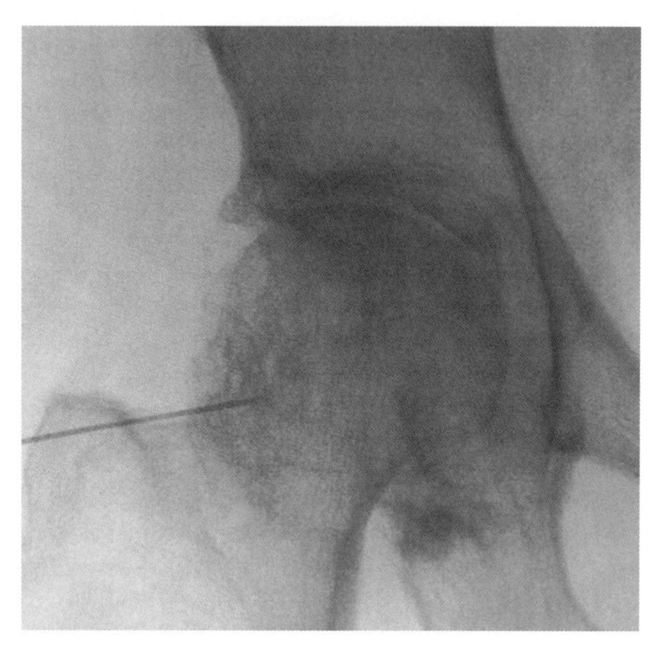

FIGURE 11–1. A bupivacaine injection into the hip joint under fluoroscopy can help define the source of knee pain.

ANTICOAGULATION NEEDS

In my experience, deep vein thrombosis (DVT) and pulmonary emboli occur less frequently in rheumatoid than in osteoarthritic patients. This may be partially due to the fact that most rheumatoid arthritis patients require the chronic use of anti-inflammatory medications, which have a mild anticoagulation effect. It might also be intrinsically related to their disease process. The reason is unclear, but it makes their anticoagulation needs different from those patients with osteoarthritis.

For all my TKA patients, I begin dosing warfarin on the night before surgery. For the rheumatoid patients I adjust the dose of warfarin during their hospital stay to an international normalized ratio (INR) between 1.5 and 2. Prior to discharge, I screen for DVT with an ultrasound examination. If it is negative, patients are discharged home on 81 mg of aspirin per day plus a return to their normal anti-inflammatory medication. I usually consider bilateral simultaneous knee patients at higher risk for DVT and maintain them on an adjusted dose of warfarin for at least 4 weeks. I make an exception for rheumatoid patients with bilateral knees who require their anti-inflammatory medication for control of rheumatoid inflammation. If bilateral ultrasounds are negative for DVT, they also are discharged on 81 mg of aspirin along with their rheumatoid medication.

FLEXION CONTRACTURE

Flexion contractures are more prevalent in rheumatoid than in osteoarthritic patients. The contracture is more likely to be due to inflammation in the soft tissues, whereas the flexion contracture of osteoarthritis is usually associated with a bony block (see Chapter 9). After studying the outcomes of a large number of patients with severe contractures, I have developed the following treatment guidelines for the rheumatoid patient.

For flexion contractures less than 15 degrees under anesthesia, I perform a normal distal femoral resection and posterior capsular stripping as needed. If the flexion contracture is between 15 and 45 degrees, I increase the distal femoral resection by 2 mm for every additional 15 degrees of correction that is necessary. I do this to a limit of a total of 13 mm to avoid compromise of the femoral origins of the collateral ligaments.

Between 45 and 60 degrees of flexion contracture, I consider preoperative manipulation and casting and always use a posterior cruciate ligament (PCL)–substituting technique. For flexion contractures greater than 60 degrees, I also consider preoperative manipulation and casting (see Fig. 9–2) and the use of a constrained articulation such as a Total Condylar III to resolve flexion gap laxity that can result from significant elevation of the femoral joint line.

For patients with inflammatory arthritis, I follow the "rule of one third." This states that intraoperative correction need only be to within one third of the preoperative contracture under anesthesia. The residual one third usually resolves with physical therapy, resolution of the inflammatory disease, and occasionally with the help of manipulation and casting. The most dramatic example I have seen was a patient with bilateral 110-degree flexion contractures. One knee was ankylosed at this degree of flexion and the other knee was fused. The techniques described above were utilized, including the use of a Total Condylar III prosthesis. At the end of surgery, the flexion contracture was corrected to 40 degrees. Following three serial casts applied under epidural anesthesia over 3 days, the patient's flexion contracture was corrected to 0.

Several additional points regarding flexion contractures should be emphasized. If there are bilateral, severe flexion contractures, both should be corrected simultaneously or there is a risk of regression of the correction on the first side until the second side is corrected.

When the capsule is closed following correction of a severe flexion contracture, the medial capsule should be advanced distally on the lateral capsule to avoid an initial extensor lag (see Fig. 8–5).

The amount of posterior slope applied when dealing with a severe flexion contracture should be 0 degrees. Every degree of slope built into the tibia creates a degree of flexion contracture or, put another way, prevents its correction.

Finally, ancillary preventive measures should be taken after surgery such as allowing the patient to have a roll under the ankle but never under the knee. A knee immobilizer at night will prevent the patient from sleeping with flexed knees and redeveloping a contracture. A "dynamic splint" can be helpful to both correct and maintain extension in refractory cases.

RHEUMATOID CYSTS

Although small juxta-articular cysts are not uncommon in osteoarthritis, they are more common in rheumatoid arthritis, and occasionally very large cysts are present on either femoral or tibial side of the joint. All cysts should always be curetted free of soft tissue and grafted with cancellous bone to seal the cyst wall from the cement interface. In my experience, failure to do this in rheumatoid patients leads to the

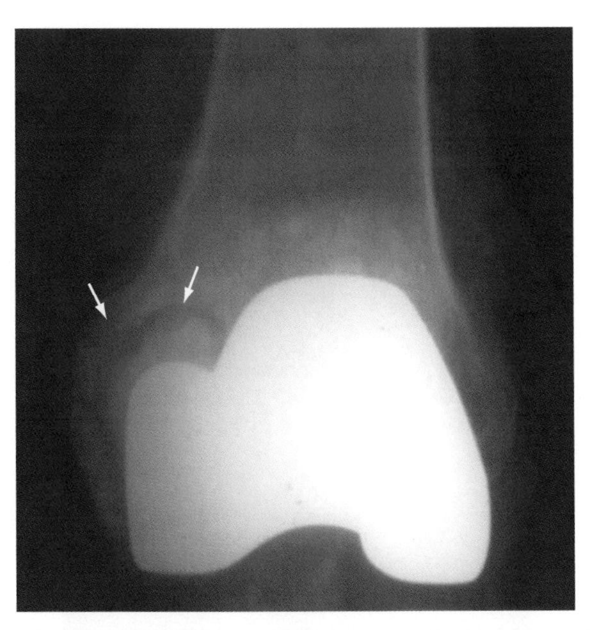

FIGURE 11–2. A large rheumatoid cyst packed with cement has demarcated and the component has loosened.

possibility of progressive demarcation at the cement-cyst interface leading to component loosening (Fig. 11–2). Examination of the tissue at the loosening interface shows histologic features consistent with recurrent rheumatoid synovium.[1]

Larger central defects can be treated with an impaction grafting technique (see Chapter 12). In this technique, morselized bone graft is packed densely around a long trial stem. When the trial stem is removed, the graft should be so densely packed as to provide structural integrity (see Fig. 12–10). Depending on the distal bone quality in the tibia, the stem of the real component can either be press fit or cemented. If the cemented technique is chosen, the canal is plugged with a cement restricter prior to application of the bone graft.

PATELLAR RESURFACING

Whether or not the patella should be resurfaced at the time of TKA remains controversial. I am convinced that there is a difference in long-term results in rheumatoid versus osteoarthritic patients when the patella is not resurfaced. In 1974, when we first had the ability to resurface both sides of the patellofemoral joint with the duopatellar prosthesis, we resurfaced the patella in only 5% of cases. Five-year follow-up showed that 10% of rheumatoid patients suffered secondary patellar degeneration (Fig. 11–3) and also had the possibility of recurrent rheumatoid synovitis in the knee (Fig. 11–4). Work in the laboratory of my associate, C. Sledge, indicated that residual cartilage in the rheumatoid patient's knee after TKA was a factor that allowed synovitis to recur.[2] Although some rheumatoid patients without patellar resurfacing have survived into their third decade after TKA, I adhere to the rule that the patella should be resurfaced in all rheumatoid patients, regardless of operative findings.

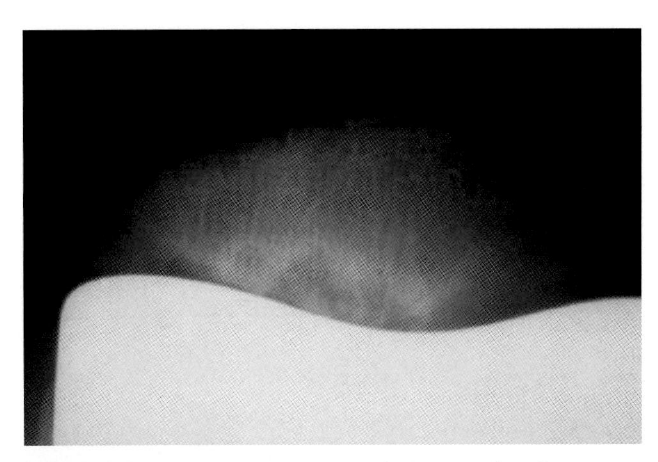

FIGURE 11–3. Loss of cartilage and cystic degeneration of an unresurfaced patella in rheumatoid arthritis.

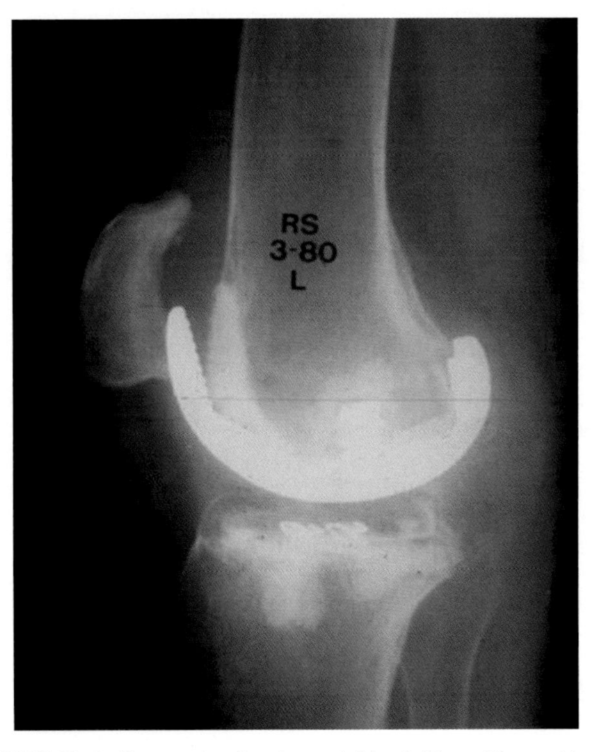

FIGURE 11–4. Recurrent active rheumatoid arthritis and femoral loosening with an unresurfaced patella.

SYNOVECTOMY AND RECURRENT ACTIVE RHEUMATOID SYNOVITIS

As mentioned above, it is possible for active rheumatoid synovitis to recur after TKA. The potential is increased if the patella has not been resurfaced and residual cartilage remains in the knee joint.

Even with TKA that includes patellar resurfacing, I have seen active rheumatoid synovitis return to the knee in at least four patients. These patients present a diagnostic dilemma. They sometimes have an acute presentation with a large effusion and an aspirate with a high cell count. In this scenario, infection is the most likely possibility, but active rheumatoid

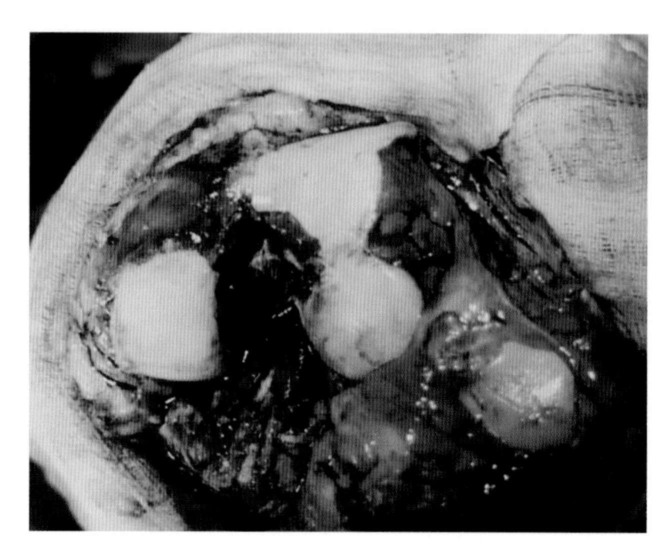

FIGURE 11–5. Active rheumatoid synovitis.

arthritis must also be considered. The cell count can be as high as 20,000 or 30,000 white cells per high-power field with a predominance of either polymorphonuclear cells or lymphocytes. The percentage of polymorphonuclear cells will not be in the high 90s as would be characteristic of infection. Cultures will be negative. Percutaneous synovial biopsy for histology may be necessary to confirm the diagnosis of rheumatoid disease. Usually this occurs in the presence of a rheumatoid flare with multiple joint involvement. Appropriate medical treatment is initiated. If infection has been ruled out, an intra-articular corticosteroid injection can quiet down the process. Occasionally, open synovectomy may be required.

This raises the question about whether synovectomy should be performed at the time of primary arthroplasty in the rheumatoid knee. I recommend that this be done universally in the patient with active synovitis at the time of the replacement (Fig. 11–5). If the disease is quiet and the synovium uninflamed, synovectomy probably is not necessary.

RISK FOR INFECTION

The risk for perioperative and late metastatic infection is greater in the rheumatoid than in the osteoarthritic patient. I have been fortunate to have avoided early infection in primary arthroplasty in rheumatoid patients, but an acceptable rate is probably 0.5% (see Chapter 14). Late metastatic infection will occur at an increased frequency owing to the immunosuppressed state of the patient because of their disease or medications and because they often have a number of remote sites of chronic infection, which can metastasize to the arthroplasty site. The most frequent sites are in the foot and lower leg. The olecranon bursa is another possible site.

NEED FOR ADEQUATE KNEE FLEXION

The rheumatoid patient requires more knee flexion than the osteoarthritic patient to have satisfactory function. All people need 60 to 70 degrees of flexion to walk on level ground. Ninety degrees of flexion is necessary for ascending most

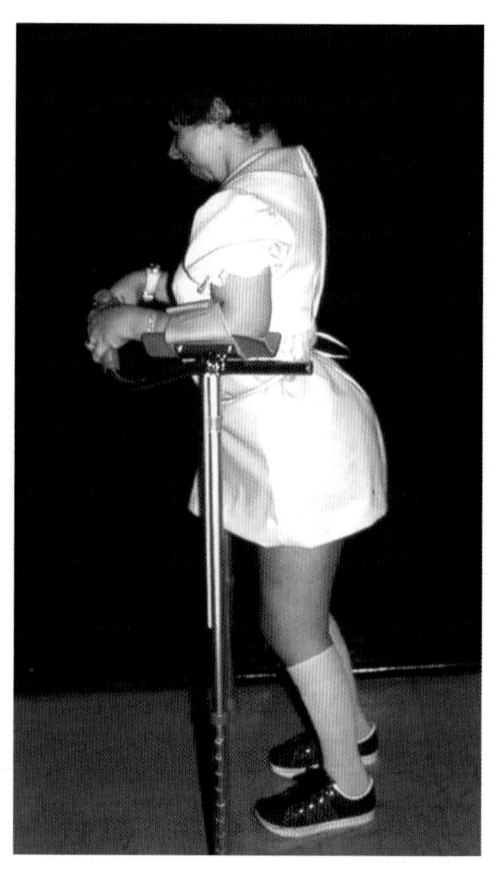

FIGURE 11–6. Platform crutches utilized by a juvenile rheumatoid patient with multiple joint involvement.

stairs. One hundred degrees of flexion is needed to descend stairs in a normal fashion. One hundred five degrees or more is necessary to rise from a standard chair without pushing up using the upper extremities.

The frequent involvement of shoulders, elbows, wrists, and hands in rheumatoid patients compromises their ability to ascend stairs or rise from a sitting position if they have inadequate knee flexion. As noted in Chapter 1, this need for flexion prompted us to adopt the PCL-retaining technique in the mid-1970s because nonsubstituting PCL-sacrificing designs from that era did not allow adequate flexion.Their upper extremity involvement also may require them to use a platform type of crutch or walker that cradles the forearm with vertical handles for grips. A platform crutch can usually be modified for use by even the most severely involved rheumatoid patient (Fig. 11–6).

OSTEOPENIA

The osteopenia associated with rheumatoid disease can present difficulties during TKA (Fig. 11–7). We first noted and reported the association of notching the anterior cortex of the femur with postoperative stress fracture in our rheumatoid patients.[3] I believe that the risk of stress fracture is great enough in the rheumatoid patient that if the cortex is significantly notched, a long-stemmed femoral component should be considered. Notching is most apt to occur when a femur that is between sizes is prepared for the smaller

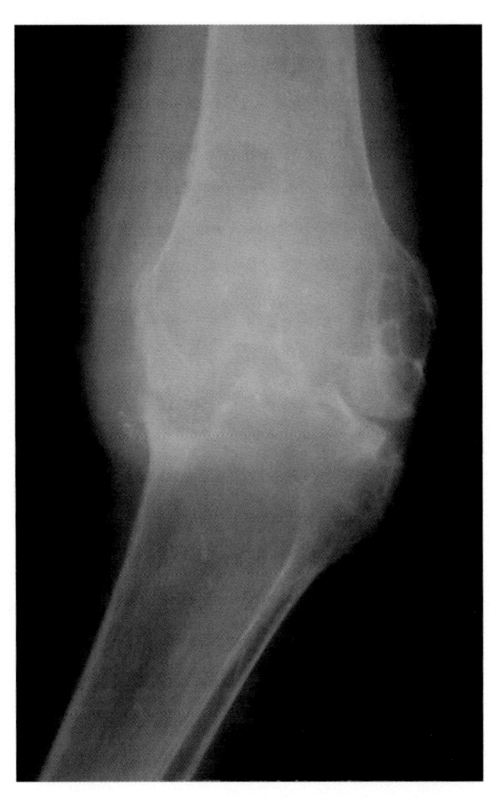

FIGURE 11–7. Severe osteopenia at risk for intraoperative and postoperative fracture.

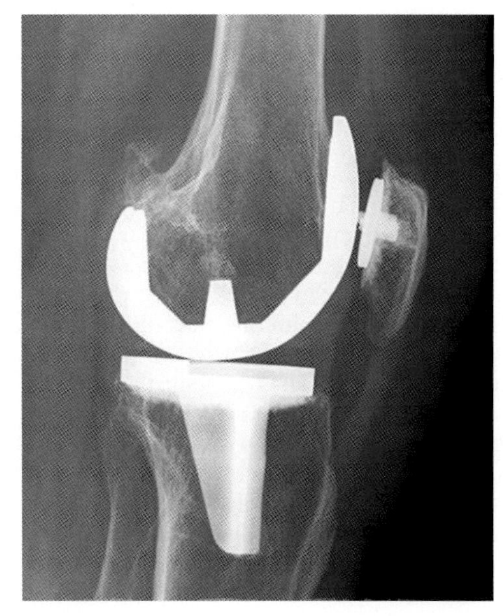

FIGURE 11–8. Nineteen-year follow-up of a rheumatoid patient with cementless femoral fixation.

component. Measures that can be taken to avoid notching are discussed in Chapters 4 and 15.

When osteopenia is severe, I have seen supracondylar fractures occur during preparation of the leg for surgery. In these cases, the hip above was stiff and the assistant holding the leg raised the leg with too much force. Similarly, I have seen supracondylar fractures occur during preparation of the leg for total hip arthroplasty in rheumatoid patients. In these cases, too great an abduction force was applied in an ankylosed hip.

Fractures can also be generated during postoperative manipulation for poor range of motion following TKA. This emphasizes the importance of assessing flexion against gravity of the replaced knee at the end of the procedure with the capsule closed so that the patient's potential is not exceeded. Early in my career when this was not appreciated, I fractured an osteopenic patella when I manipulated the TKA beyond 90 degrees in a patient whose potential was most likely less than this, since her preoperative flexion was only of 60 degrees.

Another intraoperative potential complication in the severely osteopenic rheumatoid patient is avulsion of the medial collateral ligament from its femoral origin owing to medial retraction. The avulsion usually includes the medial cortex, which separates from the soft underlying cancellous bone. As alarming as this may seem, it usually is not a clinical problem, since the soft tissue sleeve remains intact. If it occurs, I sometimes use a cancellous screw with a washer to resecure the cortex to the condyle.

Still another complication of osteopenia is intraoperative fracture of the patella. This might occur after patellar preparation including the placement of three holes for the fixation lugs. These holes are now stress risers, and a fracture can be propagated merely by retracting against the patella in a normal fashion. Again, the soft tissue sleeve remains intact. If the fragments are minimally separated, the fixation provided by the cemented patellar component across the fracture may suffice. If the fragments are separated, the surgeon must consider cerclage with wire.

Finally, in the presence of osteopenia, the surgeon must consider whether cementless fixation ever is appropriate. I am not an advocate of cementless fixation of either the tibia or patella. I do have a large experience with cementless femoral fixation in adult and juvenile rheumatoid patients, which has been universally successful (Fig. 11–8). An intraoperative decision can be made based on the primary fixation of the trial component. Because of the osteopenia, the surgeon can purposely slightly diverge the trochlear and posterior condylar resections so that as the component is inserted the bone is impacted and the fixation enhanced.

ANESTHETIC CONSIDERATIONS

Because of rheumatoid involvement of the cervical spine and temporomandibular joint, special considerations often are required to anesthetize the rheumatoid patient. Preoperative assessment by the anesthesiologist is extremely important to anticipate the individual needs of the patient. Lateral cervical spine films in maximum flexion and extension may be appropriate to evaluate the patient for C1–C2 subluxation.

Because of the many potential problems associated with the administration of general anesthesia, regional anesthesia is preferred. It can be by either the spinal or epidural route. Still, the surgeon must be prepared for the possible need for general anesthesia and intubation. The anesthesiologist should be skilled in the use of a pediatric fiberoptic laryngoscope and awake nasotracheal intubation techniques.

PCL PRESERVATION VERSUS SUBSTITUTION

The literature is controversial regarding the need for PCL substitution versus the acceptability of PCL preservation. Some articles favor PCL substitution,[4,5] while our experiences indicate that excellent minimal 10-year results can be achieved with PCL preservation.[6] I offer two hypotheses to explain the discrepancy in results.

In the PCL-sparing technique that did not fare as well, knees were implanted in an era when some laxity in the articulation was favored. The ligaments in many rheumatoid patients have a tendency to stretch out over time, leading to hyperextension, instability, and synovitis. Also during that era, an undersized inset patella often was used. This allowed for retention of residual cartilage in the knee, which provided an increased risk for active rheumatoid synovitis to recur in the knee, along with its adverse consequences.

In my own series of rheumatoid patients with 10- to 13-year follow-up, component survivorship at 10 years was 100% except for 2% of metal-backed patellae. Among 81 knees studied, the only reoperations at 10 to 13 years were for revision of a metal-backed patellar component at 6 years and a synovectomy for recurrent active rheumatoid synovitis. One asymptomatic patient had hyperextension of 5 degrees in the knee (Fig. 11–9). This finding raises the concern that late ligamentous laxity could occur in the prosthetic knee with PCL retention and is a reminder that in rheumatoid patients with ligamentous laxity preoperatively the components should be inserted on the tighter side with conservative initial bone resections.

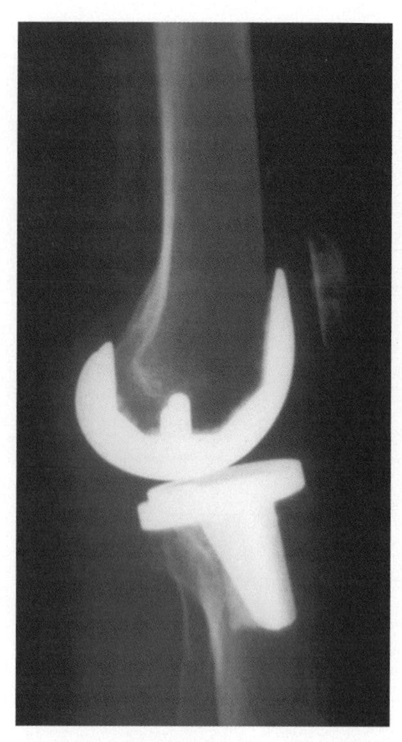

FIGURE 11–9. Five degrees of hyperextension in a rheumatoid patient.

SUMMARY

TKA in rheumatoid arthritis presents management difficulties that are unique to the disease. These include frequent ipsilateral hip involvement, bilaterality, anticoagulation needs, flexion contractures, rheumatoid cysts, the need for universal patellar resurfacing, and possibly the need for synovectomy. Rheumatoid patients are more vulnerable to both early and late infections. They need a prosthesis and technique that provides adequate flexion for activities of daily living and spare their upper extremities. Their often profound osteopenia can lead to intraoperative and postoperative fractures. Finally, their cervical spine and temporomandibular disease create challenging anesthetic considerations.

Nevertheless, given these considerations and the degree of preoperative disability suffered by the rheumatoid patient, the results of surgery can be extremely dramatic and gratifying to both patient and surgeon.

References

1. Goldring SR, Wojno WC, Schiller AL, Scott RD: In patients with rheumatoid arthritis the tissue reaction associated with loosened total knee replacements exhibits features of a rheumatoid synovium. J Orthop Rheum 1988;1:9–21.
2. Steinberg J, Sledge CB, Noble J, Stirrat CR: A tissue-culture model of cartilage breakdown in rheumatoid arthritis: quantitative aspects of proteoglycan release. Biochem J 1979;180:403–412.
3. Aaron RK, Scott RD: Supracondylar fracture of the femur after total knee arthroplasty. Clin Orthop 1987;219:136–139.
4. Laskin RS: Total condylar knee replacement in patients who have rheumatoid arthritis: a ten-year follow-up study. J Bone Joint Surg Am 1990;72:529–535.
5. Laskin RS, O'Flynn HM: Total knee replacement with posterior cruciate ligament retention in rheumatoid arthritis: problems and complications. Clin Orthop 1997;345:24–28.
6. Schai PA, Scott RD, Thornhill TS: Total knee arthroplasty with posterior cruciate retention in patients with rheumatoid arthritis. Clin Orthop 1999;367:96–106.

CHAPTER 12

Bone Stock Deficiency in Total Knee Arthroplasty

FEMORAL DEFICIENCY

Options available for reconstitution of deficient bone stock on the femoral side include bone grafting, cement alone, cement plus screw augmentation, augmented components, and custom components.

Bone Grafting

Bone grafting is appropriate for all contained defects. The graft can be in the form of morsels or solid blocks, or a combination of both. Early in my experience with rheumatoid arthritis patients, I discovered that if juxta-articular cysts were filled with cement they could eventually develop an enlarging zone of demarcation at this interface and component loosening could occur (Fig. 12–1). Histologic examination of the bone-cement interface in tissue retrieved at revision showed that the rheumatoid process had recurred at this interface, contributing to the loosening process (see Chapter 11). This finding convinced me that all juxta-articular cysts, in both rheumatoid and osteoarthritic disease, should be curetted free of fibrous tissue and grafted with cancellous bone, which usually can be obtained from the standard bone resections. Follow-up radiographs show good incorporation of bone graft in these situations.

Cement Alone

In the presence of uncontained defects, the use of long stems and cement alone sometimes can suffice to achieve adequate prosthetic fixation (Fig. 12–2). Care must be taken with this technique, however, to not distort the joint line. The most common error is elevation of the joint line combined with the use of thick tibial inserts to restore extension stability. Joint line elevation leads to patella baja and disturbance of the kinematics of the collateral ligaments (Fig. 12–3).

Cement Plus Screw Augmentation

It is important to use a method that restores the femoral joint line to its more normal location. A simple way to accomplish this has been used for many years: the incorporation of bone screws into the cement mantle. Either cortical or cancellous screws are used depending on the quality of the distal bone. The screws are allowed to protrude to the level at which they support the trial femoral component in its proper distal and varus-valgus position (Fig. 12–4). This position can be estimated by determining the level of the normal joint line based on the opposite knee and measured as the distance from a fixed bony landmark such as the lateral epicondyle. The distance is usually 2 to 3 cm distal to the epicondyle, depending on the patient's size. The proper level also can be assessed by its effect on the proximal distal positioning of the patella relative to the joint line.

Valgus knees with a deficient lateral condyle often present a problem in restoration of the joint line in a primary situation. Classically, the severe valgus knee has a deficient lateral condyle (see Chapter 6). This hypoplasia accounts for much of the valgus deformity. The surgeon must avoid resecting back to the level of the condylar deficiency because it will result in elevation of the joint line. Resection should be based on the normal medial side, resulting in the need for lateral augmentation (see Figs. 6–8 and 6–9). An effective and efficient way to accomplish this is with one or two cortical screws inserted into the sclerotic bone of the distal condyle. Properly placed screws support the trial femoral component in its proper distal and valgus positioning and perform the same function when the real component is cemented (Fig. 12–5).

I have used this method for more than 30 years without adverse effects. Concern is often raised about the use of dissimilar metals with the screw and femoral component. This concern is obviated if the screw is titanium. I believe, however, that chrome-cobalt or stainless steel screws can be used

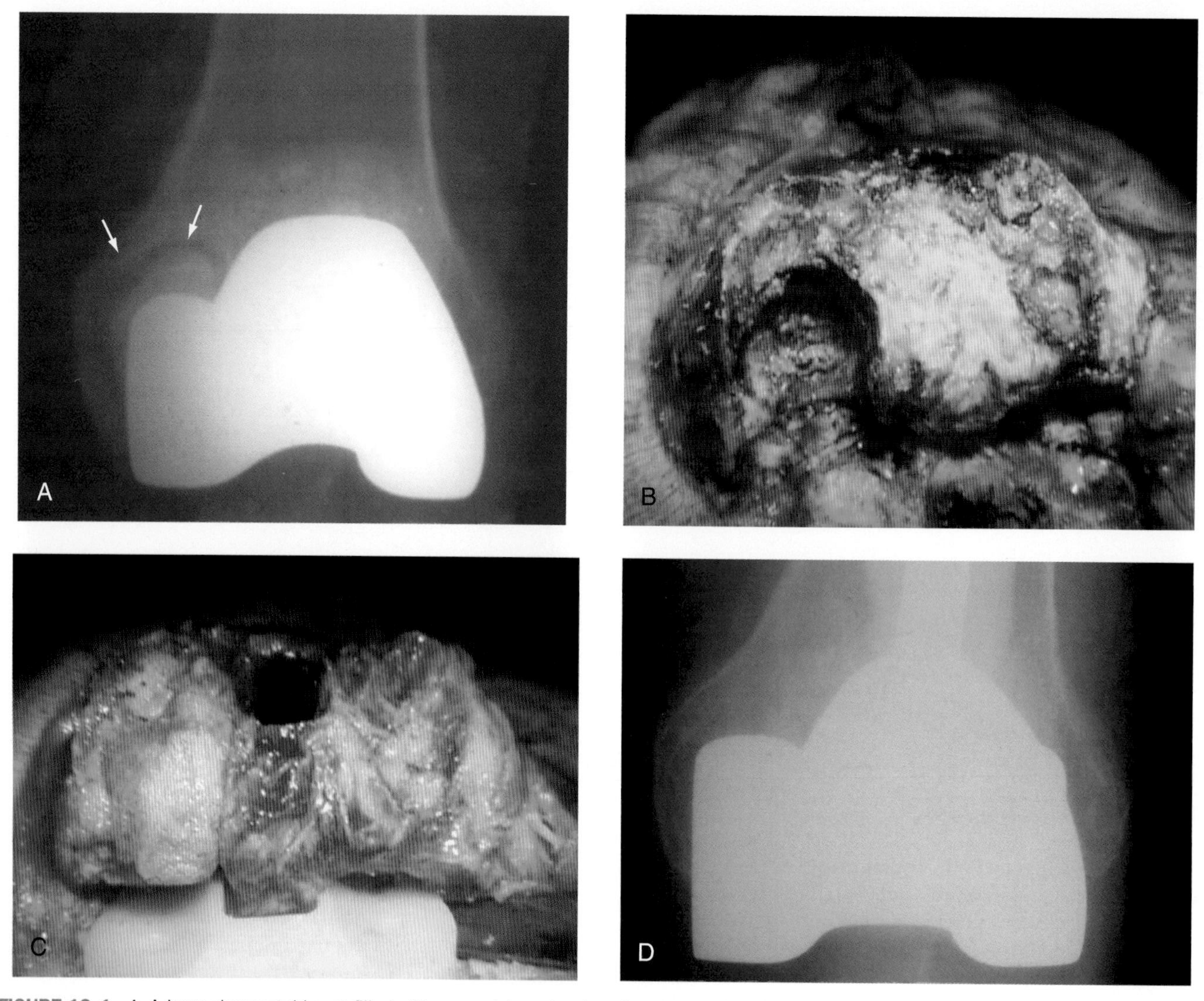

FIGURE 12–1. *A*, A large rheumatoid cyst filled with cement has developed a progressive zone of radiolucency at the interface, and the femoral component has loosened. *B*, The medial defect is large but contained. *C*, The defect is packed with a combination of morselized and bulk allograft. *D*, Five years after surgery, the graft appears to have incorporated.

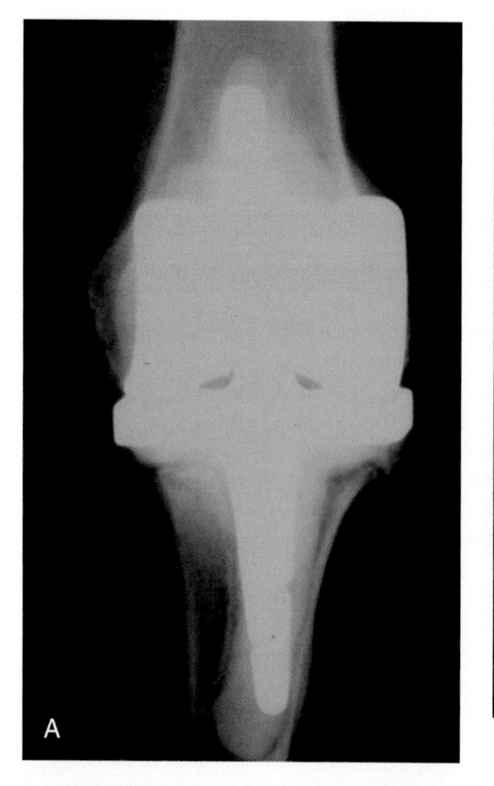

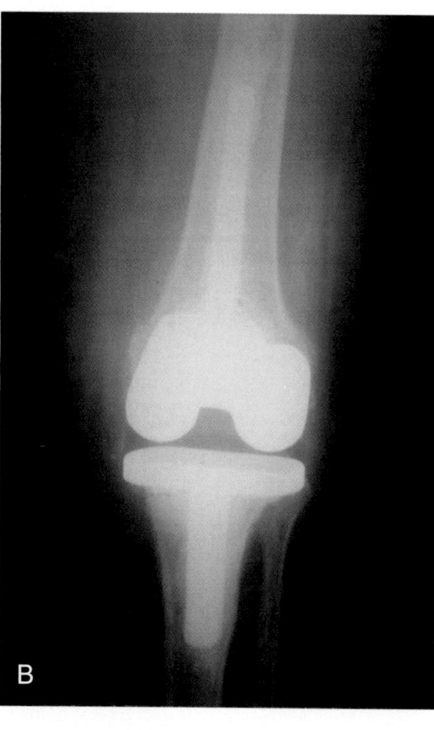

FIGURE 12–2. *A*, Failed TKA with loosening and bone stock deficiency. *B*, Revision with the use of long stems alone.

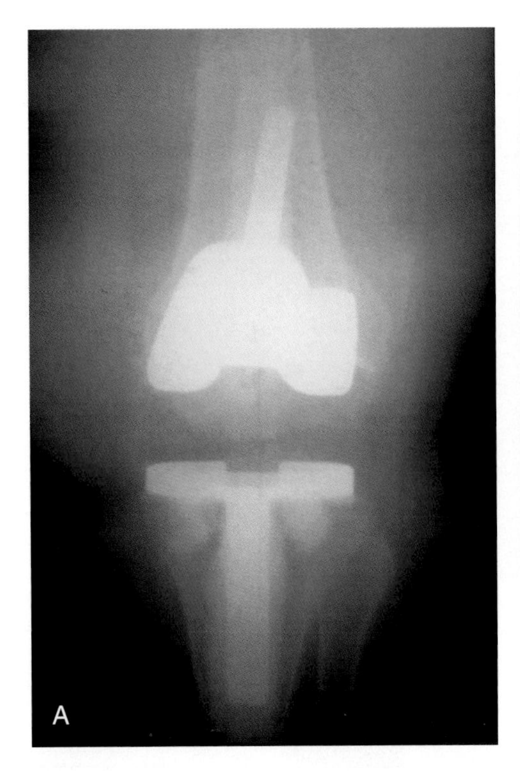

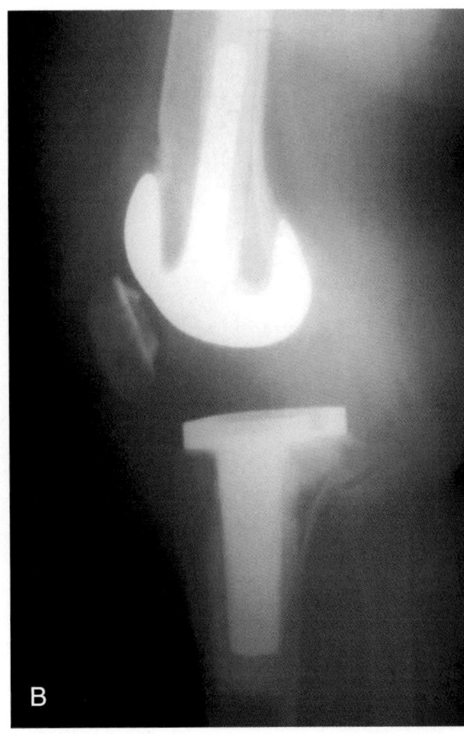

FIGURE 12–3. *A*, Failure to restore the femoral joint line at revision. *B*, Patella baja secondary to the elevated joint line.

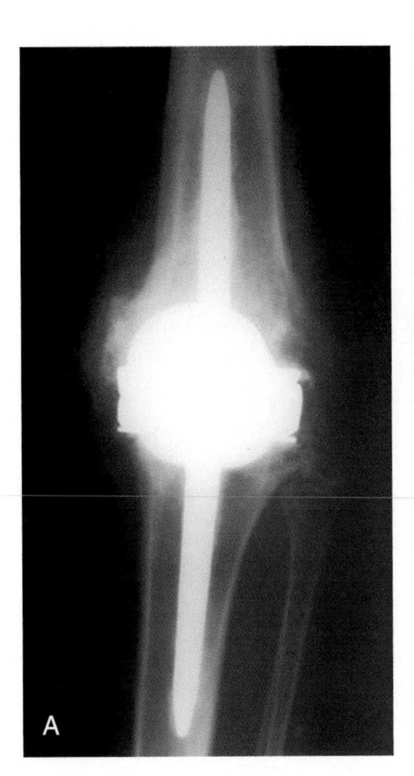

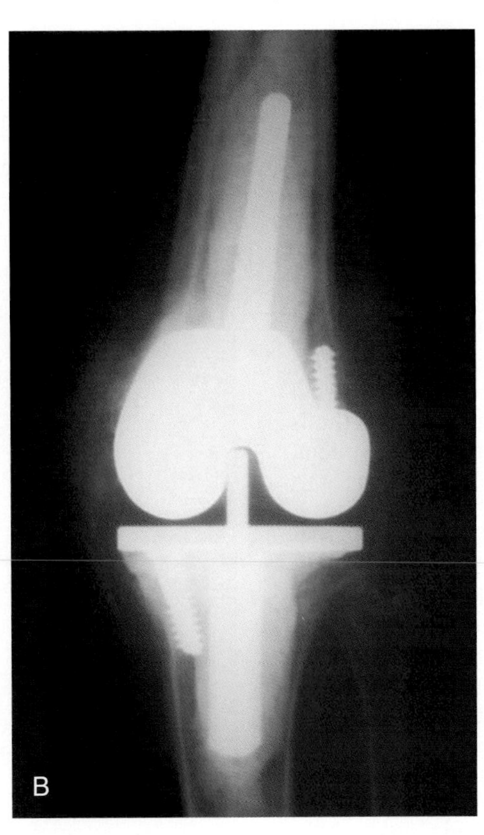

FIGURE 12–4. *A*, A loose hinge prosthesis with bone stock deficiency. *B*, Restoration of the femoral joint line and component alignment using screws as supporting templates.

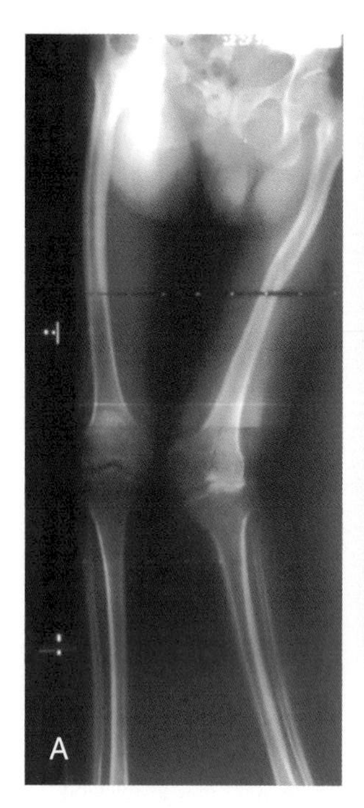

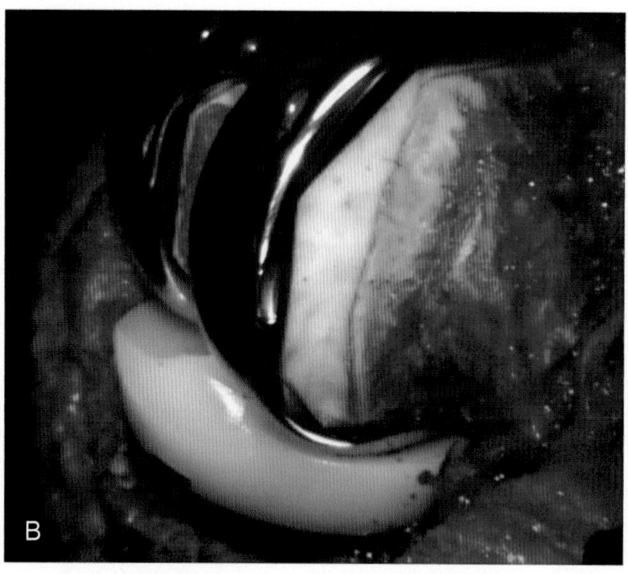

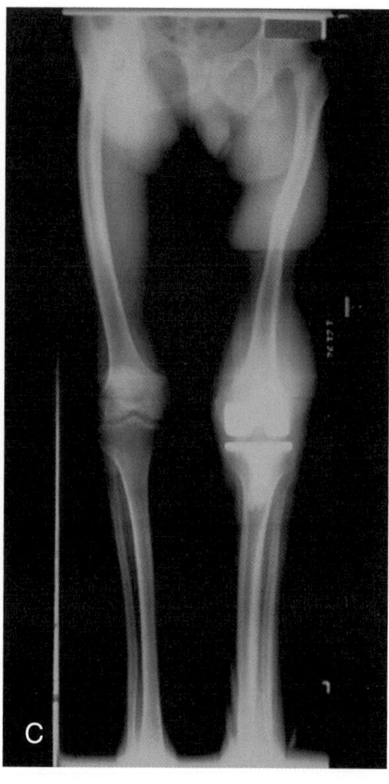

FIGURE 12–5. *A*, Severe valgus deformity with a deficient lateral femoral condyle. *B*, The lateral deficiency was augmented with a condylar screw encased in cement. *C*, Femoral component and limb alignment are restored.

safely in conjunction with a chrome-cobalt femoral component because the encompassing bone cement protects the complex from potential adverse effects of dissimilar metals in close proximity.

Augmented Components

Thomas Thornhill and I introduced femoral augmentation wedges with the Omnifit revision total knee system in the late 1980s. Modular wedges are now available with virtually all revision systems (Fig. 12–6). These can be affixed to either distal or posterior femoral condyle in various sizes. In some systems, the wedges are mechanically fixed to the femoral component, and in others, they are cemented. Both methods appear to be effective (Fig. 12–7). Depending on the system, distal wedges as thick as 20 mm and posterior wedges as thick as 12 mm are available.

Large-bulk femoral allografts are necessary for restoration of bone deficiency in extreme cases. My preferred method for their use is to affix the allograft to the host femur via the intramedullary alignment system and proceed with the bone cuts on the allograft in situ. Alternatively, the surgeon could prepare the allograft for the femoral component on a back table and subsequently couple it to the host bone via the long stem of the femoral component. The most difficult part of this technique is establishing proper femoral rotation at the host allograft junction and restoring both leg length and the position of the joint line relative to the quadriceps mechanism. I prefer to use a press-fit long stem if it can achieve excellent initial fixation. Otherwise, cemented stems are appropriate (Fig. 12–8) and are also used for most smaller bulk grafts.

TIBIAL DEFICIENCY

The same options available on the femoral side are available on the tibial side for bone stock restoration and component

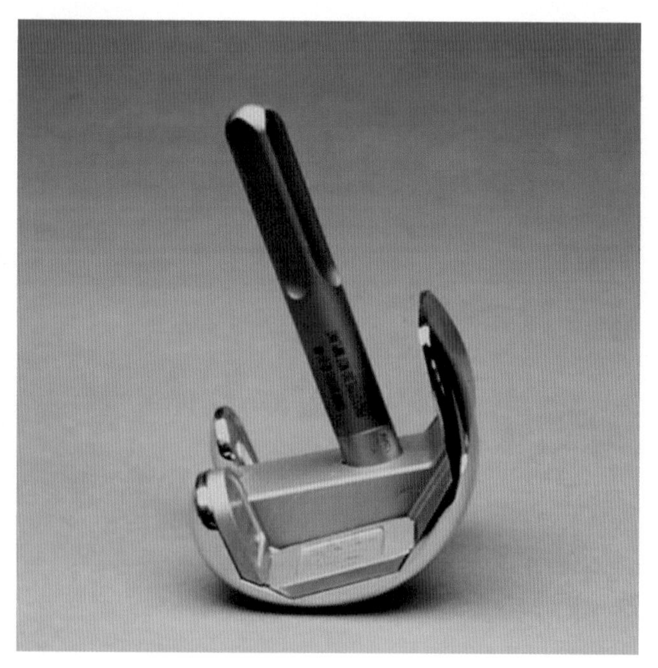

FIGURE 12–6. Modular distal and posterior augmentation wedges on a revision component.

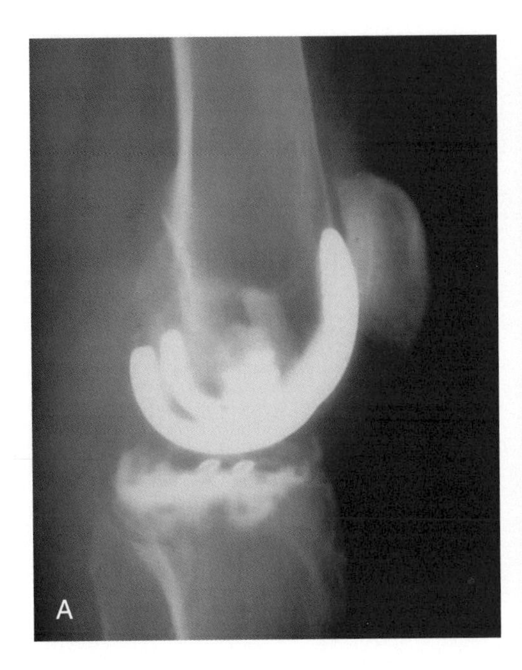

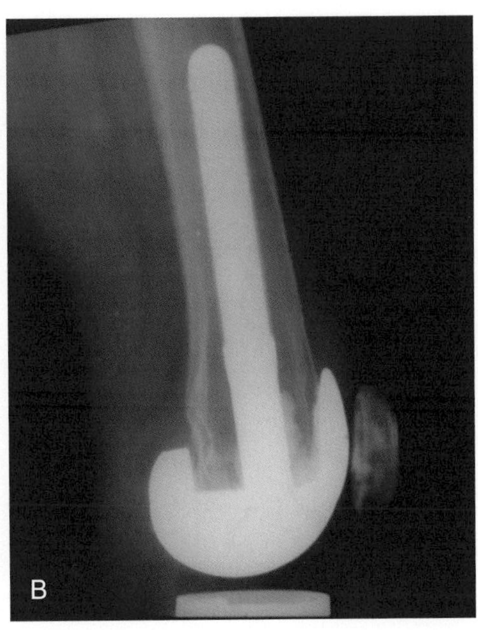

FIGURE 12–7. *A*, Failed TKA with condylar deficiency. *B*, Revision with a combination of distal and posterior femoral augmentation.

fixation. These include bone grafting, cement alone, cement plus screws, augmented components, and custom components.

Bone Grafting

As in the femur, bone graft should be utilized for all contained defects (Fig. 12–9). Any subchondral cysts that are encountered should be curetted free of fibrous tissue and grafted with cancellous bone obtained from the routine total knee resections. Larger central defects can be treated with an impaction grafting technique (Fig. 12–10). In these cases, I hand-ream the tibial canal to a level below the cyst until the tibial cortex is engaged. A trial for a modular stem of the appropriate diameter is then inserted into the canal beyond the

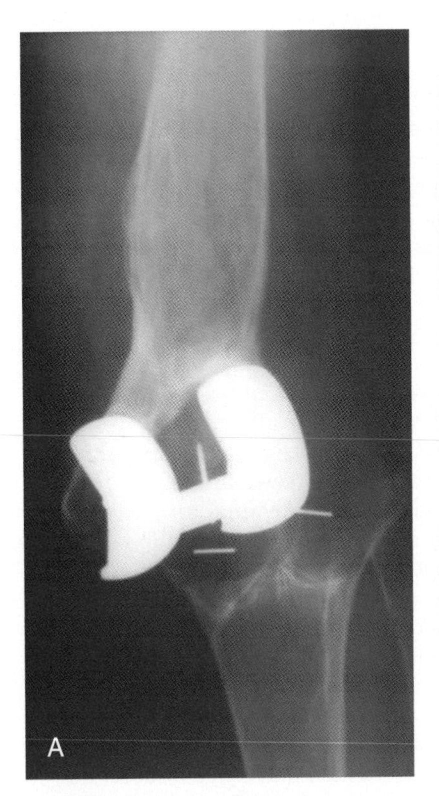

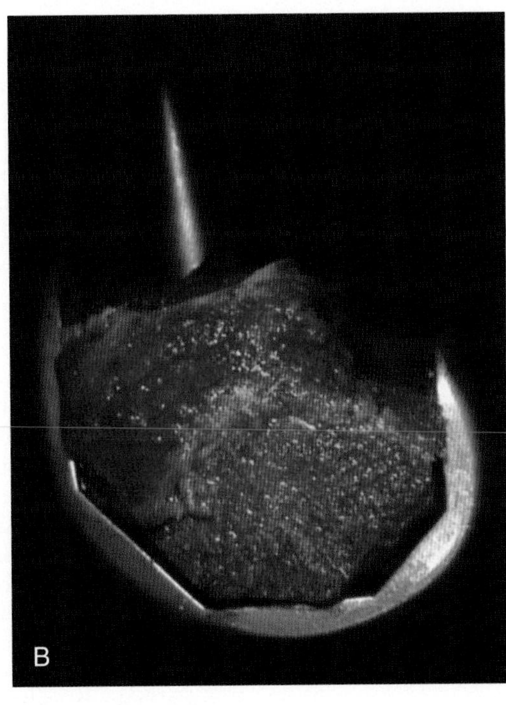

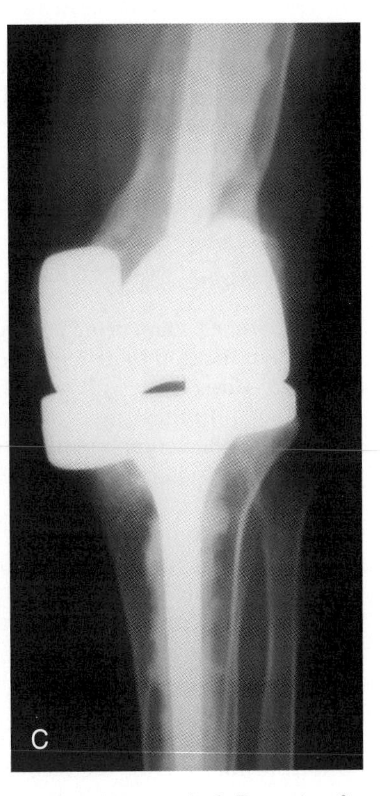

FIGURE 12–8. *A*, Failed TKA with marked loss of femoral bone stock. *B*, Use of a distal femoral allograft to restore bone stock. C, Ten years after the revision, alignment and fixation have been maintained.

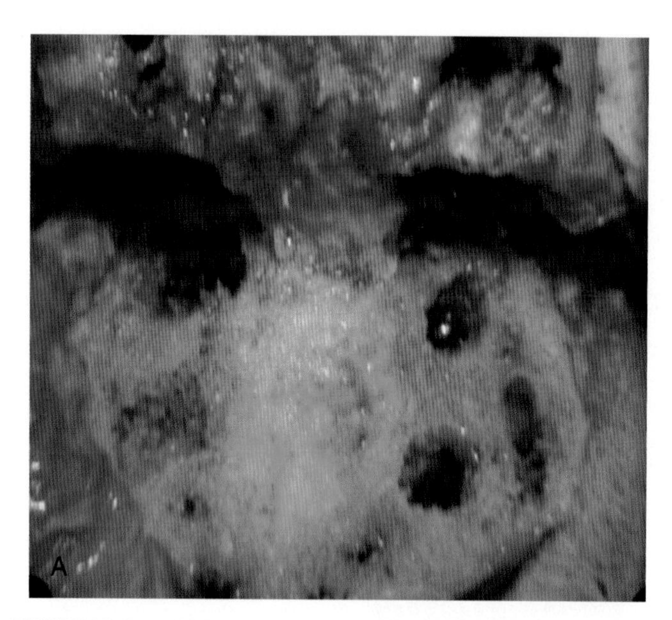

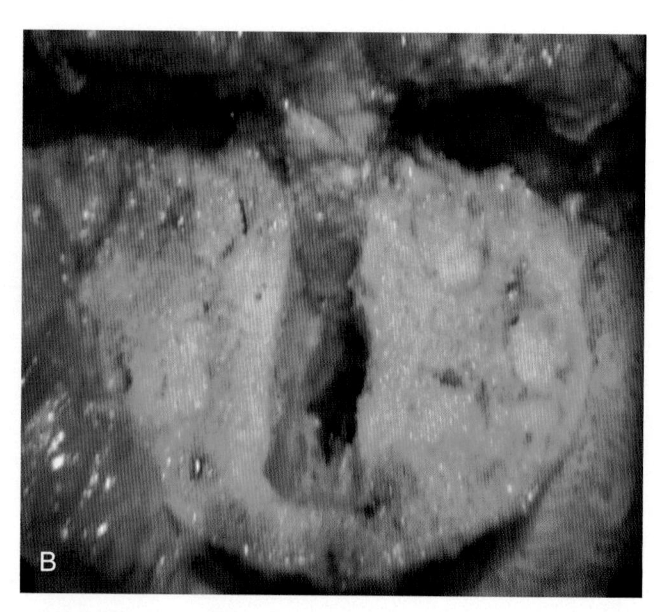

FIGURE 12–9. *A*, Multiple cysts on both the medial and lateral tibial plateaus. *B*, Autogenous grafting of the cysts utilizing bone from the standard tibial preparation.

cyst. Morselized bone is then packed around the stem into the cyst until it is fully filled.

The graft should be impacted firmly enough that when the trial stem is removed the graft has some structural integrity. A long-stemmed tibial component of the appropriate length is then utilized for the final prosthesis and passed through the grafted material. The stem can be either pressfit or cemented, depending on the quality of the tibial bone and the thickness of the diaphyseal cortex. In osteopenic cases, I prefer a cemented stem to avoid the need for one of large diameter that could lead to distal stem pain because of the mismatch in elastic modulus between a thick rigid stem and the osteopenic bone. If the stem is cemented, a smaller diameter is possible. In cemented cases, a cement restricter is placed distally before the graft is packed around the trial stem. A cement gun can be used to deliver the cement to the level of the restricter and then fill the canal in a retrograde fashion.

Cement Alone

There are times when cement alone will suffice in restoring component fixation to deficient bone. This is often true for a primary varus knee with a sloped deficient tibial plateau (Fig. 12–11). In these cases, Lotke was the first to describe shifting the tibial component laterally away from the defect to minimize its effect and to fill the residual gap with bone cement.[1]

It is helpful to be able to predict preoperatively the need for some form of augmentation. An easy way to accomplish this is to reconstruct the tibial joint line based on the normal lateral side, for example in a varus knee. A line is drawn at the level of the lateral joint line perpendicular to the long axis of the tibia and carried medially the entire width of the tibial plateau.

The distance from the bottom of the medial tibial defect upward to the level of the reconstructed joint line is then measured (see Fig. 5–10). If this distance is less than 10 mm, no augmentation is necessary. A 10-mm resection on the lateral side will decrease the deficiency to zero. If the distance is greater than 15 mm, augmentation of some form is appropriate. Between 10 and 15 mm, the surgeon has discretion whether to slightly increase the tibial resection and fill the remaining defect with cement.

Cement Plus Screw Augmentation

Cement plus screw augmentation can be considered. This method has been utilized with success for at least 30 years. Depending on the quality of tibial bone, either a cortical or a cancellous screw is inserted into the tibial plateau to be used as a template on which to support the tibial trial in proper varus/valgus alignment. During the cementing process, cement is packed around the screw and the tibial tray is supported in the proper position as the cement polymerizes. The use of a dissimilar metal for the screw and the tibial tray, again, is most likely acceptable because the junction is encased in cement (Fig. 12–12).

Bulk Allograft

In younger patients with uncontained peripheral tibial defects, the use of bulk autograft or allograft may be appropriate. The rationale is the restoration of bone stock in the younger patient for use in future revision. The disadvantage of this type of bone graft is the potential for nonunion or graft resorption with subsequent failure of the construct. Depending on the size of the defect, a large enough solid piece is occasionally provided by the distal or posterior femoral condylar resection or the tibial resection from the opposite plateau. Since the technique is being advocated for younger patients and I prefer to be conservative with my initial bone resections, I usually do not have enough autogenous graft for sizable defects. Instead, I use femoral or humeral head allografts, which have been successful in both primary and revision situations (Fig. 12–13). If there is sclerotic bone at the base of the defect, I would make

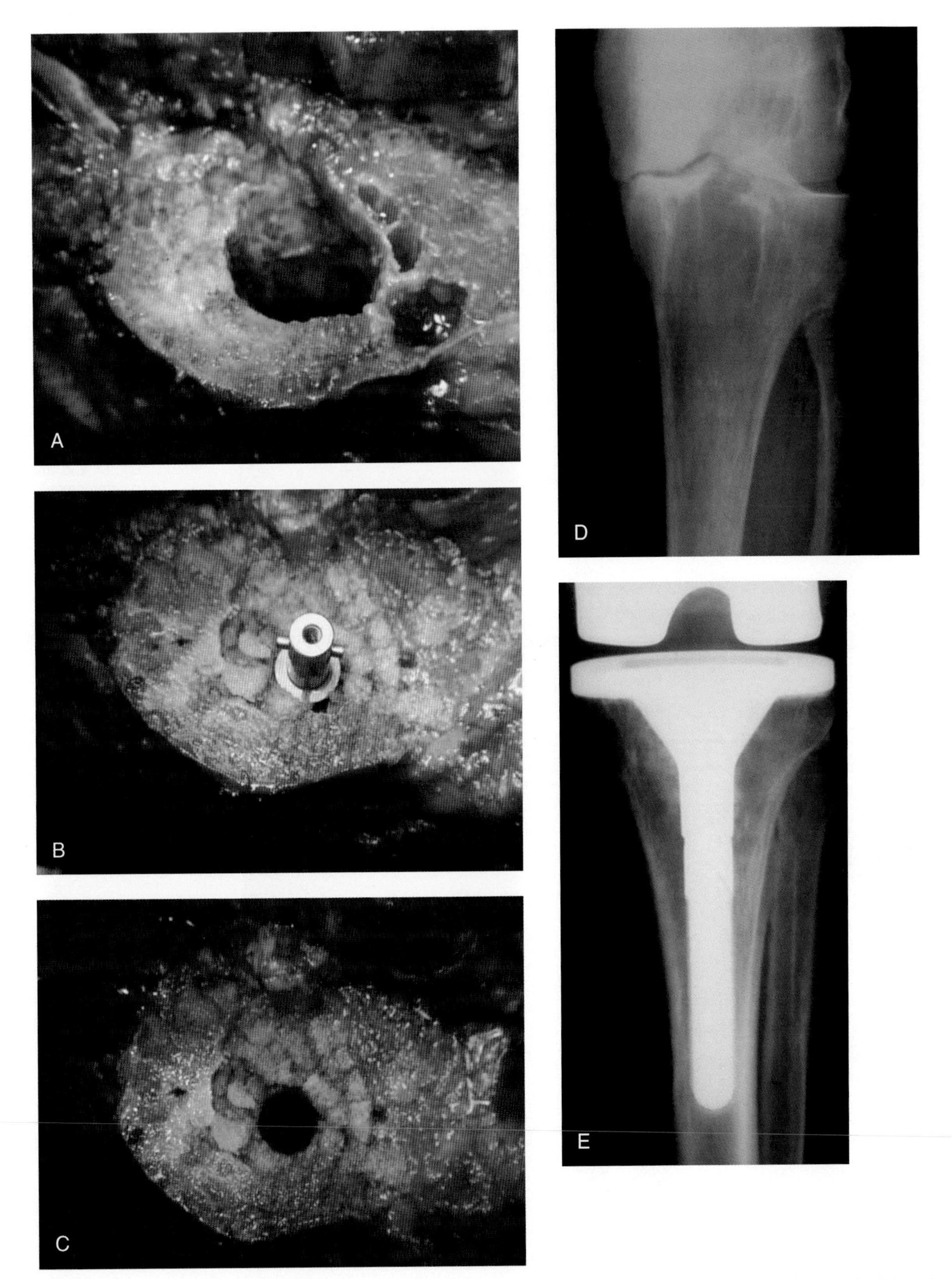

FIGURE 12–10. *A*, A rheumatoid patient with large central and multiple satellite cysts. *B*, Particulate bone graft has been packed densely around a press-fit trial tibial stem. *C*, After removal of the trial stem, the graft retains structural integrity. *D*, Preoperative radiograph showing the large central cyst. *E*, Five-year postoperative radiograph showing maintenance of the grafted material.

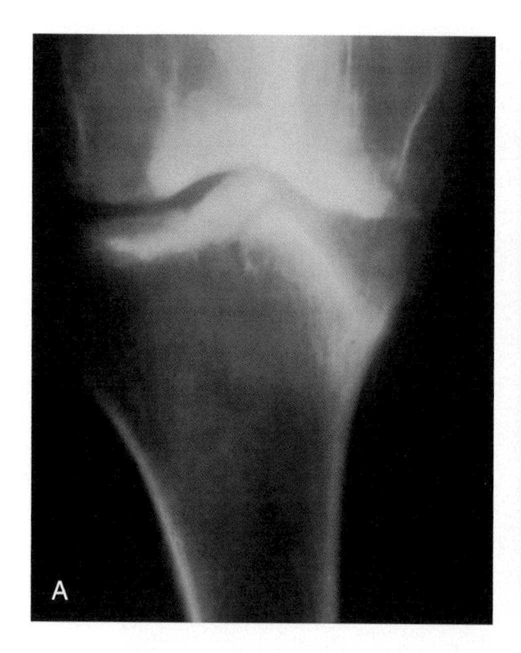

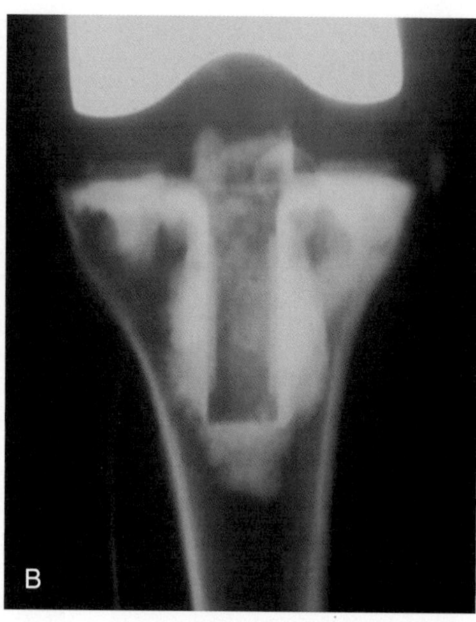

FIGURE 12–11. *A*, Varus knee with medial tibial plateau deficiency. *B*, The tibial component has been shifted laterally and the residual defect filled with cement.

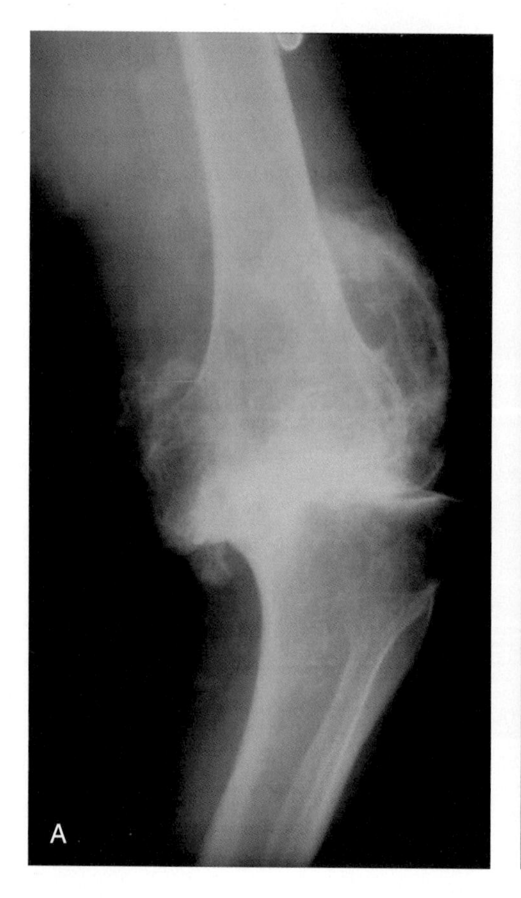

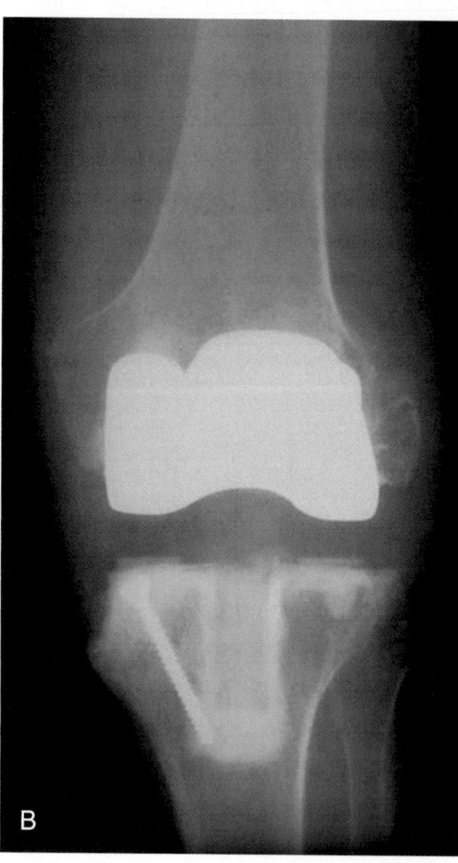

FIGURE 12–12. *A*, Preoperative radiograph of a knee with severe deformity and medial tibial deficiency. *B*, The tibial component has been shifted laterally, and a screw acts as a template to support the component in proper alignment and reinforce the cement.

multiple drill holes with a $\frac{1}{8}$-inch drill and interpose a small amount of morselized graft between the solid piece and the host. The graft is fixed to the host with at least two screws, either cortical or cancellous, depending on the density of the host bone. The screws are angled inward slightly to avoid penetrating the tibial cortex and pass into the host tibia for at least 2 cm beyond the graft host junction.

The decision must also be made whether to use a longer tibial stem to enhance component fixation and decrease the stresses across the graft. There are no established rules to guide this decision. If the graft is very secure and well supported, conventional stem length is probably sufficient. If there is any doubt about the construct, I would use an extended cemented stem of at least 3 cm of additional length.

Modular Augmentation Wedges

In the early 1980s, P. Brooks working with P. Walker and me did some laboratory studies on the amount of tibial tray deflection that might result with loading depending on whether bone deficiency was filled with cement, cement and screws, acrylic wedges, metal wedges, or custom components.[2] Brooks discovered that deflection was minimized by the use of modular wedges and custom integral components had no significant advantage over the wedges. From this work, Walker designed modular wedges to be cemented to the undersurface of metal-backed tibial trays in the Kinematic II knee system (Fig. 12–14). I implanted the first modular wedge in a severe varus knee with medial plateau deficiency in September 1984 (Fig. 12–15). Over the next 20 years, virtually all prosthetic systems offered modular wedge options in various shapes and sizes. Our initial results showed that cemented wedges functioned well.[3] Wedges can also be coupled to the tray with bolts. Angled tibial cutting jigs are available to assist in preparation of the bone. Another useful way to perform the resection is to assemble the chosen wedge onto the modular trial tray and insert the tray into the tibia until it reaches the level of the defect. The undersurface of the wedge can then be used as a template for the angle and level of the resection.

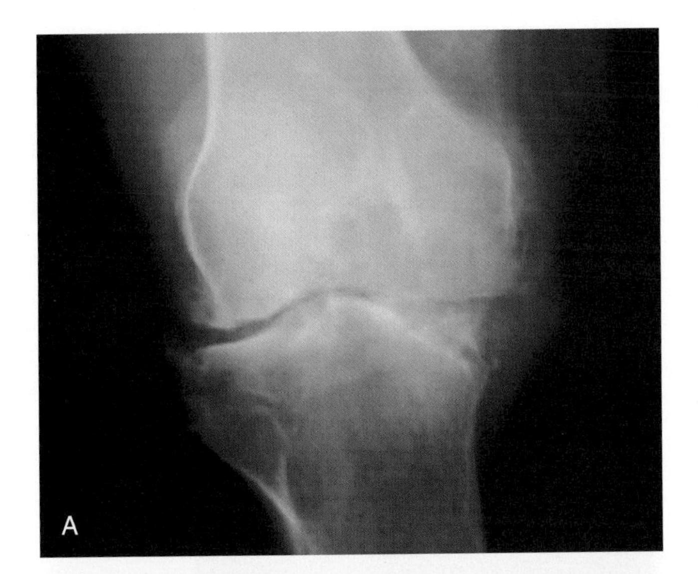

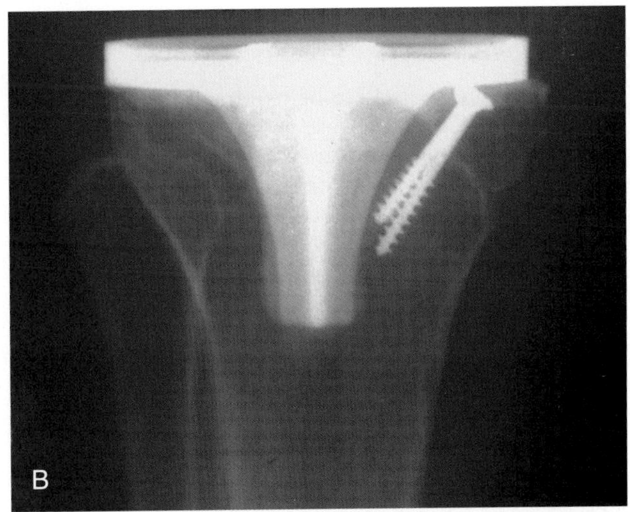

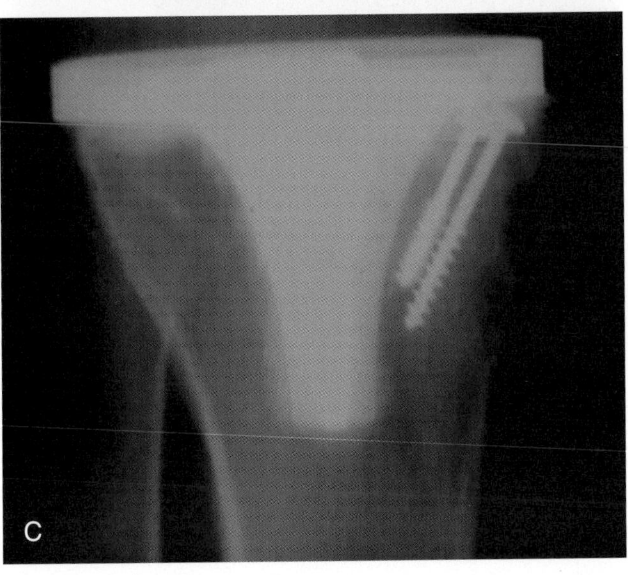

FIGURE 12–13. *A*, A 51-year-old patient with medial plateau deficiency. *B*, Restoration of bone stock using a femoral head allograft. *C*, Ten years after surgery, the graft has healed and there is no evidence of loosening.

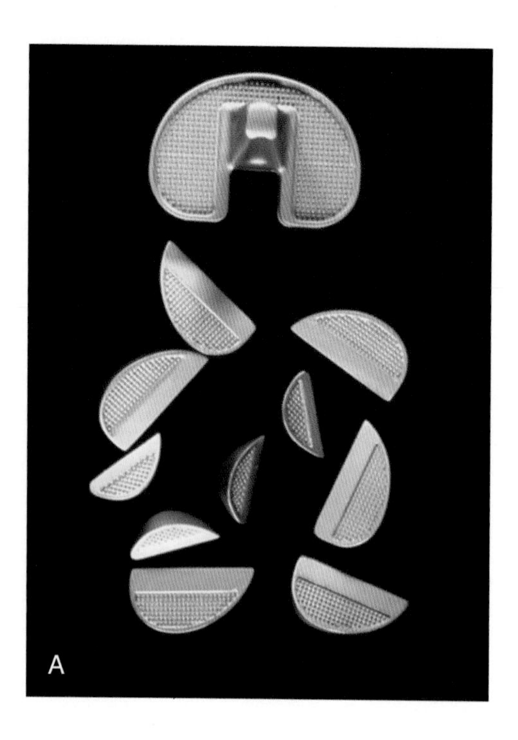

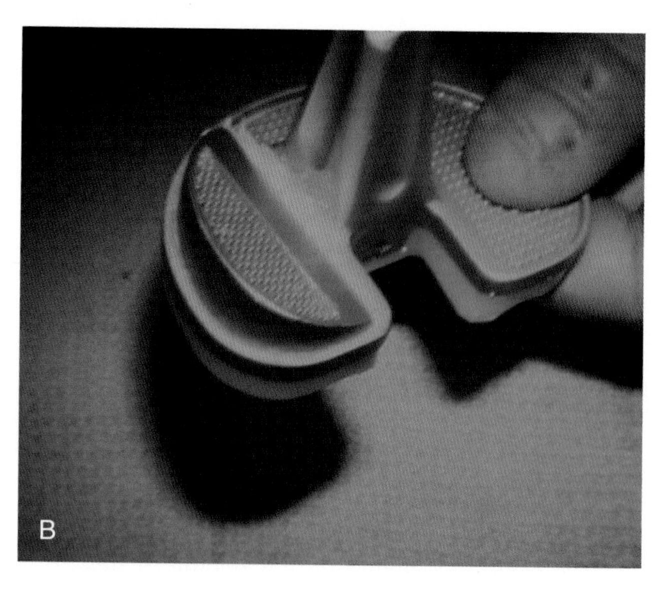

FIGURE 12–14. *A*, Modular wedges designed for the Kinematic II tibial component. *B*, The wedge is cemented to the undersurface of the tray.

Custom Components

Custom components used to be required for unusual tibial anatomy and defects. Their use is complicated by the great amount of time required for their fabrication. At the actual surgery, the defect may have changed with time or because of the extraction of prior components, possibly rendering the custom component obsolete for that case. Finally, the cost for a one-time usage is considerable.

The most frequent custom modification was the provision of an offset tibial stem, which was necessary following osteotomy or fracture (Fig. 12–16). Offset stems are now available in modular or solid forms in most total knee systems.

SUMMARY

Options are available for both femoral and tibial bone deficiency. They include bone grafting, cement alone, cement plus screw augmentation, augmented components, and custom components. On both the femoral and tibial sides of the joint, bone graft is recommended for all contained defects. Large central defects can be treated with an impaction grafting technique. Bulk grafts are appropriate for younger patients in an attempt to restore bone stock. Large femoral or tibial allografts are occasionally necessary in extreme cases.

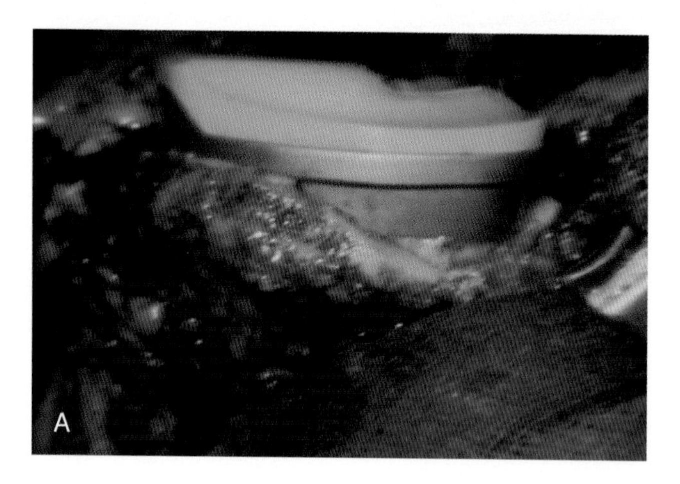

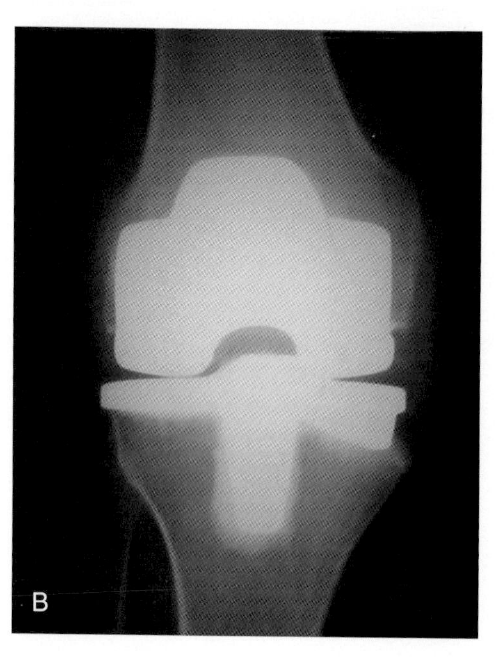

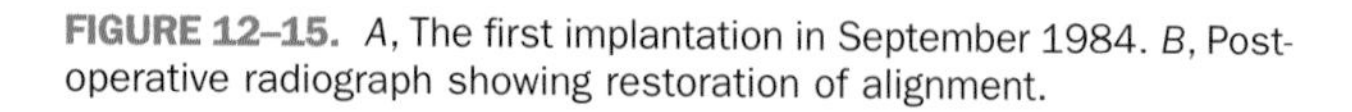

FIGURE 12–15. *A*, The first implantation in September 1984. *B*, Postoperative radiograph showing restoration of alignment.

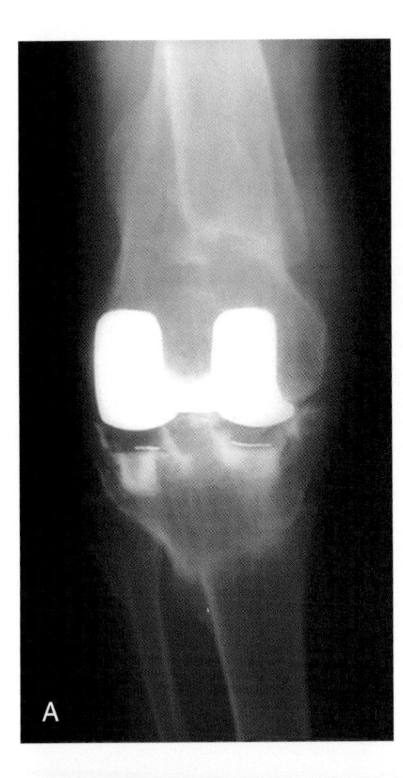

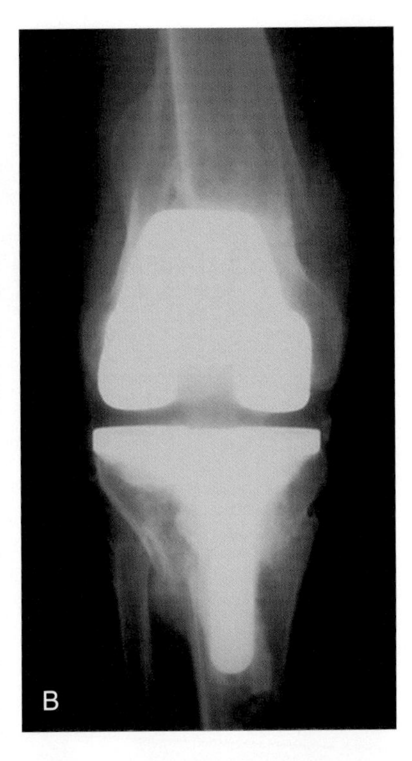

FIGURE 12–16. *A*, Failed TKA with an offset tibial shaft. *B*, A custom offset tibial stem was utilized.

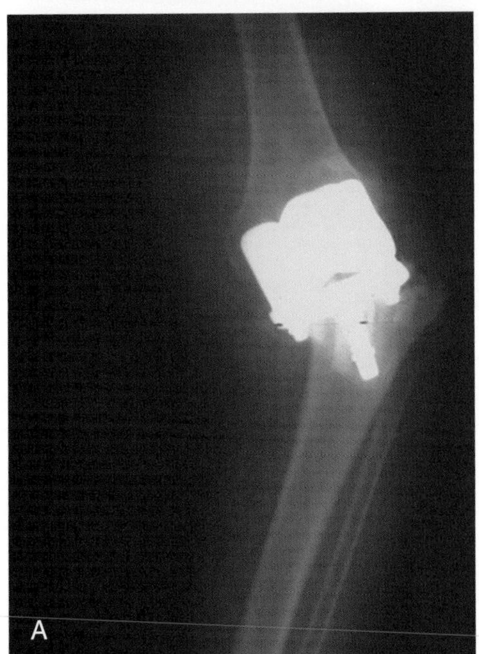

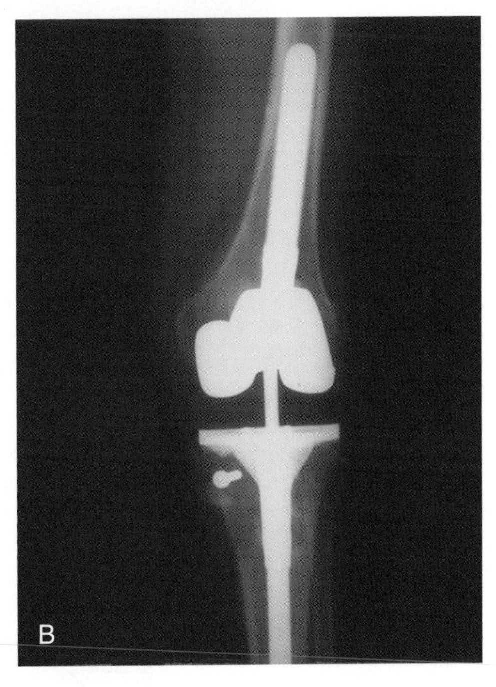

FIGURE 12–17. *A*, Failed TKA with marked loss of tibial bone stock. *B*, Restoration of alignment and stability with bulk graft, long stems, and constrained components.

Long stems and cement alone can sometimes suffice for restoration of component fixation in the presence of minor deficiencies. For some central and peripheral deficiencies, cement and screw augmentation is both inexpensive and effective. Modular wedges, stems, and inserts can address almost any problem due to bone deficiency, fixation, and stability. In a given patient, a combination of techniques may be necessary (Fig. 12–17). In this era of modularity, the need for custom components is extremely rare.

References

1. Lotke PA, Wong RY, Ecker ML: The use of methylmethacrylate in primary total knee replacements with large tibial defects. Clin Orthop 1991;270:288–294.
2. Brooks PJ, Walker PS, Scott RD: Tibial component fixation in deficient tibial bone stock. Clin Orthop 1984;183:302–308.
3. Brand MG, Daley RJ, Ewald FC, Scott RD: Tibial tray augmentation with modular metal wedges for tibial bone stock deficiency. Clin Orthop 1989;248:71–79.

CHAPTER 13

Bilateral Simultaneous Total Knee Arthroplasty

Because arthritis of the knee has a significant incidence of bilaterality, both patients and surgeons often consider the possibility of bilateral simultaneous total knee arthroplasty (TKA). I am a strong advocate of this procedure in properly selected patients, and the incidence of performing bilateral knee replacements in my practice is approximately 20% of my knee replacement patients.

THE DECISION

For me to consider bilateral simultaneous knee replacement, both knees must have significant structural damage. It is best if the patient can't decide which knee is more bothersome. In borderline cases, I ask the patient to pretend that the worse knee is normal. Then I ask if the patient would be seeing me for consideration of knee replacement on the other, less involved side. If the answer to this question is "yes," I consider the patient a potential candidate for bilateral knee replacement. If the answer is "no," I recommend operating only on the worse knee, and I expect that the operation on the second knee can be delayed for a considerable period of time.

Strong indications for bilateral simultaneous TKA are bilateral severe angular deformity (Fig. 13–1), bilateral severe flexion contracture, and anesthesia difficulties, i.e., patients who are anatomically or medically difficult to anesthetize, such as some adult or juvenile rheumatoid arthritis patients or patients with severe ankylosing spondylitis.

Relative indications for bilateral simultaneous TKA include the need for multiple additional surgical procedures to achieve satisfactory function and financial or social considerations for the patient.

Contraindications to bilateral TKA include medical infirmity (especially cardiac), a reluctant patient, and a patient with a very low pain threshold.

ANESTHETIC CONSIDERATIONS

In performing bilateral TKA, regional anesthesia is preferred. In most cases, it is in the form of epidural anesthesia with an indwelling catheter. The catheter is maintained in place for approximately 48 hours, at which time it is capped or removed, and oral narcotic medications are substituted.

ANTICOAGULATION

Anticoagulation for the prevention of deep vein thrombosis is initiated with a loading dose of warfarin on the night before surgery. The dose varies between 5 and 10 mg, depending on the size, age, and medical status of the patient. During the hospitalization, the international normalization

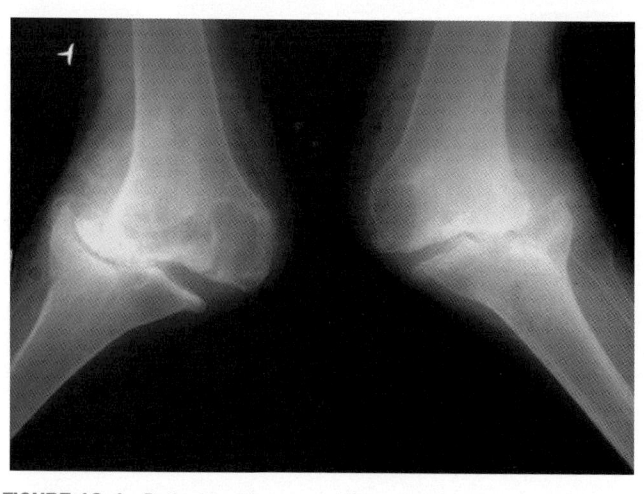

FIGURE 13–1. Patients with severe bilateral deformity are candidates for bilateral simultaneous TKA.

ratio (INR) is adjusted to between 1.8 and 2.2 by varying the warfarin dose. It generally takes 2 to 3 days for the INR to come into range, allowing the epidural catheter to be left in place for 48 hours and safely removed before the patient is too anticoagulated. Occasionally, this goal is not met, and the catheter must be kept in place (capped) until the INR drifts down into a safe range. The safe range varies somewhat among anesthesiologists.

Alternative anesthesia and postoperative analgesia might consist of a general or spinal anesthetic followed by bilateral femoral nerve blocks or intravenous patient-controlled analgesia (PCA). Postoperative pain control methods, including the preemptive use of anti-inflammatory agents and sustained-release narcotics, continue to evolve.

After the INR has been appropriately adjusted and the patient has been discharged, warfarin use continues for 4 to 6 weeks. At home or outpatient blood drawing for INR usually takes place twice a week. After the warfarin is discontinued, the patient is switched to 81 mg of aspirin daily for a minimum of 6 weeks.

Other ancillary measures that might minimize the possibility of deep vein thrombosis include use of an epidural for anesthesia, pulsatile compression stockings applied immediately postoperatively, and a continuous passive motion (CPM) machine applied immediately following surgery and alternating every 4 to 6 hours from limb to limb. Finally, early patient mobilization with standing and short-distance ambulation (even with the epidural catheter in place) is encouraged.

WEIGHTBEARING STATUS

Weightbearing status is the same for patients with bilateral simultaneous TKA whether the femoral component is cemented or cementless. Ambulation is initiated with the use of a walker. Most patients then progress to the use of two crutches and a four-point gait when ambulating more than 30 feet. I also allow full weightbearing as tolerated for short distances around the house using one crutch.

At 4 weeks, patients progress to the use of one crutch or cane outdoors for 4 more weeks with no support needed indoors and around their home. I also permit them to drive a car, if they feel ready, at 4 weeks after surgery. Full recovery generally takes 3 to 6 months, depending on the individual.

SURGICAL TECHNIQUE

Over the last several hundred bilateral simultaneous TKA procedures I have performed, I have developed a routine protocol for the surgery. Both limbs are prepared and draped at the same time. An initial dose of an intravenous antibiotic (usually 1 g of a cephalosporin) is given at least 10 minutes before inflation of the tourniquet. Surgery begins on the more symptomatic side or on the right side if neither knee is significantly worse than the other. The reason for starting on the more symptomatic side is in case one surgery has to be discontinued after only one procedure owing to anesthetic considerations.

After the components have been implanted on the first side, the tourniquet is deflated and a second dose of intravenous antibiotic is administered (usually 500 mg of a cephalosporin). After the joint capsule is closed and flexion against gravity is measured, one team completes the subcutaneous and skin closure on the first side while the other team inflates the second tourniquet and begins the exposure of the second side. When the second tourniquet is deflated, a third dose of antibiotic is given (usually 500 mg of a cephalosporin for a total dose of 2 g for both knees).

I have some concern about the potential for cross-contamination of the knee wounds that could occur when instruments used during the final stages of skin closure on the first knee are maintained on the field and used on the second knee. For this reason, I sequester the skin closure instruments from the first side and hand them off the table after they are used. Surgical gloves are changed when a team member from the first side moves to the second side.

LENGTH OF THE INCISIONS

Patients will notice if the skin incisions on their knees differ in length. For this reason, I try to measure them and keep them the same length. If, however, the patient points out such a difference to me at the bedside, I am prepared with an immediate response. I inform the patient that we had to do a little more work on the longer side.

PREEMPTIVE ADVICE TO PATIENTS

Since patients undergoing bilateral simultaneous TKA rarely comment that their knees are identical during the immediate postoperative period, I remind them that one knee will usually feel better than the other and progress faster. I tell them to think of this knee as their "better" knee rather than to call the other knee their "worse" knee.

PATIENT SATISFACTION

In my practice, 99% of patients report to me after their complete recovery that they are glad they did both knees at the same time. Almost all volunteer to be patient advocates for this technique and to speak with preoperative patients considering bilateral TKA. I maintain a list of such patients to give to preoperative candidates wishing to speak with someone who has been through the experience.

A patient who has any uncertainty about proceeding with bilateral surgery should have only one knee done at a time. In this situation, I space the knees at least 3 months apart and encourage the patient to delay the second side even further. In many cases, the second side receives a "reprieve," becoming more tolerable after the first side has been operated on.

BILATERAL REVISION

I do not recommend undertaking bilateral revision knee arthroplasty unless one side involves a relatively minor procedure such as an insert exchange.

Revision arthroplasties often involve intramedullary instrumentation and reaming on both the femoral and tibial sides of the joint. The use of an intramedullary tibial align-

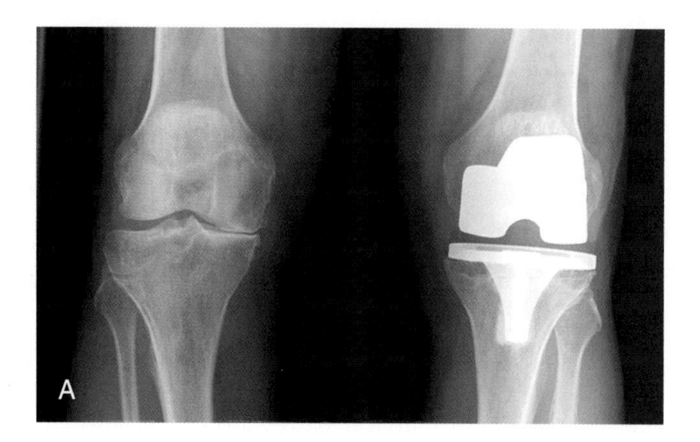

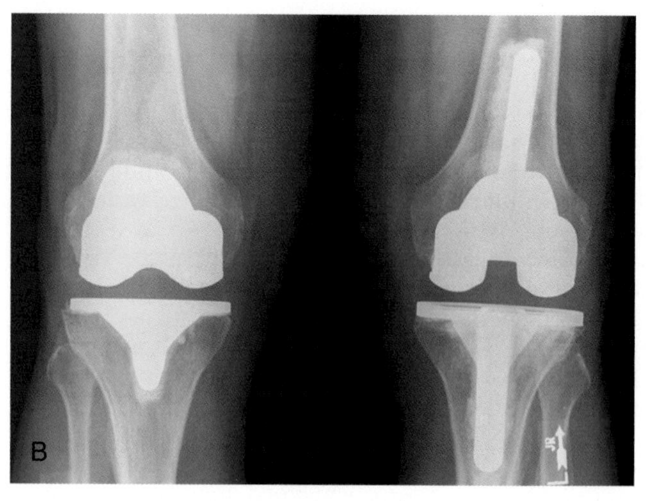

FIGURE 13–2. *A*, A patient requiring both primary and revision arthroplasty. *B*, The primary side was operated on first, and autogenous bone resections were used on the revision side.

ment device should be avoided even in simple primary bilateral knee arthroplasty to minimize the potential for fat embolization if instrumentation involves four bones during the same period of anesthesia.

BILATERAL PRIMARY/REVISION SURGERY

I am not opposed to performing bilateral TKA that involves a primary on one side and a revision on the other. This situation is especially attractive if the primary arthroplasty is straightforward and the bone resections obtained from the primary side can be utilized as autogenous bone graft for defects on the revision side (Fig. 13–2). Alternatively, if the hospital has the facilities to store bone graft under appropriate conditions and temperature, the procedures could be staged and the graft from the first side saved for use at the time of revision on the second side.

SUMMARY

I am an advocate of bilateral simultaneous primary TKA. Approximately 20% of my patients undergo this procedure. In reviewing more than 500 such cases, I saw a low level of patient morbidity coupled with a high level of patient satisfaction as long as proper patient selection and surgical techniques were utilized.

CHAPTER 14

Sepsis and Total Knee Arthroplasty

Sepsis following total knee arthroplasty (TKA) is a disastrous complication. I have been most fortunate in my career that so far, after more than 4000 primary TKAs, none of my patients has experienced an early deep infection. I have seen late "metastatic" infection to primary TKAs at a rate that is 0.5% at average 10-year follow-up after 3000 consecutive primary TKAs. What follows has been gleaned from my experience treating my own patients with late infection, as well as other patients with septic knees who have been referred to me.

PERIOPERATIVE PROPHYLACTIC MEASURES

It is preferable to prevent an infection rather than to have to treat one. Prophylactic measures can be taken before, during, and after surgery to minimize the chance for infection.

All patients should be screened preoperatively for potential sites of active infection that could spread to the knee. The most common are oropharyngeal and urologic. Any patient with a chronic infection such as sinusitis or pharyngitis should be cleared by an otolaryngologist prior to their surgery. Similarly, patients with chronic dental infection in need of reconstructive procedures should have these performed prior to the arthroplasty.

It is not unusual to encounter a female patient with a history of recurrent urinary tract infection. A urinalysis and urine culture should be obtained preoperatively on all patients.

Any active urinary tract infection should be treated, and chronic problems should be cleared by a urologist. If a preoperative urine culture is positive but there are few white cells in the sediment and the patient is totally asymptomatic, the surgery need not be canceled. A repeat "clean-catch" or catheterized specimen can be helpful to clarify whether antibiotic treatment of the infection is necessary. In the presence of a positive culture of greater than 100,000 colonies and benign sediment in an asymptomatic patient, I will often start oral antibiotics preoperatively and obtain the catheterized specimen in the operating room prior to the arthroplasty.

PREOPERATIVE GERMICIDAL SKIN SCRUB

All my patients are instructed to use a chlorhexidine germicidal skin scrub (e.g., Hibiclens) twice a day for 2 days prior to their surgery. In theory, this should decrease the colonization of bacteria on the patient's skin and decrease the chance for contamination.

SURGICAL PREPARATION AND DRAPING

It has been my practice to prepare the entire extremity including the foot for TKA. The foot is draped out of the surgical field, of course, but I am more comfortable with this area being surgically prepared in the event of any breakdown in the drapes that cover the foot. I use a surgical stockinette over the prepared foot up to the level of the tourniquet. The stockinette has a double layer. The outer layer is cut, and the incision is defined with a marking pen. The inner stockinette is then cut and reflected medially and laterally for a few centimeters. The skin incision is drawn out, and then the entire field is sealed, including the foot, with a povidone-iodine–impregnated adhesive drape. Care is taken to not actually touch the skin during this draping procedure, and fresh outer gloves are applied after it is completed (see Chapter 4).

LAMINAR AIR FLOW VERSUS ULTRAVIOLET LIGHTS

I am often asked by ex-fellows or residents whether laminar air flow or ultraviolet (UV) light is better. I operate at two different hospitals; ultraviolet lights are used at one and vertical laminar air flow is used at the other. The incidence of infection in my patients is zero at both institutions. Each method has its advantages and has been shown to be an effective deterrent to infection. The UV light method is less expensive and requires all operating room personnel to cover up to shield their eyes and skin, which may decrease the potential for the shedding of bacteria by personnel. The fact that UV lights are potentially "sterilizing" the field during the procedure is reassuring when I am performing sequential bilateral TKAs. When I am using laminar air flow for bilateral arthroplasty, I sequester the instruments that are used on the first knee during the skin closure and pass them off the operating field after they have been used. A change of outer gloves is also performed between the procedures (see Chapter 13).

INTRAVENOUS ANTIBIOTICS

Intravenous antibiotics have long been shown to decrease the incidence of perioperative orthopedic wound infection. I commonly use a second-generation cephalosporin, giving 1 g intravenously at least 10 minutes prior to inflation of the tourniquet. A second gram is administered at the time the tourniquet is deflated in order to maximize the concentration of antibiotic in the evolving wound hematoma. The antibiotics are continued every 8 hours for three additional doses. When patients are "allergic" to penicillin, I still administer the cephalosporin, unless the allergy has been one of anaphylaxis. A test dose is given with caution and under surveillance by the anesthesiologist. If it is well tolerated, the standard protocol is utilized. Although there is said to be a cross-over in sensitivity between penicillin and cephalosporins of as much as 15% in terms of allergy, in hundreds of cases over the past 20 years using this protocol, I have not yet seen this cross-over. This test dose, therefore, allows a "penicillin-sensitive" patient to receive a cephalosporin in the future, should that be appropriate.

PROPER SKIN INCISION

Prior skin incisions about the knee must be respected. The knee does not tolerate multiple parallel incisions, especially a medial incision made parallel to an old lateral incision (see Chapter 15). If skin breakdown were to occur, infection would be likely. My standard incision is approximately 15 cm long. It begins 5 cm above the patella centered over the shaft of the femur, crosses the medial one third of the patella, and ends 10 cm distally at the medial aspect of the tibial tubercle. In general, when prior incisions are present, it is best to use the most lateral incision that allows arthroplasty or the most recent incision that healed without difficulty (see Chapter 15). Medially based flaps are safer than laterally based flaps. In questionable cases, the skin incision can be made with the tourniquet deflated. If the wound edges appear poorly vascularized, the surgery can be aborted and plastic surgical consultation obtained. I have used tissue expanders successfully on one occasion when a patient with a 20-degree valgus deformity had adherent lateral skin that followed a posttraumatic split thickness skin graft.

WOUND CARE

Following the skin incision and arthrotomy, I always sew in wound towels along the capsule that protect the subcutaneous tissue from debris and from drying out under the operating room lights. The towels are irrigated with an antibiotic solution of bacitracin and a combination preparation of neomycin sulfate, polymyxin B sulfate, and bacitracin zinc or gramicidin. When these towels are removed at the end of the procedure, it is always impressive to see how healthy the tissues appear compared with the brown, dried-out appearance of the subcutaneous tissues when wound towels have not been used (Fig. 14–1).

Infection is often a result of wound necrosis secondary to compromise of blood supply to the skin and subcutaneous tissue. For this reason, in a lateral retinacular release, it is beneficial, if possible, to preserve the lateral superior genicular artery (Fig. 14–2). Infection can also be the result of breakdown of the wound due to a large hematoma. To minimize this possibility, I deflate the tourniquet prior to closure of the wound to check for significant bleeding points.

During rehabilitation, if the capsular closure loses its integrity, a wound problem can also occur. For this reason, I prefer an interrupted capsular closure with a strong monofilament suture. My preference is No. 1 polydioxanone (PDS).

The use of suction drains following TKA is controversial. The studies that support the contention that they are unnecessary involve only several hundred cases. In my opinion, a review of a thousand consecutive cases without the use of a drain would reveal at least one significant complication such as wound breakdown, necrosis, secondary infection, or even compartment syndrome that cost the patient and society more than the price of a thousand standard suction drains. These drains do their most important work during the first several hours after surgery. I always discontinue their use on the morning after surgery. If for some reason the output is excessive, I flex the knee for 30 minutes and clamp the drains. If excessive output continues, I would consider removing the drains. The wound is then observed carefully over the next 24 hours, and if necessary, the patient can be brought back to the operating room to control any bleeding. In my experience of more than 4000 consecutive knee surgeries, this has never been necessary.

The skin closure is one of the most important parts of TKA. It must be meticulously performed with the skin edges accurately opposed. I prefer the modified Donati suture (Fig. 14–3). This is a vertical mattress suture that is subcuticular on the lateral side (the side more prone to skin necrosis). Interrupted closure is preferred over a running subcuticular stitch because the length of a knee incision increases as much as 40% from extension to flexion. This movement puts a repetitive strain on the subcuticular suture. A continuous suture also prevents the removal of a few localized stitches to deal with a superficial wound separation or infection.

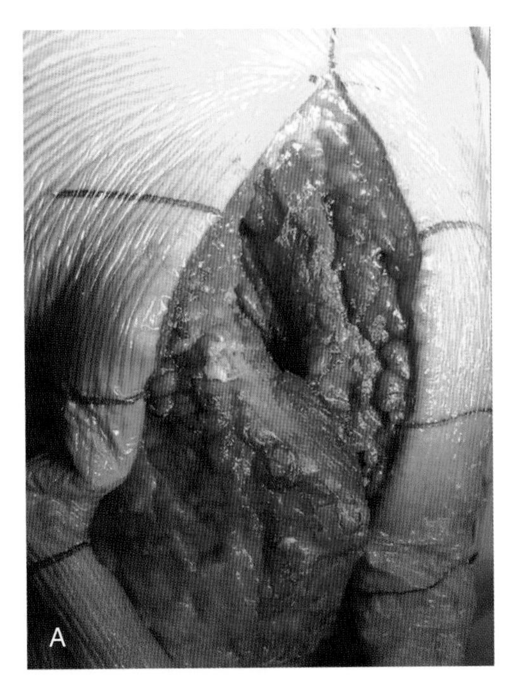

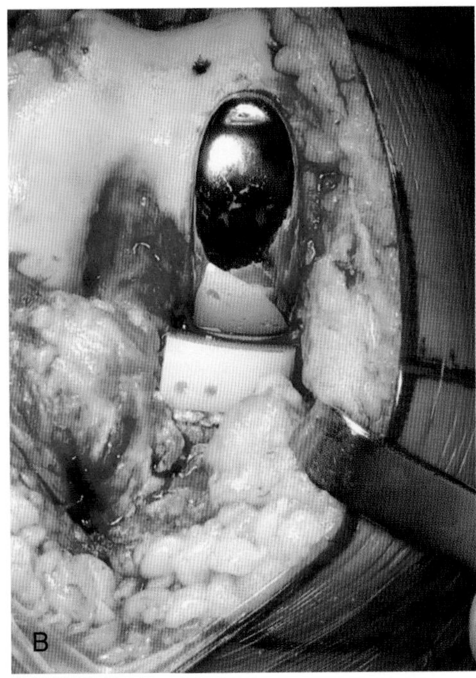

FIGURE 14–1. *A*, If unprotected by moist wound towels, the subcutaneous tissues dry out during surgery. *B*, Moist wound towels keep the tissue healthier and more resistant to infection.

Any perioperative wound problems should be dealt with aggressively to prevent the chance for secondary infection (see Chapter 15). If wound drainage persists after 48 hours, my preference is to perform a sterile preparation on the area and apply benzoin and Steri-Strips to reseal the wound. If the problem fails to resolve, I take the patient back to the operating room for treatment. The knee joint is separately aspirated for cell count and culture. Antibiotics (hopefully prophylactic rather than therapeutic) are initiated after the culture has been obtained. The few sutures in the local area are removed, the wound is irrigated, and minor débridement is performed. The wound is then reclosed with interrupted vertical mattress sutures. Prophylactic antibiotics are continued for several days until the wound appears totally sealed and benign. If the joint aspiration is positive with a high cell count or positive culture, major débridement and lavage of the knee joint will be necessary.

FIGURE 14–2. The lateral superior genicular vessels (arrow) should be preserved whenever possible for their blood supply to the patella and overlying skin flap.

SKIN NECROSIS

If skin necrosis occurs, the goal is to keep the problem superficial. To allow the capsular closure to seal, all flexion exercises are stopped and the knee is protected in a knee immobilizer. The size of the necrosis is assessed, along with the extent of any drainage. At least five treatment options exist. The most common is to allow the skin beneath the eschar representing the necrosis to granulate in. This is appropriate if the wound remains dry and the necrotic area is only millimeters in width. If the patient has pliable skin, the second option is to excise the area of necrosis and perform a primary closure. A third option is to excise the area and perform a split-thickness skin graft. This usually would be a late procedure, taking place after the deep tissues are well healed. If the necrotic area is very large and the wound breaks down with capsular dehiscence, a gastrocnemius flap is necessary. A fifth option is considered in a rare situation. If the patient has undergone an extensive lateral release associated with a medial arthrotomy, the patella itself may be avascular. A technetium bone scan showing no activity whatsoever in the patella is confirmatory. In such a case, a patellectomy can be considered as a way to gain enough skin and capsular tissue for a primary closure.

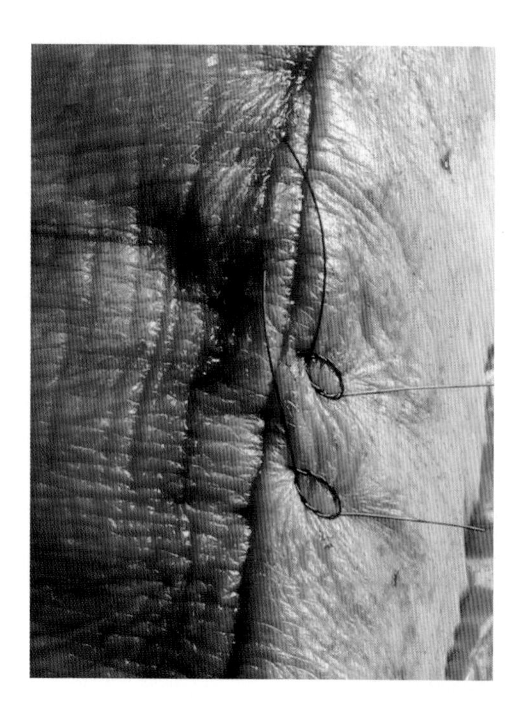

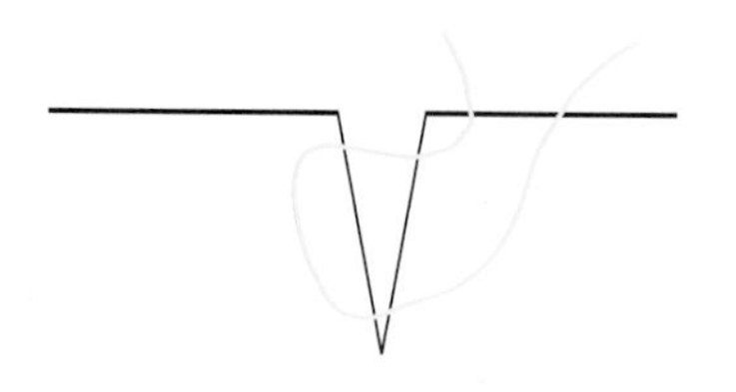

FIGURE 14–3. A modified Donati interrupted suture protects the lateral skin flap from necrosis.

POSTOPERATIVE PROPHYLACTIC MEASURES

Late metastatic infection to the knee may be prevented if patients, physicians, and dentists are well educated as to its potential. Patients are informed of this possibility as part of their preoperative education and are given a letter prior to discharge that documents the need for prophylactic antibiotics surrounding dental procedures and other medical procedures such as cystoscopy and colonoscopy. The American Heart Association Guidelines are utilized. For dental procedures, amoxicillin 2 g is given 1 hour prior to the procedure. For other surgical procedures, the physician involved chooses the appropriate antibiotic. Whether premedication for routine dental procedures should continue after 2 years is controversial. If there are no intolerance or allergy issues, I recommend premedication indefinitely.

CLASSIFICATION OF INFECTIONS

Infections following TKA can be classified in at least three ways. The first is early versus late infections. The second is splitting infections into those resulting from operative seeding versus late hematogenous infection. The third is acute versus chronic infections.

The classification of an infection as early versus late is helpful in determining whether the surgeon's personal infection rate is satisfactory, and if not, where the source of higher infection originates. I would characterize an early infection as occurring within the first 3 months of surgery. A late infection would first manifest itself at least a year following the surgery. Obviously, there is an overlap between early and late. Some "late" infections could be smoldering low-grade infections that actually started early, with a history of persistent pain and swelling following the operation. Early infection rates should be less than 1%, and high-volume centers report rates roughly between 0.3% and 0.5%. As of this writing, after more than 4000 consecutive primary TKAs, I have not had a patient experience an early deep infection. This is due to significant good fortune but also to the prophylactic measures discussed above.

The second classification method describes whether the infection is due to operative seeding or late metastatic infection from a remote source. If it comes from operative seeding, the surgeon must pursue the source to minimize the recurrence of this complication. If the infection comes from late metastatic seeding from a remote source, this source must be located so that the problem does not recur after resolution of the knee infection itself. It may also signal a deficit in patient education or education of the patient's treating physicians about the possibility of metastatic infection and need for prophylactic measures for certain procedures such as dental work or cystoscopy.

Whether the infection is acute or chronic is the most important classification in terms of the type of treatment to be instituted. Other factors that determine treatment are the status of the wound (is it sealed or draining?), the bone-cement interface (is it pristine or demarcated?), the organism (is it sensitive to multiple antibiotics or resistant to most?), and the medical status of the patient (is the patient able to withstand major surgery or surgeries?).

Workup of the septic TKA involves the search for another site of infection when the infection is late from a remote source. It also includes assessment of the sedimentation rate and C-reactive protein. The knee should be aspirated for cell count and differential along with aerobic and anaerobic culture and fungal cultures (if suspected). The cell count and differential are extremely important. If the bacteria are difficult to incubate in the laboratory, a high cell count with a negative culture can still be diagnostic for infection. For example, if the cell count is 80,000 with 98% nucleated cells, infection is certain, even in the face of a

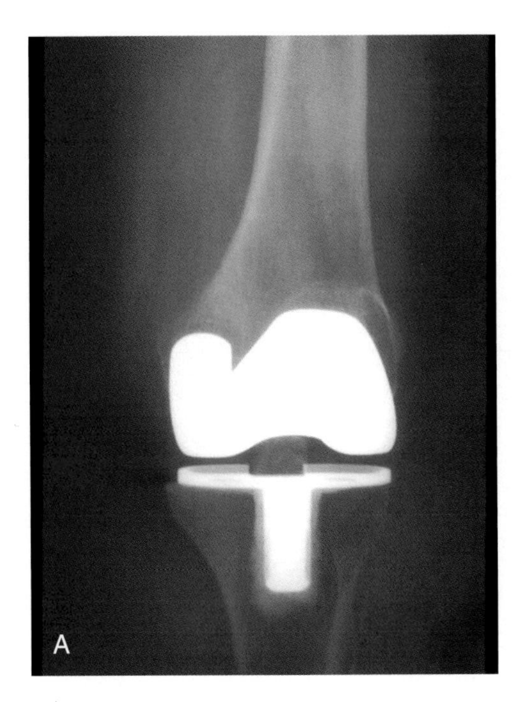

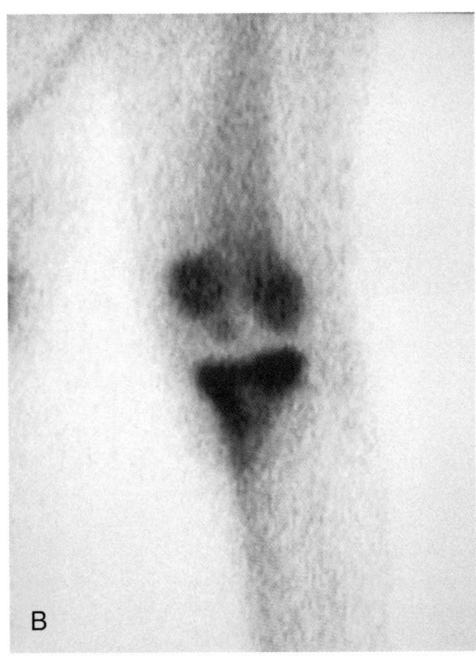

FIGURE 14–4. *A*, A plain radiograph in a patient with metastatic infection shows no sign of loosening. *B*, A bone scan in the same patient shows focal increased uptake and contraindicates retention of the components.

negative culture. On the other hand, a positive culture that could be a contaminant can be ruled nonpathogenic if the cell count is less than 100 cells per high-power field with few nucleated cells. These results are, of course, correlated with the clinical picture along with the sedimentation rate and C-reactive protein level. If routine tests fail to define the diagnosis, a percutaneous synovial biopsy specimen for histologic study as well as culture can be helpful.

Plain radiographs are useful to assess the presence or absence of bone-cement demarcation. A demarcated interface always requires removal of the prosthetic components. A pristine interface means that the knee can possibly be treated by retention of components, depending on other factors discussed below. A technetium bone scan may be of use (Fig. 14–4). If retention of the components is being considered and a bone scan shows a focal area of markedly increased uptake in a knee well over a year after surgery, bone involvement is likely and components probably should be removed.

TREATMENT OPTIONS

At least seven treatment options exist for septic TKA. All involve the use of 4 to 6 weeks of intravenous antibiotics. The first is closed treatment with repeated aspiration or arthroscopic lavage. The second consists of open débridement with synovectomy, retention of components, and exchange of a modular insert (if present). The third includes débridement, synovectomy, and immediate prosthetic exchange. The fourth involves débridement, synovectomy, and delayed prosthetic exchange. The fifth is débridement, synovectomy, and permanent resection arthroplasty. The sixth consists of débridement, synovectomy, and fusion of the knee. The seventh option requires amputation of the limb as a lifesaving procedure for overwhelming sepsis.

Closed Treatment

It is unusual for closed treatment to be indicated, but it is appropriate in certain circumstances. These might be in the presence of an infection with an acute presentation (24 to 48 hours), an intact wound, a sensitive organism, an intact bone-cement interface, and a poor operative risk due to concomitant medical conditions. If the patient can withstand arthroscopic lavage under local anesthesia, this may be an appropriate adjunct.

Open Synovectomy, Débridement, and Insert Exchange

Indications are similar to those for closed treatment, except that anesthesia is a reasonable risk for the patient. The infection can also be chronic, as long as the wound is intact, the organism is sensitive to standard antibiotic therapy, the bone-cement interface is pristine, and bone scans are negative for focal areas of increased uptake.

Primary Prosthetic Exchange

Primary prosthetic exchange might be indicated in the presence of an acute or chronic infection with an intact wound and a demarcated bone-cement interface. I prefer the organism to be highly sensitive, such as a streptococcus highly sensitive to penicillin. I have had success in four such cases. An additional indication would be a patient who is a poor operative risk for multiple surgical procedures.

Delayed Prosthetic Exchange

The most common and appropriate treatment for TKA infection is delayed prosthetic exchange. The infection can be acute or chronic with an intact or draining wound and a demarcated bone-cement interface (or a positive bone scan). With luck the organism will be sensitive to standard antibiotic therapy.

Delayed Exchange Protocol

Protocols for delayed exchange will evolve with time. What follows is the basic protocol that I have used for the past 20 years with good success.

The joint suspected of being infected is aspirated for cell count with differential and aerobic and anaerobic culture. As mentioned above, the cell count gives extremely important information. Serial cell counts can also help follow the progress of the treatment.

After the cell count and culture have been obtained, the patient is started on an intravenous antibiotic chosen by the infectious disease consultant as broad spectrum or the most likely choice of antibiotic if, for example, the infection is thought to be metastatic from a urinary tract infection. If the patient is not systemically ill, it is reasonable to delay the arthrotomy and débridement for 24 to 48 hours to allow initial treatment of the periarticular tissues and help the surgeon determine healthy versus unhealthy tissue at the time of débridement. It is also helpful to wait for 48 hours to obtain final culture reports and sensitivities so that if an inappropriate antibiotic was chosen initially, it can be changed to the one with greatest efficacy.

At surgery, a standard medial parapatellar arthrotomy is performed with a proximal quadriceps snip or release if necessary to facilitate patellar eversion. Thorough débridement and synovectomy are performed along with component removal. If possible, any retained bone cement should be removed. The joint is thoroughly cleansed with pulsatile lavage using at least 2 L of fluid. An antibiotic-laden cement spacer is then fabricated to fill dead space, keep the femur and tibia distracted, and make reimplantation surgery less difficult. Depending on the size of the gap between the femur and the tibia, two to four bags of cement are mixed. The most common antibiotic added is tobramycin using 600 mg per bag of cement. The cement spacer is applied with the tourniquet deflated. This purposely interferes with bone-cement interface fixation so that the spacer is more easily removed at the time of reimplantation. A pseudo-stem is fabricated on the undersurface of the spacer to go into the tibial metaphysis so that the spacer will not tend to migrate beyond the periphery of the bone and possibly impinge on soft tissues. It is most important to prevent the spacer from extruding anteriorly and injuring the quadriceps mechanism. After the bolus of cement is applied to the gap between the femur and the tibia with the stem into the tibial canal, the knee is distracted and held in approximately 5 degrees of valgus and 10 to 15 degrees of flexion. During this time, the assistant shapes the spacer to stay within the confines of the bony anatomy and to remove any excessive cement. At this time as well, a pseudo-trochlea is formed at the front of the spacer to articulate with the ventral surface of the patella and allow the patella to remain mobile (Fig. 14–5).

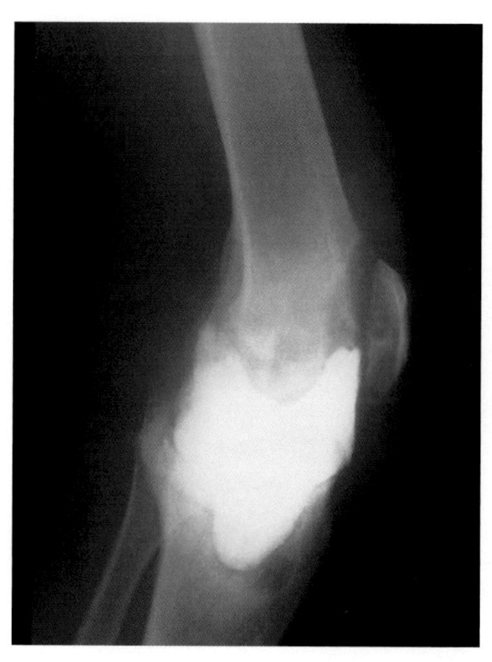

FIGURE 14–5. An antibiotic-laden cement spacer with a pseudo-trochlea and tibial system.

After polymerization of the cement, two outflow drains are inserted and brought out through separate stab wounds laterally. The knee is closed in two layers. Monofilament suture is used in both. I prefer No. 1 PDS for the capsule and deep vertical mattress sutures of 3-0 nylon for the skin and subcutaneous tissue. To assure accurate coaptation of the skin edges, some simple sutures can be placed between the mattress sutures. The closure is also reinforced with Steri-Strips. The knee is then placed in a standard knee immobilizer so that access can be obtained to the wound at any time for inspection. Alternatively, a fracture type of brace can be used to stabilize the limb.

The appropriate intravenous antibiotic is continued for 6 weeks. If all goes well, reimplantation will occur at 4 weeks, allowing 2 more weeks of intravenous antibiotics with the new components in place.

Some surgeons are experimenting with loosely reimplanting an acrylic, antibiotic-laden prosthesis or a metal-to-plastic prosthesis as a spacer that allows better pain relief, stability, and range of motion. I have no experience with this technique.

The outflow drains are discontinued at 24 hours. The incision is inspected at 48 hours or sooner if there is significant drainage from the wound. The patient is allowed to ambulate with two crutches or a walker with partial weight-bearing as tolerated. The nylon skin sutures are removed between 10 and 14 days after surgery. The patient is discharged home with intravenous antibiotics administered there until the patient is readmitted approximately 4 weeks after explant surgery for reimplantation. Three or four days prior to reimplantation, the knee is reaspirated for repeat cell count and culture. Cultures most likely will be negative because of the antibiotic coverage. Obviously, if they are positive, the reimplantation cannot occur and re-débridement is necessary. With the cultures most likely negative, the cell count is of great importance in determining whether to proceed with reimplantation. For example, if an initial cell count of 80,000 prior to removal of components is at 60,000 three and a half weeks postoperatively, reimplantation should not occur, and re-débridement is necessary. If the cell count has fallen below 5000 white cells per high-power field, reimplantation can proceed. At this surgery, new cultures are obtained from soft tissue and bone, and frozen sections are sent from the periarticular tissue to assess the cell count. If there are fewer than five white cells per high-power field, reimplantation can proceed. If the cell count is greater than 15 white cells per high-power field, consideration must be given to re-débridement. Antibiotics are again mixed with the bone-cement as for the cement spacer. The intravenous antibiotics are continued for 2 more weeks for a total of 6 weeks of therapy. Suppressive antibiotics are given for a period of time in some cases as recommended by the infectious disease consultant. Occasionally, some patients with a chronic focus of infection will require suppression for life, such as penicillin VK 250 mg twice a day for an oropharyngeal focus.

Resection Arthroplasty

Resection arthroplasty is usually an interim procedure as described above in a delayed exchange protocol. Very rarely, permanent resection arthroplasty is appropriate. For example, I have one patient who was referred with a chronic draining sinus and three different gram-negative infecting organisms. No cement spacer was utilized. The knee was immobilized in a cast for 6 weeks following the resection, and the patient developed a stable, well-aligned resection that allowed painless weightbearing with a walker. The patient was elderly and otherwise homebound and was satisfied with the result.

Knee Arthrodesis

Knee arthrodesis is usually saved for failure of delayed exchange, especially when associated with loss of the extensor mechanism. Techniques of knee fusion continue to evolve from the use of external fixation devices to plating or intramedullary rod fixation. It must be realized that, although this is a recommended salvage for failure of delayed exchange, it does not guarantee that the infection will be eradicated, as chronic osteomyelitis can persist even after a successful fusion. For this reason, I am not an advocate of buried intramedullary rods that are not accessible after bony fusion.

Amputation

I had one patient progress to the need for amputation as a life-saving procedure. She was a diabetic with chronic renal failure on dialysis. She developed septicemia from an infected A-V shunt and seeded her knee arthroplasty. Gangrene ensued in her foot below this knee, and she underwent an above-knee amputation. Patients must be cautioned that in extremely rare cases amputation may be a possibility.

SUMMARY

Infection associated with TKA is a devastating complication. It is crucial to prevent this complication so that treatment will be unnecessary. The incidence of early primary infection should be less than 0.5%. The incidence of late metastatic infection will be approximately 1% at 10-year follow-up. In my practice, the incidence of early infection is zero at this time after more than 4000 primary arthroplasties. I attribute this to a combination of good fortune and the implementation of the measures described in this chapter. My personal incidence of late metastatic infection after 3000 consecutive primary arthroplasties at average 10-year follow-up is 0.5%. Most of these patients have rheumatoid arthritis with some deficiency in their immune system. Sources of metastatic infection have included pneumonia, urinary tract infection, infected foot ulcers, infected dentition, and diverticulitis. There are at least seven treatment options, all incorporating 6 weeks of intravenous antibiotics.

CHAPTER 15

Staying Out and Getting Out of Trouble During Total Knee Arthroplasty

Many problems or mishaps can be encountered during routine and not-so-routine total knee arthroplasty (TKA). In this chapter, I address several of these and offer potential solutions.

CHOOSING THE CORRECT INCISION

Wound necrosis following TKA can be a minor inconvenience or a major disaster that can lead to secondary infection and potential loss of the knee replacement. Necrosis is most likely to occur in the setting of a knee with prior incisions. It is imperative, therefore, for the surgeon to respect old incisions about the knee and choose the right incision for the arthroplasty. Unlike the hip, the knee does not tolerate parallel incisions or crossing incisions (Fig. 15–1). The ideal skin incision for a knee without prior surgery is vertical and relatively straight (see Chapter 4). I prefer an incision that is approximately 15 cm long and begins over the mid-shaft of the femur, crosses the medial third of the patella, and ends just medial to the tibial tubercle. In the early 1970s, a routine skin incision was parapatellar, curving around the medial border of the patella to create a laterally based skin flap. A certain number of patients suffered some necrosis at the apex of the flap, and this led us to straighten the incision. The vascular supply to the skin about the knee appears to be much more tolerant of medially based flaps than laterally based flaps. The knee most vulnerable to necrosis is one that has a long prior lateral incision that is followed by a parallel, more median incision (Fig. 15–2).

When parallel incisions are necessary, the surgeon should make the bridge between the two incisions as wide as possible or consider utilizing the lateral incision and elevating a medial based flap for a medial arthrotomy. If the alignment of the arthritic knee is in valgus, this may be an excellent indication for a lateral arthrotomy where the patella is everted medially.[1]

In general, in the presence of prior incisions, the surgeon should use the most lateral one that is viable or the most recent one that successfully healed. In unclear situations, a "sham" or "delayed incision" technique can be considered.

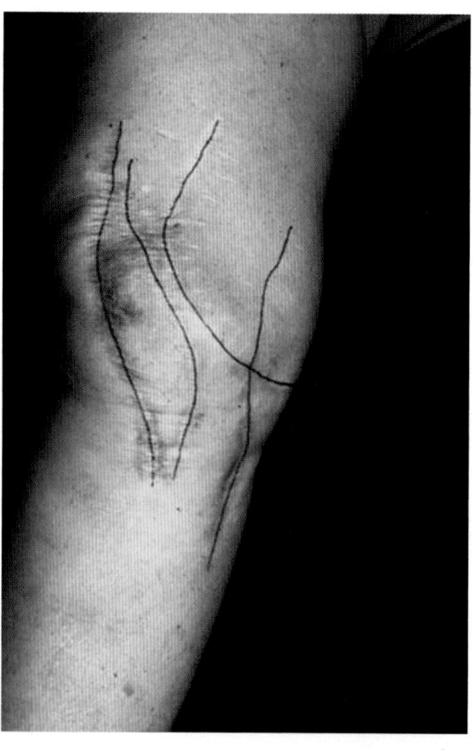

FIGURE 15–1. The knee does not usually tolerate multiple parallel or crossing incisions.

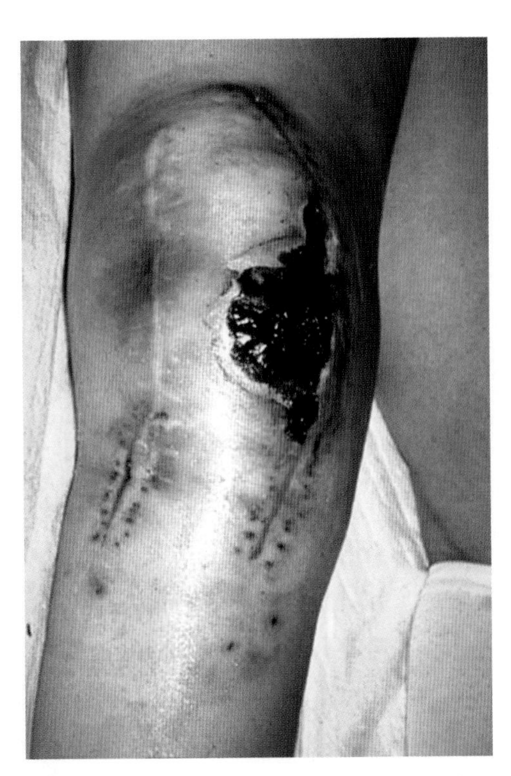

FIGURE 15–2. Skin necrosis occurring after a medial incision was made parallel to an old lateral incision.

The "sham" incision was advocated by my associate, F. Ewald. In this technique, the skin incision is made and the flaps are elevated in preparation for the arthrotomy. A tourniquet, if utilized, is deflated or uninflated. The medial and lateral skin edges are carefully inspected for active bleeding. If blood flow is equivocal, the procedure is aborted and consultation obtained with a plastic surgeon.

The "delayed incision" technique was advocated by J. Insall. The skin incision is made, the skin flaps are elevated for the arthrotomy, then the wound is closed regardless of the clinical appearance. Assuming no skin necrosis has occurred, the knee arthroplasty is carried out through the same incision 4 to 6 weeks later. It is thought that this technique not only tested the viability of the skin flap but also promoted increased collateral circulation secondary to the healing process.

Tissue expanders have been recommended in the presence of tight adherent skin and subcutaneous tissue.[2] I have used this technique in only one patient but with an excellent result.

Figures 15–3*A* to 15–3*F* show diagrams of the most frequently encountered prior knee incisions accompanied by a diagram of the most likely approach I would utilize in each case.

DEALING WITH SKIN NECROSIS

When skin necrosis occurs, I believe it is extremely important to keep the skin sealed for as long as possible and allow the capsular closure to seal as well. To help accomplish this, I stop all range-of-motion exercises and immobilize the knee in a splint that is easily removable so I can inspect the wound on a daily basis. If the wound remains completely dry for 10 days, I start range-of-motion exercises and assess the size of necrosis, which should have fully declared itself by this time. If there is any drainage from around the area of necrosis that does not slow and cease within several days of surgery, a plastic surgery consult is obtained for immediate intervention.

There are several options for the treatment of skin necrosis about a TKA. If the area is small and dry, it can be left to granulate in beneath the eschar. If the area is relatively small and the skin pliable, it can be excised and closed primarily.

Once the joint capsule is sealed, the area could also be excised and a split thickness skin graft applied. If the area is extensive and the joint unsealed or exposed, a gastrocnemius muscle flap may be required, followed by a split thickness skin graft.

I have twice encountered a situation in which patellectomy allowed resolution of a significant skin necrosis problem. Both cases involved severe preoperative deformities in patients in whom an extensive lateral release had been performed with sacrifice of the lateral genicular vessels. In both cases, a bone scan showed no uptake in the patella, indicating it was avascular.[3] Since the patella is always more than 2 cm thick, removing it might provide sufficient laxity in the capsule and skin to allow for primary closure of both layers as it did in both these cases.

DRAINING A WOUND

Persistent wound drainage following TKA should not be tolerated. I change the operative dressing on the second postoperative day. If any wound drainage is present, I carefully inspect the suture line for gaps in the skin closure. If present, the skin is cleaned with povidone-iodine and alcohol and then benzoin is applied along its edges followed by Steri-Strips to reseal the wound. This maneuver might have to be repeated for another day or two. Flexion exercises are suspended until the wound is dry for 24 hours. If drainage still persists, I believe that treatment should be aggressive and the patient returned to the operating room for minor wound débridement, irrigation, and primary closure.

To be sure that the drainage does not represent a deep problem, the knee joint is aspirated through a remote site. The fluid is sent for cell count, differential, and aerobic and anaerobic cultures. Oral prophylactic antibiotics are begun; I usually use a second-generation cephalosporin, 500 mg 4 times a day. I always close knee wounds with interrupted nylon sutures (see Chapter 4). In the operating room, the knee area is sterilely prepared and draped. Two or three sutures are removed from around the area of drainage. A subcutaneous culture is obtained. The wound is thoroughly irrigated and a primary closure performed with interrupted 3-0 nylon vertical mattress sutures. The skin edges are freshened by removal of 1 or 2 mm of tissue, if necessary. The procedure is performed under local anesthesia using 1% lidocaine. Flexion exercises are suspended for 1 or 2 days until it is apparent that the wound is now sealed.

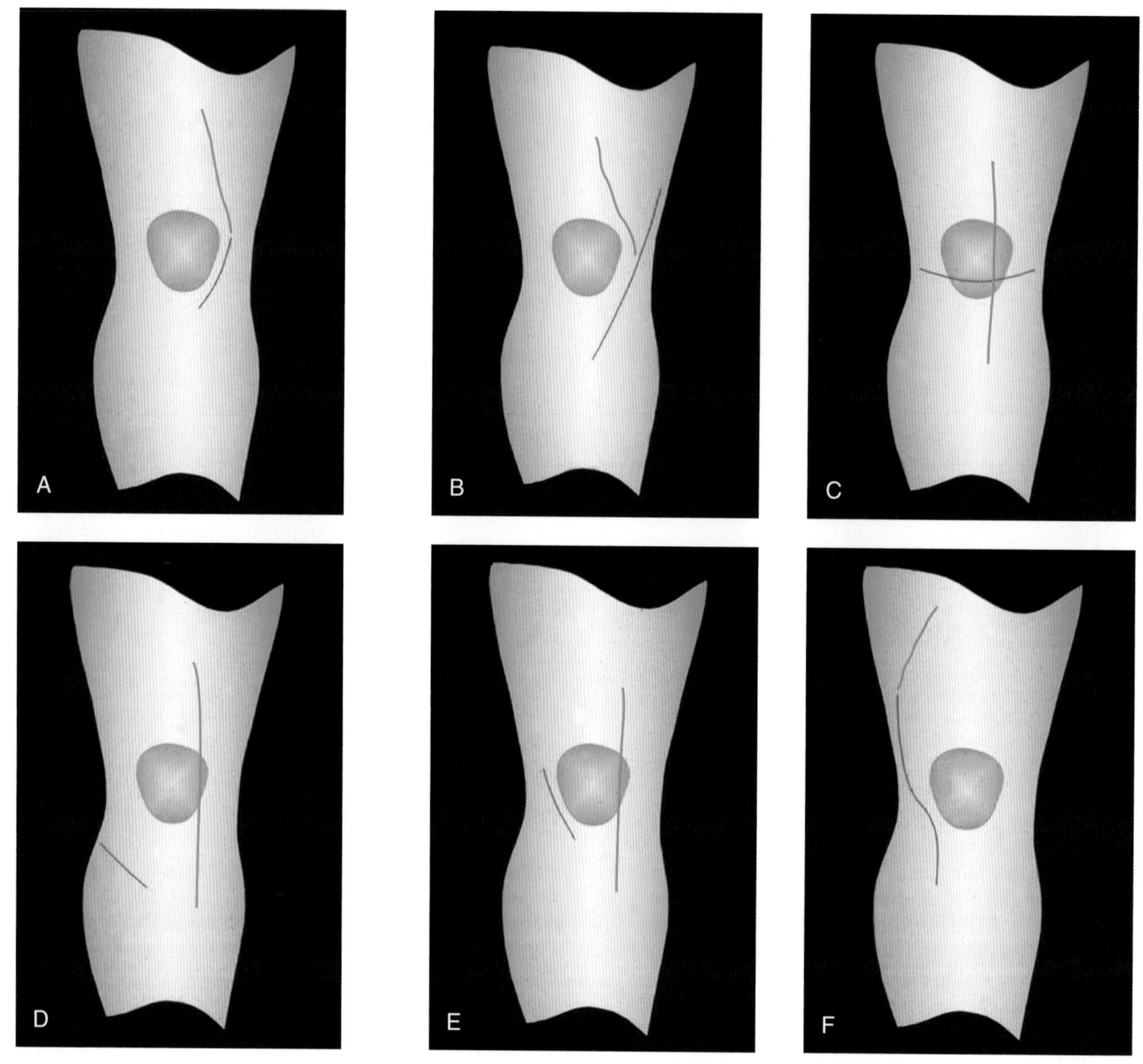

FIGURE 15–3. *A*, A short oblique medial incision can be extended to a longer median parapatellar incision. *B*, In a prior long oblique medial incision, only the distal half is utilized. *C*, Transverse old incisions usually can be ignored. *D*, A prior short oblique Coventry incision usually can be ignored. *E*, After a short oblique prior lateral arthrotomy, the incision should be shifted medially to widen the skin bridge. *F*, A long prior lateral parapatellar incision must be respected and utilized.

DEALING WITH EXCESSIVE SUCTION DRAINAGE

It is somewhat controversial whether or not a TKA should be drained. I remain an advocate of low suction drains for the first 24 hours after surgery to minimize wound swelling. The published studies indicating that drains may not be necessary are based on only several hundred cases. I firmly believe that in 1000 or more cases, there will be a rare complication due to not using a drain that will cost more in actual dollars to heal the wound than would have been spent on drains for all 1000 patients.

When drains are used, there will sometimes be reports in the first few postoperative hours that the drainage is excessive. I have a simple treatment algorithm that seems to work well. We have all observed the fact that when the tourniquet is deflated, the knee bleeds less in flexion than it does in extension. If the drain output is large, therefore, simply flex the knee for 30 minutes and the output usually slows. If this method fails or is too painful for the patient, I clamp the suction drain for 30 minutes. If this is insufficient, I clamp and unclamp the drain for several cycles. In extremely rare, persistent cases, I remove the drain and apply a moderate compression dressing. Persistent bleeding may, of course, be due to a latent bleeding disorder or one created by the method of prophylactic anticoagulation; these possibilities must be checked.

TREATING A LARGE HEMATOMA

A large hematoma following TKA can be extremely painful, inhibit postoperative rehabilitation, and can, if treated improperly, lead to significant morbidity. The key to successful resolution is the maintenance of an intact wound without drainage or neurovascular compromise. Coagulation parameters should be checked if warfarin is being used for deep venous thrombosis prophylaxis and is responsible for coagulopathy. The most common scenario is a very elderly patient sensitive to this medication. In my own practice, I rarely use low-molecular-weight heparin for anticoagulation because of the high incidence of wound bleeding with this medication.

If a significant hematoma has developed, the knee should be immobilized and ice applied for at least the first 24 hours. The wound should be inspected daily. If it remains intact and there is no neurovascular compromise or compartment syndrome, flexion exercises are started gently and slowly after several days. Some of these patients may fall into the rare category of those requiring later manipulation, but this is preferable to overly aggressive early physical therapy leading to wound healing difficulties.

Evacuation of the hematoma is rarely required, but indications for this include intractable pain, loss of wound integrity, neurovascular deficit, and compartment syndrome. I have yet to aspirate a wound hematoma although this is a reasonable conservative initial attempt to decompress an extremely painful knee. When active treatment of a hematoma is required, I think it will almost always involve return to the operating room for evacuation of the hematoma, irrigation of the wound, attempt to control the bleeding source if possible, and primary wound closure. I have not yet needed to proceed with this form of treatment in my own practice but recommend it when indicated. Perhaps my universal use of postoperative drains has minimized this complication.

TREATING PATELLAR TENDON AVULSION

The key is to avoid patellar tendon avulsion in the first place. I am fortunate to have no personal experience with this complication, but I am prepared to treat it if necessary. Prophylaxis involves anticipating the problem and taking two important measures during exposure: the first is the early use of an inverted V-quadriceps release or quadriceps snip,[4,5] and the second is the placement of a smooth $\frac{1}{8}$-inch pin into the tubercle to arrest the propagation of a tendon avulsion (see Fig. 10–2).

If the tendon were to avulse, several treatment options are possible. The surgeon should have taken care during the initial exposure to preserve an intact medial capsular sleeve on the tibia. This sleeve should remain well anchored to its tibial attachment. A side-to-side repair of the tendon to this intact medial capsule will reconstitute the integrity of the distal quadriceps mechanism. This repair would then be supplemented by some form of anchoring mechanism of the tendon to its original attachment on the tubercle. If this seems insufficient, the third step is to harvest the semitendinosus tendon, maintaining its attachment to the tibia and bringing it up to the inferior pole of the patella on the medial side of the tendon and then down to the lateral aspect of the tubercle. The repair should then be protected for a minimum of 4 weeks. Its initial integrity should be tested by flexing the knee against gravity and recording the amount of flexion that does not overstress the repair. Postoperative flexion would then be limited to 10 degrees less than this recorded amount for the full 4 weeks. Although quadriceps setting exercises are permitted, the patient should not be allowed to perform a straight-leg exercise or actively extend the knee from a flexed position during this interval.

Late repair of a patellar tendon rupture consists of use of the semitendinosus or allograft reconstruction. I have used the patella/patellar tendon/tubercle technique with some success but prefer the Achilles tendon allograft, fixing a small piece of the retained os calcis into the medial aspect of the tubercle and over-sewing the Achilles tendon on top of the patellar tendon and patella to the quadriceps tendon. Allograft reconstructions must be implanted as snugly as possible and immobilized in extension for a minimum of 6 weeks.

AVOIDING MEDIAL COLLATERAL LIGAMENT INJURY

The most vulnerable times for a medial collateral injury are during the proximal medial capsular exposure, the excision of the posterior half of the medial meniscus, the distal and posterior femoral condylar resections, and the proximal medial tibial resection.

As the proximal medial tibial sleeve is developed, it is important to keep the scalpel blade tangential to the tibial bone. If not, an angled blade can inadvertently sever fibers of the deep medial collateral ligament.

A second vulnerable time is during the completion of the medial meniscectomy (Fig. 15–4). If the medial third of the meniscus is grasped and pulled laterally into the joint to complete the meniscectomy, it can pull the medial collateral

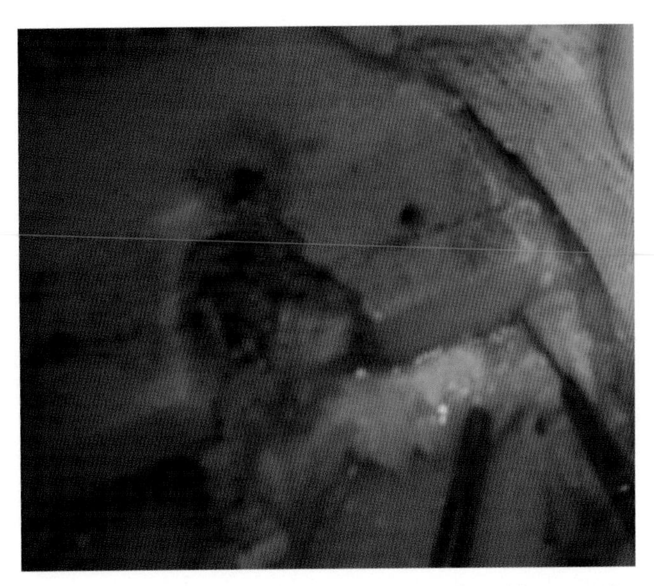

FIGURE 15–4. It is possible to injure the medial collateral ligament when excising the middle third of the medial meniscus.

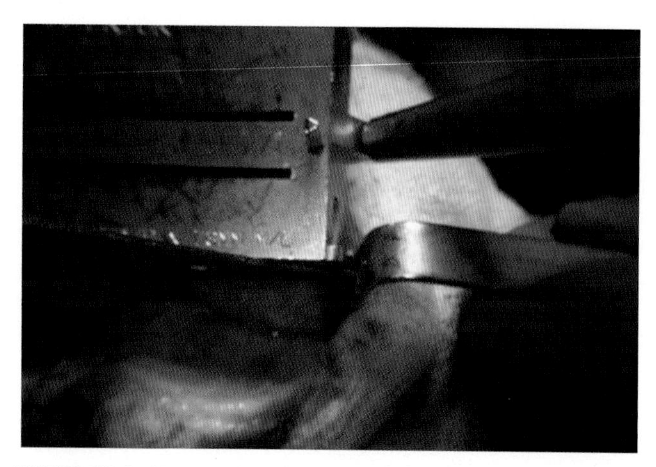

FIGURE 15–5. The medial collateral ligament should be protected by a retractor when a saw is used to resect the posterior femoral condyle.

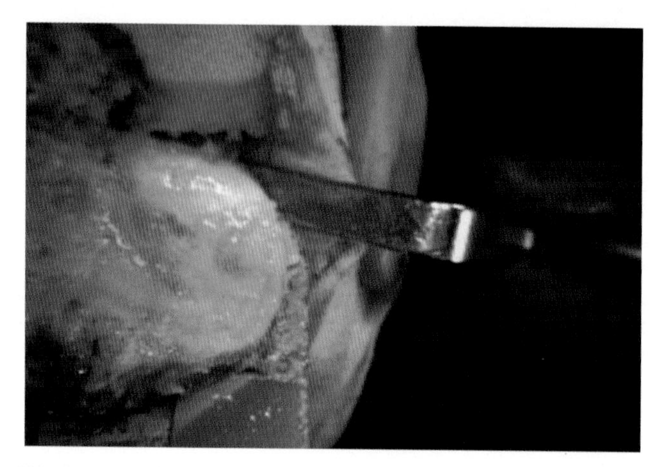

FIGURE 15–6. The medial collateral ligament should also be protected during resection of the medial tibial plateau.

ligament with it. If the surgeon does not carefully define the junction between the rim of the meniscus and the collateral ligament, a tangential rent can be created.

A third vulnerable time is during preparation of the femur, specifically, the posterior condylar resections. The surgeon fails to appreciate the extent of the excursion of the moving saw blade, or the saw cuts out medially as it engages sclerotic bone. Protection is achieved by placing a retractor at least 1.5 cm wide at the precise level of the posterior femoral resection (Fig. 15–5). The assistant holding that retractor will invariably report feeling the vibrations of the saw blade against the retractor.

A final vulnerable time is the proximal tibial resection on the medial side. The medial plateau in a varus knee is always sclerotic and the saw blade frequently cuts out of this hard bone. Just as in the femoral preparation, a retractor should be placed at the level of the tibial resection to protect the ligament (Fig. 15–6).

ADDRESSING MEDIAL COLLATERAL LIGAMENT INJURY

Ideally, the injury will be detected prior to the bone resections. If so, the resections should be very conservative to allow a thicker insert to tense what ligament remains intact. The valgus angle should also be diminished to overall alignment of 3 degrees of anatomic valgus or less to minimize stress on the remaining medial collateral ligament or on the repair. A primary repair of the cut ends (anatomic, if possible) is carried out using the technique recommended by Krackow.[6] If possible, the posterior cruciate ligament is retained for its medial stabilizing force. The repair should be accomplished in the presence of a trial tibial insert 2 mm thinner than the final insert to be placed. Postoperatively, the repair is protected by a stabilizing brace for 6 weeks. Range-of-motion exercises are permitted along with quadriceps strengthening exercises. If the patient is very elderly (certainly if over 80 years of age) I might use a Total Condylar III constraint to internally brace the repair and allow it to be protected indefinitely.

AVOIDING AND RESOLVING POPLITEUS IMPINGEMENT

Popliteus impingement can occur when the tendon subluxates over a retained lateral osteophyte or a prominent metallic posterior femoral condyle (Fig. 15–7).[7]

The subluxation usually occurs between 40 and 90 degrees of flexion and may not be detected during surgery unless tested for with the capsule closed. This is because the everted quadriceps mechanism artificially externally rotates the tibia during flexion and the impingement is avoided. It presents as an audible and visible clunk during passive flexion of the knee, and the source may not be immediately apparent. The diagnosis can be made by palpating the popliteus insertion on the femur during flexion and feeling the subluxation. The problem is cured by release of the popliteus tendon from its femoral origin. If

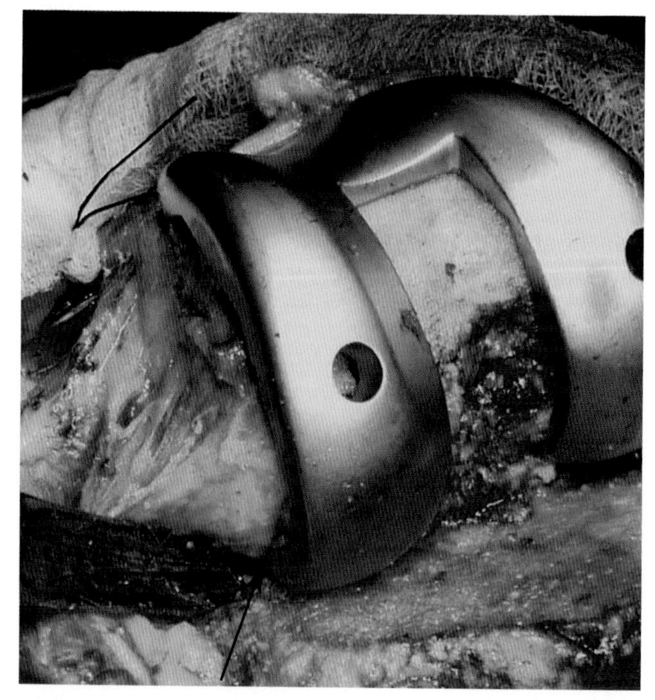

FIGURE 15–7. The popliteus tendon can impinge on an overhanging metal posterior femoral condyle.

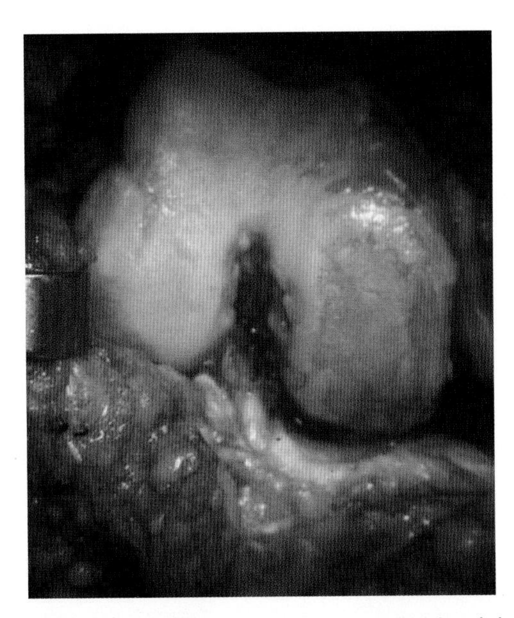

FIGURE 15–8. The female femur tends to be taller than it is wide.

it is not detected until the postoperative period, it can be resolved by arthroscopic release of the tendon.

The popliteus syndrome can be initially avoided by taking two measures. The first is to use a straight osteotome after femoral preparation to clear any retained osteophytes or uncapped lateral bone (see Chapter 4).

The second measure is to avoid oversizing the femoral component in the mediolateral dimension. This is more likely to occur in a female because the female femur tends to be larger in the anteroposterior (AP) dimension relative to the mediolateral dimension than the male femur is (Figs. 15–8 and 15–9).[8] Occasionally this will lead to the properly sized AP dimension being too wide in the mediolateral dimension, and the femur must be downsized (see below).

A final word about the popliteus tendon: on occasion I resect it because it is large and partially dislocated into the posterior aspect of the lateral compartment. Usually, a

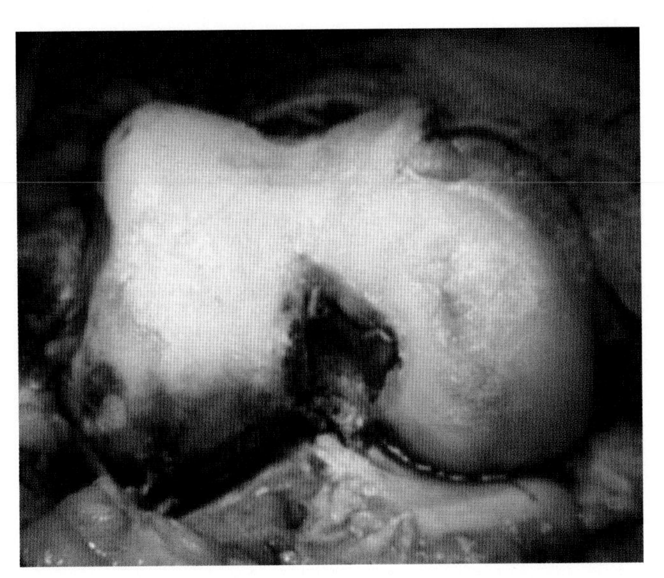

FIGURE 15–9. The male femur tends to be wider than it is tall.

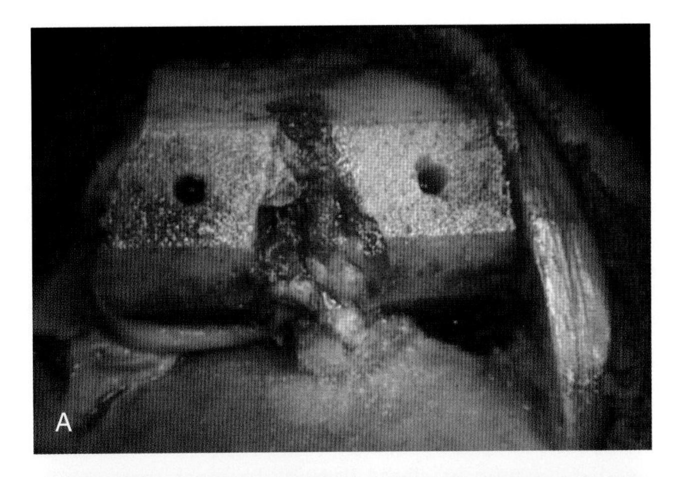

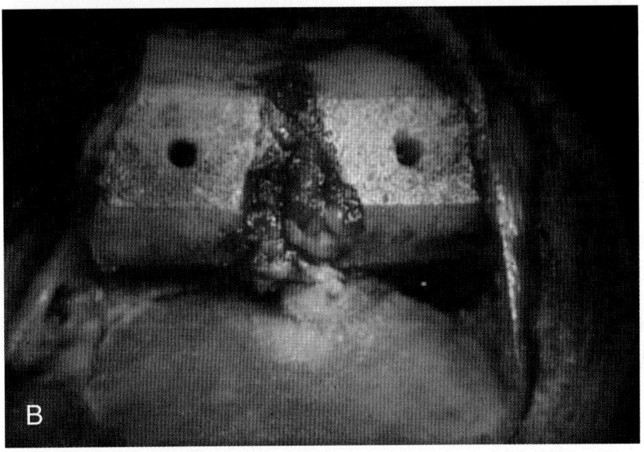

FIGURE 15–10. *A*, This popliteus tendon is very thick and prominent and could impinge in the lateral joint space. *B*, A tangential resection of the popliteus tendon has relieved any possible impingement.

tangential, rather than a complete, resection of the tendon suffices to debulk it and relieve any potential impingement (Fig. 15–10).

CHOOSING AMONG FEMUR SIZES

Femurs come in a variety of sizes and shapes, and there are intrinsic differences between male and female anatomy. It has also been my experience that the femur in Asians tends to be larger in the mediolateral dimension relative to the AP dimension. When choosing between sizes, the smaller should be selected to avoid "stuffing" the joint. A trochlear flange that is proud of the anterior cortex will diminish quadriceps excursion. Metallic condyles that overhang the bone on either side can also diminish quadriceps excursion and cause capsular discomfort.

The surgeon basically has two options when choosing between sizes. The first is to size from anterior down. The surgeon measures off the anterior cortex and accepts the fact that more than an anatomic amount of posterior condyle will be resected.

A way to effectively half-size a femur from anterior down is to locate the pinholes for the AP cutting jig of the larger size but then apply the smaller size AP cutting apparatus via these pinholes. In most systems, this will essentially accomplish a half-size alteration in the AP cuts. The difference in the AP dimension of most systems from size to size on the femur is 4 to 5 mm. Thus, a half-size change will take approximately 2 mm more from the anterior resection and 2 mm more from the anatomic posterior resection.

The main consequence of sizing from anterior down is the increased posterior condylar resection. This results in a larger flexion gap. Thicker polyethylene is then needed to regain flexion stability. More distal resection will then be necessary in the presence of the thicker polyethylene to allow full passive extension. The net effect is elevating the joint line approximately 2 mm in both flexion and extension. There is a slight kinematic consequence, since joint line elevation leads to some mid-flexion laxity. The 2-mm difference, however, is not usually clinically significant.

The second option when choosing between sizes is to cut the distal femur in slight flexion. In most systems, the trochlear flange already diverges about 3 degrees away from the neutral position of the posterior condyles. By adding 3 more degrees of flexion to the distal cut, the trochlear flange now diverges by 6 degrees. This allows a smaller size femoral component to be utilized without distorting the joint line and the amount of posterior condylar resection.

The diverging trochlear eliminates the possibility of notching of the anterior cortex. I use a special distal condylar cutting block that accommodates to the pins for the regular cutting block and allows me this option (Fig. 15–11).

There are no adverse consequences of cutting the femur in slight flexion unless the articulating surfaces of the femur and tibia do not allow for hyperextension without causing impingement or loss of metal-to-plastic contact. Most posterior cruciate retaining systems allow more than enough articular hyperextension (Fig. 15–12). The one I use allows at least 30 degrees. Posterior cruciate substituting designs, however, with a stabilizing post do not accommodate as much hyperextension between articulating surfaces. Some designs allow no hyperextension, while others allow up to 10 or 12 degrees. The surgeon should be aware of this number in the system being used. For example, if the system allows only 5 degrees of hyperextension before post impingement occurs, 3 degrees of femoral flexion cannot be combined with 5 degrees of posterior tibial slope. The result will be deleterious post impingement and accentuation of post and back-side wear (see Chapter 2).

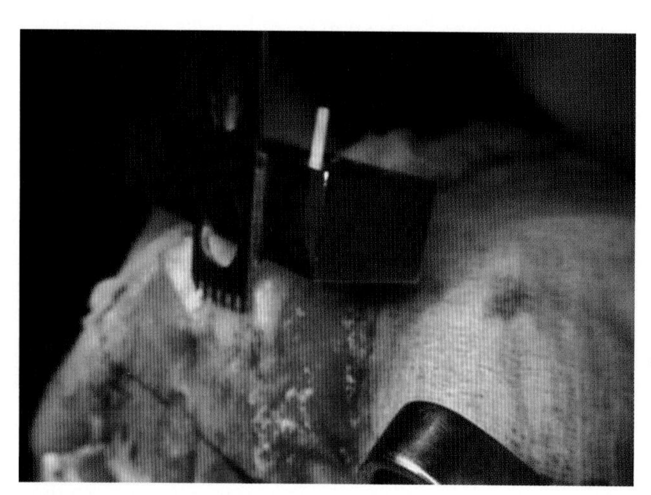

FIGURE 15–11. A distal femoral recut guide can apply a few degrees of flexion to the resection.

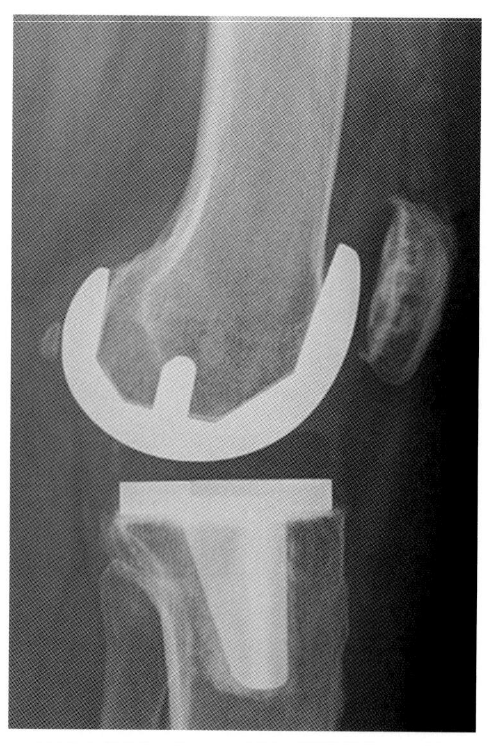

FIGURE 15–12. When the femur has been cut in flexion, the articulating surfaces of the prostheses must be allowed to hyperextend without consequence.

SUMMARY

Many complications can occur during TKA and in the immediate postoperative period. The most frequent of these are addressed in this chapter.

References

1. Keblish PA: The lateral approach for total knee arthroplasty. J Knee Surg 2003;16:62–68.
2. Manifold SG, Cushner FD, Craig-Scott S, Scott WN: Long-term results of total knee arthroplasty after the use of soft tissue expanders. Clin Orthop 2000;380:133–139.
3. Wetzner SM, Bezreh JS, Scott RD, et al: Bone scanning in the assessment of patellar viability following knee replacement. Clin Orthop 1985;199:215–219.
4. Garvin KL, Scuderi G, Insall JN: Evolution of the quadriceps snip. Clin Orthop 1995;321:131–137.
5. Scott RD, Siliski JM: The use of a modified V-Y quadricepsplasty during total knee replacement to gain exposure and improve flexion in the ankylosed knee. Orthopedics 1986;8:45–48.
6. Krackow KA, Thomas SC, Jones LC: Ligament-tendon fixation: analysis of a new stitch and comparison with standard techniques. Orthopedics 1988;11:909–917.
7. Barnes CL, Scott RD: Popliteus tendon dysfunction following total knee arthroplasty. J Arthroplasty 1995;10:543–545.
8. Chin KR, Dalury DF, Zurakowski D, Scott RD: Intraoperative measurements of male and female distal femurs during primary total knee arthroplasty. J Knee Surg 2002;15:213–217.

CHAPTER 16

Reoperation After Total Knee Arthroplasty

The specific incidence of and causes for reoperation after total knee arthroplasty (TKA) continue to change with time. In the early experience with hinge and condylar knees, reoperations were most frequently required for prosthetic loosening, knee instability, and sepsis. Fifteen to 20 years ago, patellofemoral complications accounted for up to 50% of reoperations.[1] With improved prosthetic designs and better surgical technique, reoperations are becoming less frequent. Polyethylene wear is now the leading cause for reoperation, while prosthetic loosening, instability, and patellofemoral problems are rare.

In this chapter, the incidence and causes of reoperation after 2000 consecutive posterior cruciate ligament (PCL)–retaining primary TKAs followed for a mean of 11 years are discussed. Some causes are obviously prosthesis specific. Nevertheless, my personal experience gives an overview of the complications most likely to be seen today in an arthroplasty practice.

FEMORAL COMPONENT LOOSENING

In the early experience with these 2000 consecutive knees, hybrid fixation was popular.[2] Seven hundred eighty-six of the femoral components were implanted without cement, while 1214 were cemented. Among the cementless components, only one had clinically loosened. This patient had a dysplastic femur with an additional 5-degree valgus bow that was not visible on her short radiographs (Fig. 16–1*A*).

The patient's mechanical axis, therefore, was in 5 degrees more valgus than was apparent on a short film. Over a 4-year period, the femoral component loosened and subsided into valgus. She required revision with a long-stem femoral component inserted in 5 degrees of varus to counteract her metaphyseal deformity (Fig. 16–1*B*). Ironically, her opposite knee was one of the two loose cemented components among the series and required the same treatment with a varus long stem. While the cementless femur failed at 4 years, the cemented femur loosened at 15 years. This time difference might reflect the probability that cemented femoral fixation is more forgiving to adverse forces across the fixation interface than a cementless component is.

FRACTURED FEMORAL COMPONENTS

An interesting complication seen in the early series of cementless femoral components is the occurrence of stress fracture of one metal condyle. Although somewhat prosthesis specific, fracture has been reported with other designs.[3] There were seven such cases among the 786 cementless porous coated components. All but one occurred in active men weighing between 90 and 140 kg and involved the larger component sizes. All fractures occurred in otherwise well-fixed components at the junction between the distal medial condyle and the posterior medial chamfer (Fig. 16–2) except in the female patient who had a fracture at the anterior medial chamfer. All presented with accelerated medial polyethylene wear due to abrasion from the rough edge of the fracture line. The fracture was missed preoperatively in most cases and only apparent in retrospect on some lateral roentgenograms.

Examination of all seven retrieved components showed that the stress fracture was initiated at the porous surface on the inside of the component. This would imply that the force causing the fracture was one of expansion of the posterior condyle away from the trochlear flange as the bone was loaded. By way of contrast, a compression force on the posterior condyle implicated in femoral component loosening might occur as a patient ascends a stair or rises from a chair.[4] No fractures were seen in cemented components. Subsequently, the femoral component used in this series

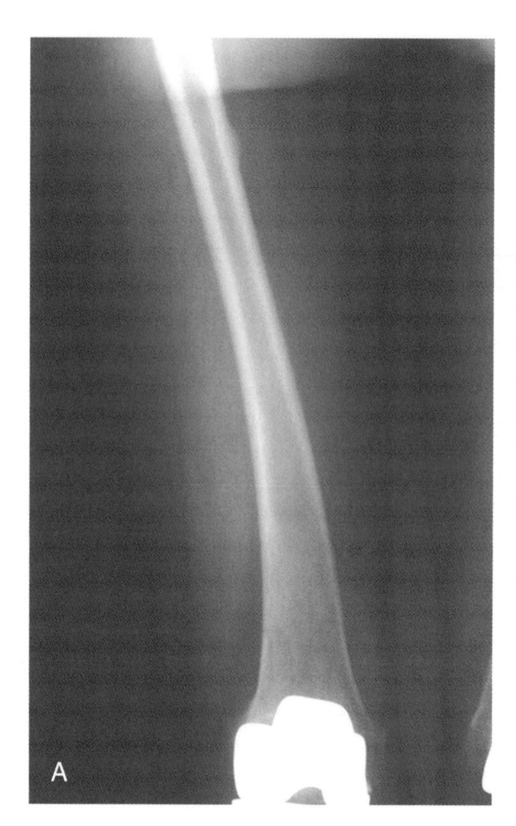

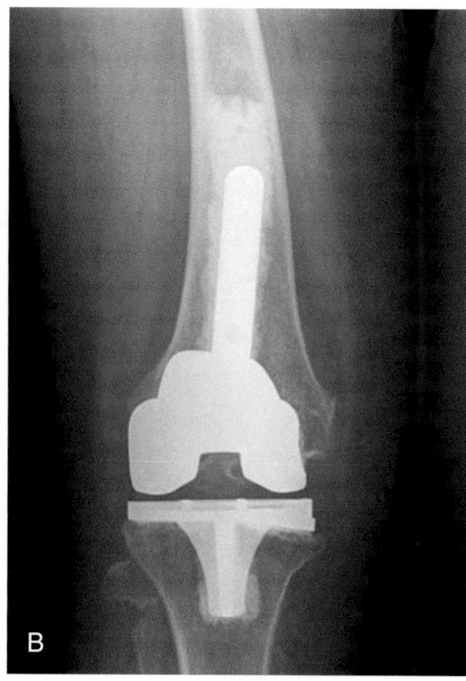

FIGURE 16–1. *A*, A femoral shaft with a significant valgus metaphyseal bow not visible on standard short roentgenograms. The femoral component failed by subsiding into increased valgus. *B*, Salvage at revision by the use of a 5-degree varus stem to offset the 10-degree valgus femoral shaft deformity.

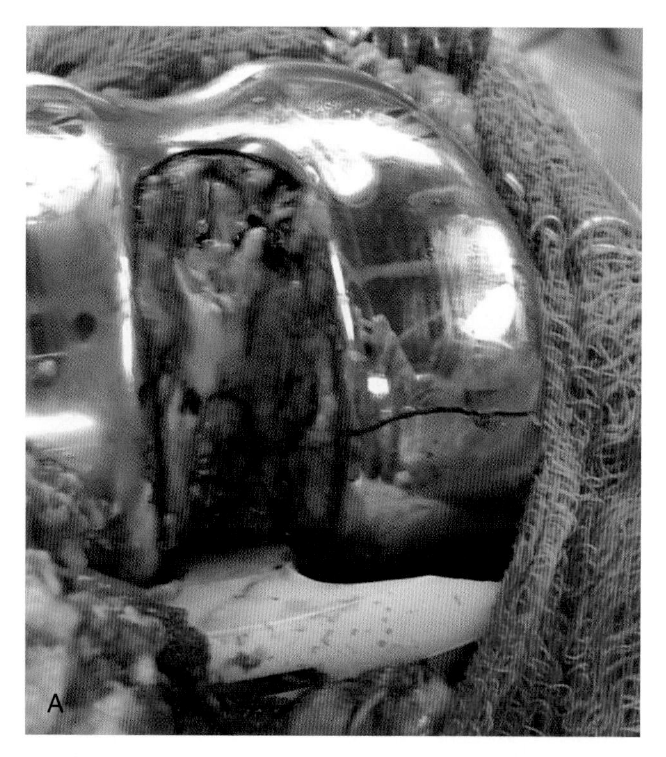

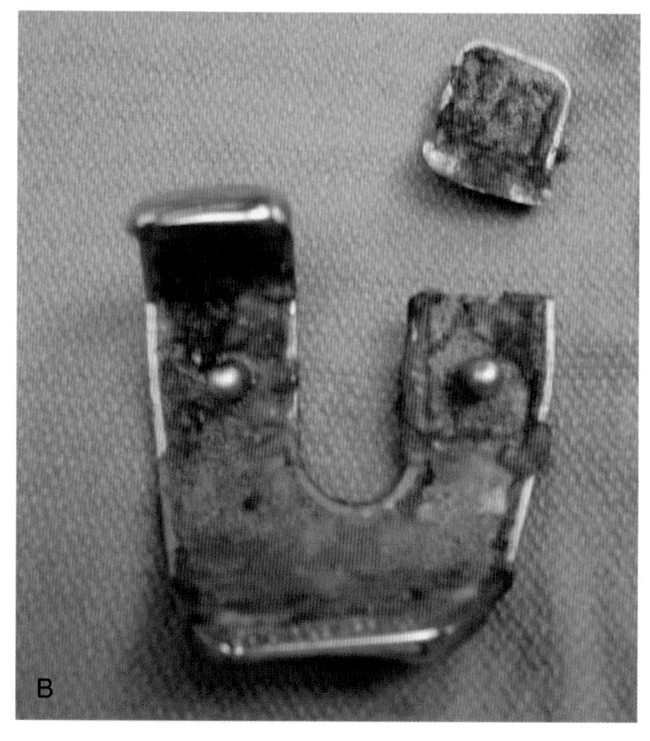

FIGURE 16–2. A fractured femoral component.

was redesigned and reinforced at the chamfers, and no fractures have been seen since that time.

TIBIAL COMPONENT LOOSENING

Tibial component loosening (among cemented components) also was infrequent. Among the 2000 consecutive knees, cementless tibias were implanted in only 38, or approximately 2% of patients, and never with ancillary screw fixation. Among these 38 knees, three loosened, for an incidence of 8%. Eighty-seven knees were implanted with the so-called hybrid technique. In these knees, the plateau was cemented but the tibial keel was not. One of these 87 knees loosened. Hybrid tibial fixation was initially attractive as a bone-sparing technique. There has been only one tibial loosening, however, among the 1875 fully cemented tibias, and several long-term follow-up studies have shown an increased incidence of tibial radiolucent lines or loosening with the "hybrid" technique.[5] Most surgeons now fully cement all tibial components.

Advocates of cementless tibial fixation prefer and succeed with ancillary screw fixation. There are long-term concerns with this technique, however, in regard to potential screw migration as the tibial tray normally undergoes some long-term subsidence. This movement would allow well-fixed screws to begin to penetrate the undersurface of the polyethylene, and the screw holes in the tray would allow ingress of wear debris to the bone with subsequent osteolysis. Examples of both these complications have been described in the literature.[6]

METAL-BACKED PATELLA

When tibial components adopted metal-backing in the late 1970s and early 1980s, the same rationale was used to metal-back the patella. The metal-backing was to add support to the polyethylene and decrease focal forces across the fixation interface. It would also allow for the application of a porous surface for bone ingrowth, permitting cementless fixation. In the mid-1980s, failures of metal-backed patellae were reported due to accelerated polyethylene wear with early designs.[7] In retrospect, it was appreciated that the application of a metal backing diminished the polyethylene thickness to such an extent that accelerated wear would occur especially if the patella tracked asymmetrically (usually with some lateral tilt). In this series, 7 of the 87 implanted metal backed patellae failed as a result of wear. Most surgeons now avoid metal-backed patellae except of the mobile-bearing variety, for which the same high incidence of failure has not been reported.[8]

ALL-POLYETHYLENE PATELLAR REPLACEMENT

Since the mid-1980s a three-pegged all-polyethylene patellar component has become the state of the art. Among the 1723 all-polyethylene patellae in this series, none has been revised for wear or patellar instability. There have been three traumatic fractures, but all were treated conservatively and did not require surgery.

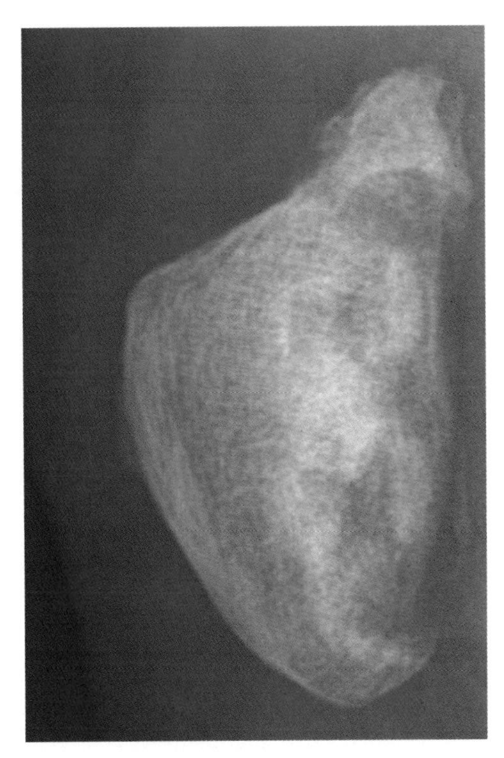

FIGURE 16–3. An asymptomatic avulsion fracture of the superior pole of the patella.

A small number of avulsion fractures were seen that usually involved a few millimeters of the superior pole of the patella (Fig. 16–3). Most often, these were incidental findings at routine follow-up. Occasionally, they were symptomatic for approximately 6 weeks during which time the patients were advised to avoid high forces across the patellofemoral articulation such as ascending stairs and rising from a sitting position without arm support.

There were four reoperations due to patellar complications. Three involved shearing-off of the three lugs from an early design. The junction between the lug and the patellar component was reinforced, eliminating this complication. The cause of the complication also involved the presence of an abnormal shearing force due to imbalance in the quadriceps mechanism. The conformity of the articulation would tend to keep the patella located in the trochlear groove, while the soft tissue imbalance would attempt to pull the patella toward the lateral side.

A fourth reoperation involving a cemented three-pegged all-polyethylene patella was a rare case of patellar loosening. This patient had undergone a lateral retinacular release, and examination of the patellar bone at reoperation showed signs of osteonecrosis, possibly contributing to the loosening.

THE UNRESURFACED PATELLA

Among the 2000 consecutive primary TKAs, 175 patellae were left unresurfaced. In this series, there were specific indications for not resurfacing the patella.[9,10] At mean 15-year follow-up, four of these patients had required secondary resurfacing at 1, 5, 10, and 12 years, respectively, after initial arthroplasty. Only two of the four patients experienced complete relief of their pre-resurfacing pain, emphasizing the point that the unresurfaced patella invites reoperation even if it may not be the source of persistent discomfort.

Because the complications of resurfacing with a cemented three-pegged all-polyethylene patella are so rare, most surgeons now consider not resurfacing only young, active, osteoarthritic male patients who fulfill specific selection criteria and only after a careful discussion with them of the pros and cons of not resurfacing. There are regional and individual exceptions to this viewpoint, where leaving the patella unresufaced is common.

POLYETHYLENE INSERT WEAR

Polyethylene wear has now become the most frequent cause of reoperation after TKA. In this series of 2000 consecutive knees at mean 11-year follow-up, wear complications have necessitated reoperation in 47 knees. This gives an incidence of 2.3% at 11 years, or slightly over 0.2% per year of follow-up. Twenty-nine of the inserts exhibited wear with synovitis and osteolysis. Eleven had insert wear with synovitis only. Seven had insert wear without symptoms. These seven were detected at routine follow-up screening and exchanged electively within a year following detection. In two cases, residual varus alignment was corrected by the use of a custom angle bearing to modify the alignment. One bearing was angled at 3 degrees and the other at 5 degrees (Fig. 16–4).

Osteolysis was extremely rare in knees implanted in the 1980s. Its incidence began to slowly climb in the early 1990s, peaked in 1995, and then subsided. The reasons are unclear. Multiple factors are most likely responsible including increased top-side conformity, oxidation due to gamma irradiation in air, polyethylene resin changes, and others.

MISCELLANEOUS CAUSES FOR REOPERATION

Recurrent Hemarthrosis

Recurrent hemarthrosis is an unusual complication, with four cases requiring open synovectomy among the 2000 knees. An additional number of incidences of acute late bleeding occurred that did not require surgery.[11]

Recurrent Rheumatoid Synovitis

Recurrent rheumatoid synovitis also is an unusual complication, with four documented cases seen following TKA that included resurfacing of the patella. In these four cases, infection was ruled out because their presentation often simulated that of metastatic infection. Medical treatment of a rheumatoid flare can help relieve the synovitis. Occasionally, a steroid injection is appropriate. Rarely, an open synovectomy may be necessary and was curative in the three cases in which it was employed.

Stiffness Requiring Arthroscopic Manipulation

This specific need for reoperation comes from a desire to improve postoperative range of motion in a select group of patients who have passed the time when closed manipulation might still be effective. There were five such cases among these 2000 knees. Four of the five patients gained and maintained sufficient flexion or extension following the procedure for them to consider it a success.

Laxity After Total Knee Arthroplasty

Six knees required surgical intervention owing to late onset knee instability. Three were associated with trauma, and three developed insidiously over many months. The three trauma cases involved falls. Two of the patients were status postpatellectomy with persistent quadriceps weakness and episodes of giving-way. The third patient had muscle weakness and imbalance due to syringomyelia. All three were treated with thicker inserts. The neurologic deficit progressed in the syringomyelia patient, and falls were repeated until she became wheelchair bound. Thicker inserts stabilized the two patellectomized knees, although one required revision of the femoral component and insert to a posterior-stabilized topography.

The three atraumatic cases involved preoperatively varus knees that slowly drifted back into varus, associated with lateral laxity. All three knees had been slightly undercorrected with reference to their mechanical axis and most likely had some residual lateral laxity that then progressed as the varus recurred. They were treated with thicker inserts and a medial release to improve ligament balance (Fig. 16–5).

Ganglion Cysts

Two patients required reoperation to excise a ganglion cyst that arose from the tibiofibular joint.[12] Neither cyst appeared to communicate directly with the knee joint. One of the cysts intermittently caused symptomatic peroneal nerve compression. The source of the cysts was identified by injecting methylene blue into the mass and following the dye to the tibiofibular joint. The joint was excised with a rongeur, and neither cyst had recurred at 4 and 8 years, respectively. A third patient required excision of a popliteal cyst involving the semimembranous bursa.

SUMMARY

Table 16-1 shows all the operations reported among these 2000 consecutive knees at mean 11-year follow-up (range, 3–19 years). At that point, there had been 116 reoperations for an incidence of 5.8% at mean 11 years, or approximately 0.5% per year. Insert wear was the most frequent cause, with 47 reoperations, or 2.3%, at 11 years. These reoperations account for 40% of the total. The next most frequent cause was metastatic infection. Sixteen had been recorded coming from various remote sites. There were no early primary infections in this series. Other reasons for reoperation in decreasing incidence of frequency were the following: seven cases of worn metal-backed patellae and broken femoral components; five cases of stiffness requiring arthroscopic manipulation; four cases each of recurrent hemarthrosis, recurrent rheumatoid synovitis, and unresurfaced painful patellae; and three cases each of loose cementless tibias, shear-off of patellar lugs, traumatic laxity, atraumatic lateral

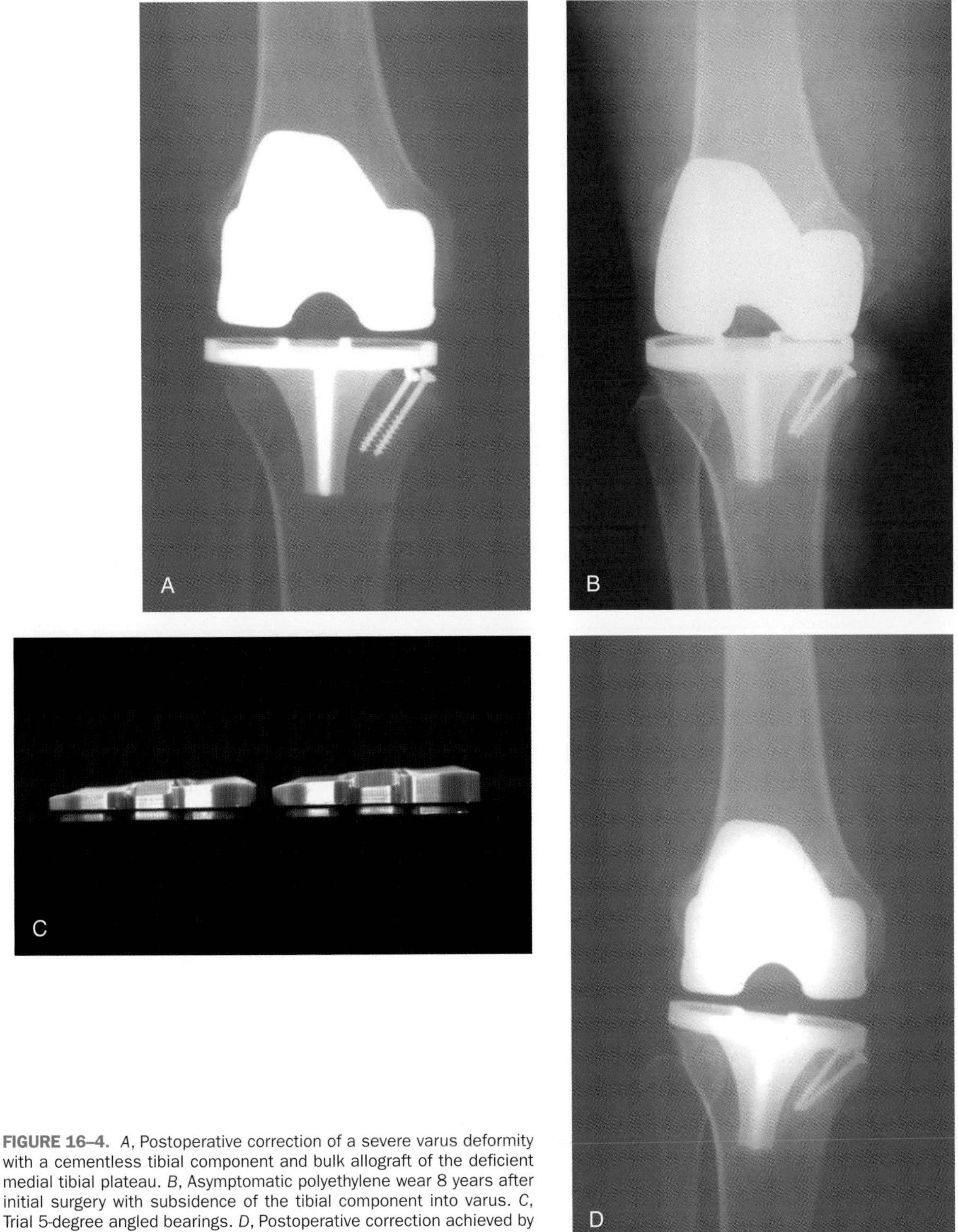

FIGURE 16–4. *A*, Postoperative correction of a severe varus deformity with a cementless tibial component and bulk allograft of the deficient medial tibial plateau. *B*, Asymptomatic polyethylene wear 8 years after initial surgery with subsidence of the tibial component into varus. *C*, Trial 5-degree angled bearings. *D*, Postoperative correction achieved by the angled-bearing insert exchange.

laxity, and ganglion cyst. There were two loose cemented femurs, one loose cementless femur, one loose cemented tibia, one loose hybrid tibia, one traumatic tibial fracture involving the tibial component, and one case of patellar loosening associated with osteonecrosis.

A review of these reasons for reoperation indicates that cemented and cementless femoral components, cemented tibial components, and cemented three-pegged all-polyethelene patellar components have excellent longevity. Components needing attention are metal-backed patellae, cementless tibias, and polyethylene inserts. Two of these—the metal-backed patella and the cementless tibia—are no longer used in most practices. The tibial insert polyethylene remains as the only significant factor needing attention. This factor is being addressed several ways, including the increased use of mobile-bearing articulations that can

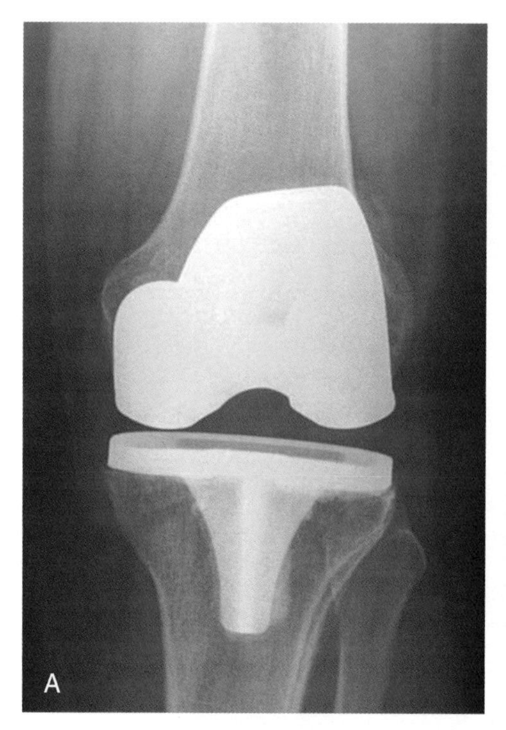

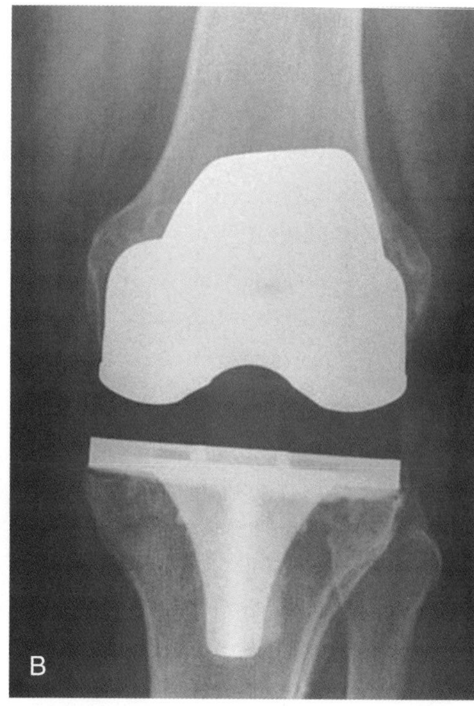

FIGURE 16–5. *A*, Recurrent varus with secondary lateral laxity. *B*, Stabilization achieved with a thicker insert and a medial release to balance the lax lateral side.

TABLE 16–1 116 REASONS FOR REOPERATION ON 2000 KNEES (MEAN 1-YEAR FOLLOW-UP)

- 47 insert wear problems
- 29 insert wear with lysis (most implanted in 1995)
- 7 insert wear without symptoms
- 16 metastatic infections
- 7 metal-backed patellar wear
- 7 broker femoral components
- 5 stiffness requiring arthroscopic manipulation
- 4 recurrent hemathrosis
- 4 recurrent rheumatoid synovitis
- 4 unresurfaced patellar pain
- 3 loose cementless tibias
- 3 traumatic laxity
- 3 atraumatic lateral laxity
- 3 ganglion cysts
- 3 shear-off of patellar lugs
- 2 loose cemented femur
- 1 loose cementless femur
- 1 loose hybrid tibia
- 1 traumatic tibial fracture
- 1 patellar loosening (associated with AVN?)

provide high top-side conformity without imparting constraint to the insert tray interface. Some surgeons are also making more use of nonmodular metal-backed or all-polyethylene tibial components to eliminate the possibility of back-side wear. Finally, all manufacturers are pursuing improvements in the quality and fabrication of polyethylene and modular locking mechanisms to maximize polyethylene performance.

In summary, TKA has a high initial success rate. Patients can expect a successful outcome at 1 year after surgery in up to 99% of cases and the need for reoperation at a rate of approximately 1% per year over the first 15 years.

This chapter was modified from Scott RD: Re-operation after total knee arthroplasty. In Bono JV, Scott RD (eds): Revision Total Knee Arthroplasty. New York, Springer Verlag, 2005, pp 3–9.

References

1. Brick GW, Scott RD: The patellofemoral component of total knee arthroplasty. Clin Orthop 1988;231:163–178.
2. Wright JR, Lima JRN, Scott RD, Thornhill T: Two to four year results of posterior cruciate sparing condylar total knee arthroplasty with an uncemented femoral component. Clin Orthop 1990;260:80–86.
3. Whiteside LA, Fosco DR, Brooks JG Jr: Fracture of the femoral component in cementless total knee arthroplasty. Clin Orthop 1993; 286:160–167.
4. King TV, Scott RD: Femoral component loosening in total knee arthroplasty. Clin Orthop 1985;194:285–290.
5. Schai PA, Thornhill TS, Scott RD: Total knee arthroplasty with the PFC System. J Bone Joint Surg Br 1998;80:850–858.
6. Berger RA, Lyon JH, Jacobs JJ, et al: Problems with cementless total knee arthroplasty at 11 years followup. Clin Orthop 2001; 392:196–207.
7. Bayley JC, Scott RD, Ewald FC, Holmes GB: Failure of the metal-backed patellar component after total knee replacement. J Bone Joint Surg Am 1988;70:668–674.
8. Buechel FF, Rosa RA, Pappas MJ: A metal-backed rotating-bearing patella prosthesis to lower contact stress: an 11-year clinical study. Clin Orthop 1989;248:34–49.
9. Levitsky KA, Harris W, McManus J, Scott RD: Total knee arthroplasty without patellar resurfacing. Clin Orthop 1993;286:116–121.
10. Kim BS, Reitman RD, Schai PA, Scott RD: Selective patellar nonresurfacing in total knee arthroplasty. Clin Orthop 1999;367:81–88.
11. Kindsfater K, Scott RD: Recurrent hemarthrosis after total knee arthroplasty. J Arthroplasty 1995;10 Suppl:S52–S55.
12. Gibbon AJ, Wardell SR, Scott RD: Synovial cyst of the proximal tibiofibular joint with peroneal nerve compression after total knee arthroplasty. J Arthroplasty 1999;14:766–768.

CHAPTER 17

Unicompartmental Knee Arthroplasty

In theory, unicompartmental knee arthroplasty (UKA) is an attractive alternative to osteotomy and total knee arthroplasty (TKA) in selected osteoarthritic patients. Advantages of UKA over osteotomy include a higher initial success, fewer early complications, greater longevity, better cosmetic limb alignment, easier conversion to TKA, and the potential to perform bilateral procedures on the same day. Later conversion of osteotomy to TKA is potentially complicated by many factors (see Chapter 10).

Advantages of UKA over TKA include the preservation of both cruciate ligaments, resulting in more normal knee kinematics and potential for a higher level of performance. Bone stock is preserved in the opposite and patellofemoral compartments, allowing easier conversion to TKA should this be necessary. Initial reports from my institution did not confirm that UKA conversion was necessarily an easy procedure.[1] A later report, however, showed that if the UKA was done in a conservative fashion, conversion was easy and results were the same as those for primary TKA.[2] Potential revision problems involved in osteotomy, TKA, and UKA conversion are listed in Table 17–1. In UKA, the only potential revision problem should be medial tibial plateau deficiency treated with bone graft or metal wedge augmentation (see Chapter 12).

Despite these arguments, UKA has been a controversial procedure since its introduction in the early 1970s. Initial reports were discouraging regarding UKA in medial compartment osteoarthritis.[3,4] A few years later, R. Santore and I published more favorable results using the unicondylar prosthesis.[5] We studied 100 knees with 2- to 6-year follow-up. There had been three reoperations, for an incidence of revision of roughly 1% per year at this short follow-up. The average flexion was 114 degrees, significantly better than any contemporary report using bicompartmental arthroplasty. When the same series was followed at 5 to 9 years (mean 7 years), there had been seven revisions, for a revision rate continuing at 1% per year.[6] The total condylar experience at that time for the same follow-up also showed a revision rate of 1% per year.[7] Armed with this information, our enthusiasm for unicompartmental arthroplasty began to grow. We felt that when the knee was exposed for arthroplasty and the patient fulfilled the criteria for unicompartmental replacement, it was reasonable to perform this procedure on these patients. By the early 1980s, approximately 10% of my patients with osteoarthritis underwent unicompartmental replacement.

Reasons for failure of UKA included patient selection, prosthetic design, and surgical technique. We learned the lesson that patients with lateral compartment arthritis and a lax medial collateral ligament (MCL) could not be stabilized by a unicompartmental procedure (Fig. 17–1). We also began to see failures in obese patients. These were due to either

TABLE 17–1 REVISION PROBLEMS SEEN IN OSTEOTOMY, TKA, AND UKA CONVERSION

	Tibial Osteotomy	TKA	UKA
Unusable prior incision	+	–	–
Poorly accessible prior hardware	+	–	–
Joint line angle distortion	+/–	+/–	–
Malunion	+/–	–	–
Nonunion	+/–	–	–
Patella baja	+/–	+/–	–
Offset tibial shaft	+/–	–	–
Deficient femoral bone	–	+	–
Deficient patellar bone	–	+	–
Deficient lateral tibial bone	+/–	+	–
Deficient medial tibial bone	+/–	+	+/–

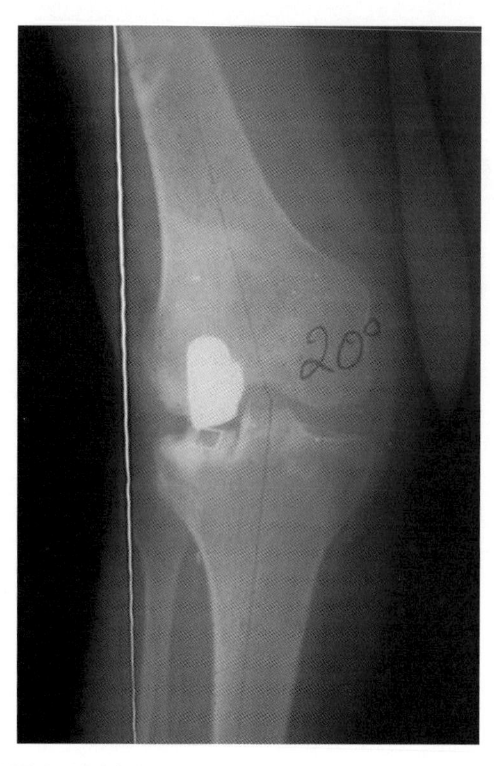

FIGURE 17–1. UKA failed to restore stability to this severe valgus knee with medial collateral ligament laxity.

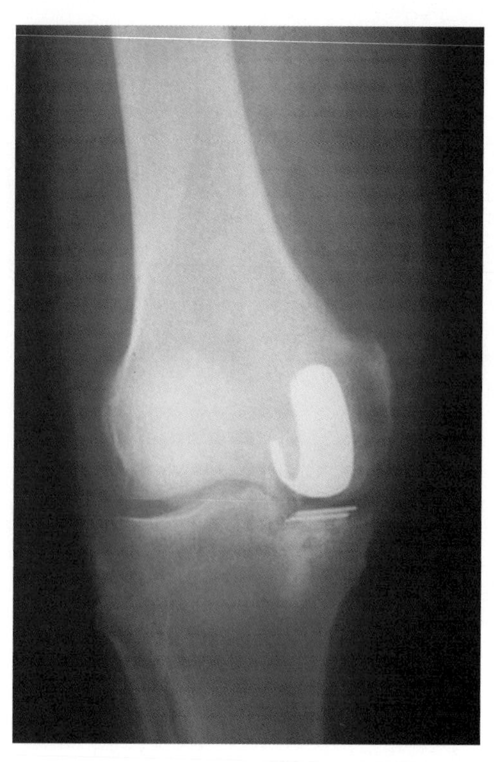

FIGURE 17–2. Subsidence of the femoral component in a heavy patient.

tibial or femoral loosening. We saw some femoral component loosening by subsidence into the subchondral bone (Fig. 17–2). The force across the knee in level gait is approximately three times body weight. This force is ideally distributed evenly to the medial and lateral compartment over the surface area provided by each compartment. The pounds per square inch increases if more pounds and fewer square inches are covered by the prosthetic components. The relatively small size of early UKA components, therefore, made them vulnerable to loosening in heavy patients.

To address this issue, Peter Walker and I redesigned the unicondylar prosthesis to the Brigham unicompartmental knee in 1981 (Fig. 17–3). The femoral component was made 5 mm wider to better cap the subchondral bone and resist subsidence. The tibial component was a nonmodular, metal-backed component with a composite thickness starting at 6 mm (Fig. 17–4). The articulation was flat-on-flat to diminish stress on the polyethylene and increase surface contact. We used this prosthesis exclusively for the next 8 or 9 years. The specifics of its design and surgical technique taught us more important lessons about unicompartmental arthroplasty.[8]

Because the articulation was flat-on-flat, it became apparent that imprecise surgical technique was unforgiving. If the component articulating surfaces were not parallel during weightbearing, edge-loading would occur, leading to accelerated wear of the polyethylene (Fig. 17–5). We also learned that mediolateral and rotational congruity between the components must be assessed in extension rather than flexion. Through the classic median parapatellar approach with patellar eversion, the tibia is artificially externally rotated in flexion owing to the force of the everted quadriceps. Normally, of course, the tibia tends to internally rotate in flexion. If component congruency is assessed in flexion, it will give an inaccurate view of component congruency when the quadriceps is relocated and the patient bears weight in extension.

Modes of failure during this era were most frequently secondary to wear, loosening, and degeneration of the opposite compartment. The flat-on-flat articulation highlighted the problem of edge-loading as a cause for wear. The specific design of the Brigham nonmodular metal-backed tibial component also showed the importance of having an adequate thickness of polyethylene in the articulating area. The "6-mm" Brigham tibial component consisted of a 2-mm-thick titanium metal backing with 4 mm of polyethylene. The coupling of the polyethylene to the tray was designed in a manner that provided this full 4 mm in the middle 60% of the articulation, but only 2 mm of polyethylene in the anterior and posterior 20% of the components. Although most of these 6-mm components survived for at least 6 or 7 years after implantation,[9] a significant number began to wear through by the end of the first decade (Fig. 17–6). This complication occurred when the articulating pattern of the arthroplasty replicated the preoperative articulating pattern of the arthritic knee. As described by White and colleagues,[10] this is most frequently an anteromedial wear pattern. This pattern would bring the femoral component onto an area of the tibial component with only 2 mm of polyethylene thickness and often at the right-angle metallic junction between the 2- and 4-mm depths.[11]

We now realize that all fixed-bearing UKA designs are subject to this wear pattern. Attempts to address this issue by providing fixed bearings with more conforming articulations failed because the increased constraint transmitted too much

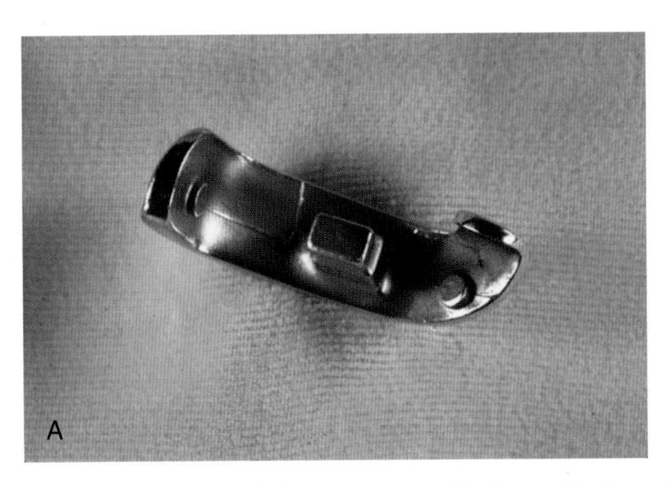

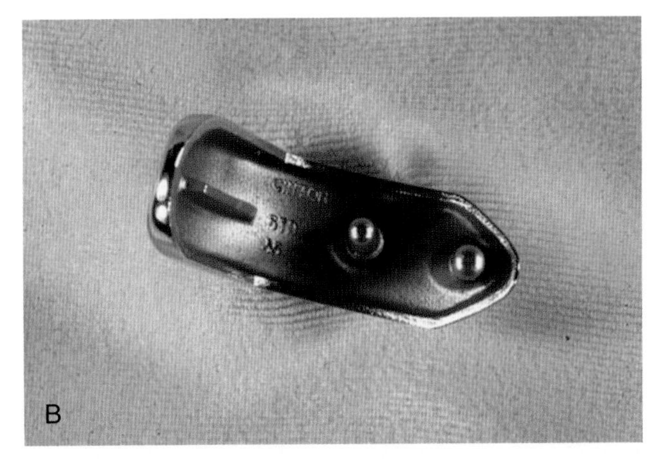

FIGURE 17–3. *A*, The relatively narrow runner of the Unicondylar femoral component made it vulnerable to subsidence. *B*, The Brigham knee was 5 mm wider to better cap the subchondral bone and resist subsidence.

force to the fixation interface. Failures were seen on both the femoral and tibial sides, and there was an increased incidence of tibial radiolucent lines with more conforming articulations.[12] If a conforming insert is used to address topside wear, the system must be one of a mobile-bearing design to eliminate the adverse effects of constraint on the fixation interface.[13]

Degeneration of the opposite compartment is a second mechanism of failure in UKA designs implanted today. This complication is usually late, occurring after the first decade, unless the UKA was overcorrected (Fig. 17–7). The ideal corrected alignment following medial unicompartmental replacement is probably somewhere between 2 and 5 degrees of valgus. Varus malalignment of the limb secondary to medial unicompartmental arthritis is best corrected by removal of peripheral osteophytes from the femur and tibia that tent-up the MCL and medial capsule (Fig. 17–8). Adequate passive correction of the deformity is usually achievable after osteophyte débridement (see Chapter 18).

CLASSIC SELECTION CRITERIA

In 1989, S. Kozinn and I reported on the ideal candidate for unicompartmental arthroplasty. Criteria included an elderly patient, noninflammatory osteoarthritis, a mechanical axis

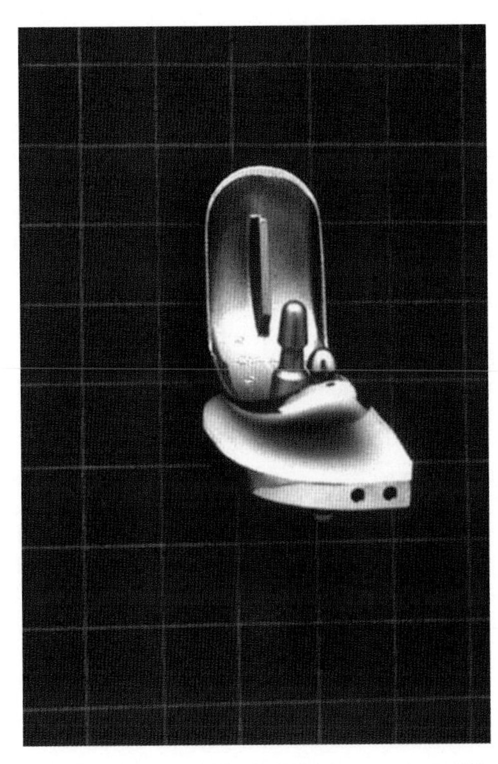

FIGURE 17–4. The 6-mm metal-backed tibial component of the Brigham knee had only 2 mm of polyethylene in parts of its articulating surface.

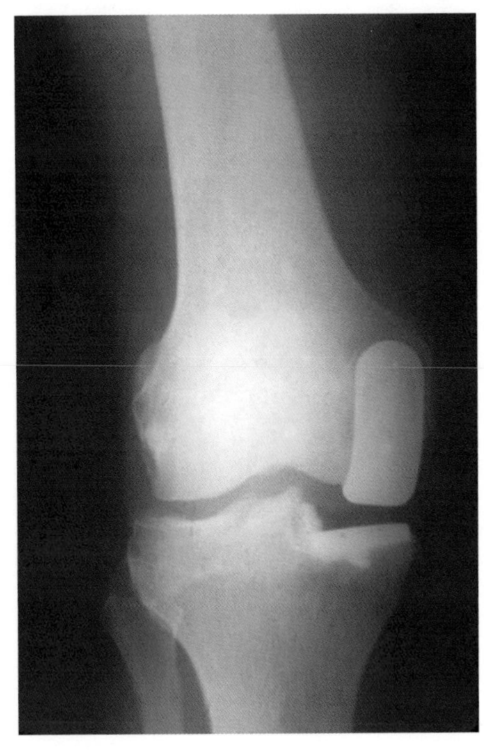

FIGURE 17–5. Poor surgical technique can lead to edge-loading of a flat-on-flat articulation.

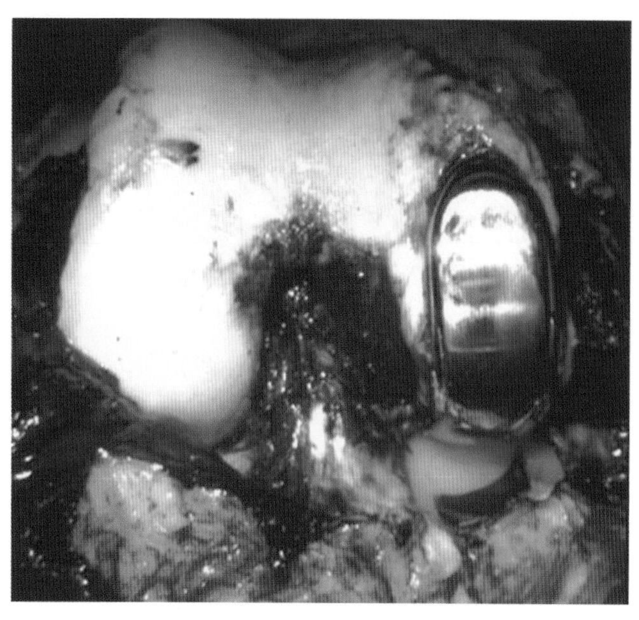

FIGURE 17–6. Wear-through of a composite 6-mm Brigham UKA.

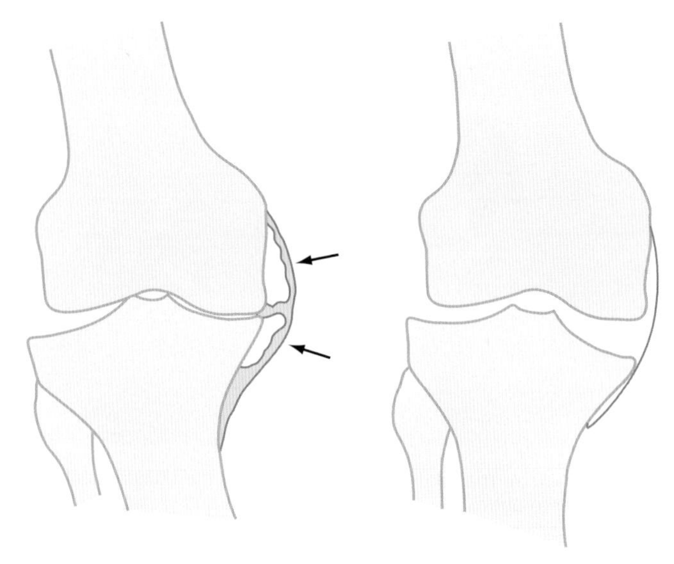

FIGURE 17–8. *A*, Peripheral osteophytes tent-up the medial collateral ligament and medial capsule. *B*, Removal of peripheral osteophytes allows passive correction of the deformity.

deformity of less than 10 degrees of varus or 5 degrees of valgus, an intact anterior cruciate ligament (ACL) without mediolateral subluxation, a flexion contracture less than 15 degrees, a body weight less than 80 to 90 kg, and patellofemoral changes not greater than grade II or III.[14] Several years later, Stern and colleagues studied their osteoarthritic patient population and found that 6% of patients fulfilled all these selection criteria.[15] Coincidentally, approximately 6% of the knee arthroplasty market received unicompartmental replacement. This percentage remained relatively stable until the advent of minimally invasive surgery at the beginning of the 21st century. Enthusiasm for the procedure began to grow quickly, perhaps to a point where some perspective was lost regarding indications for the procedure.

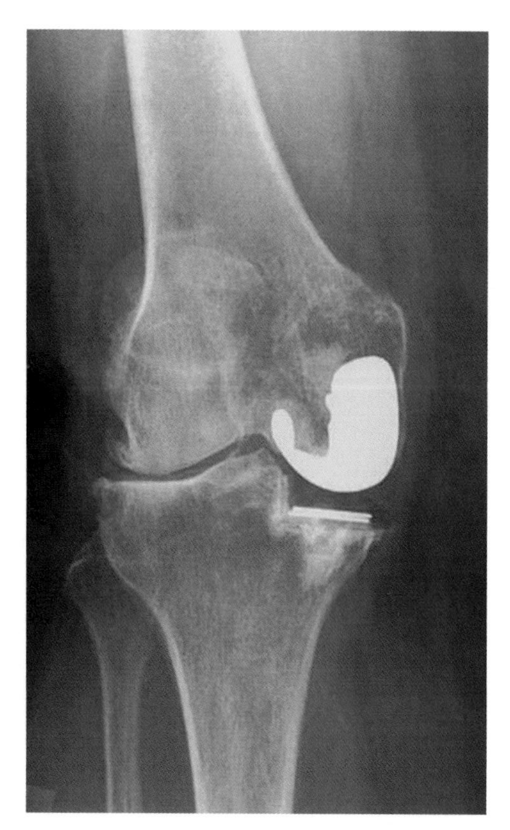

FIGURE 17–7. Secondary degeneration of the lateral compartment 24 years after the initial surgery.

My own perspective changed somewhat when we examined our second decade survivorship in unicompartmental devices implanted in the mid-1970s.[6] Although the reoperation rate progressed for the first decade at roughly 1% per year of follow-up, the need for revision surgery appeared to grow faster in the second decade than that seen for bicompartmental replacement. This made me question the advisability of performing UKA in patients with approximately 15 to 20 years of life expectancy. These patients would have a greater statistical chance of requiring no further surgery throughout the remainder of their lifetime with TKA rather than UKA. Using this rationale, I began to stratify my UKA candidates into two categories. The first would be a middle-aged patient, especially female, and the second would be an octogenarian. I began to think about the procedure as the first arthroplasty in middle-aged patients that would buy them 10 or more years of longevity with an easy conversion to TKA when that was inevitably necessary in later life. They would benefit from a high initial success, few early complications relative to high tibial osteotomy (HTO), an acceptable cosmetic appearance relative to HTO, preservation of both cruciate ligaments relative to TKA, and an easier revision in comparison with both HTO and TKA.

Advantages for the octogenarian would include faster recovery, less blood loss, less medical morbidity, and a less expensive procedure to be borne by the health care system. Given the life expectancy and activity level of octogenarians, the UKA would be unlikely to require revision in their lifetime.

We have reported a small experience with UKA in patients under the age of 60 years.[12] There were only 28 knees in the study with a 2- to 6-year follow-up. Ninety percent had good to excellent results, but there had been two revisions in heavy, active males due to femoral component loosening. This series was generated at a time when we were using conforming femorotibial geometry, which we now know can promote too much stress at the fixation interface. This prosthetic design issue diminishes the significance of this series.

MINIMALLY INVASIVE UKA

At this writing, minimally invasive UKA (MIU) is fueling a trend toward increasing the number of UKAs.[16] The advantages of this technique include less time in hospital with a faster recovery and faster return to work and recreational activities. This reopens the potential indications for UKA to all age groups from middle-aged on. Disadvantages include the fact that the technique for UKA is demanding in the first place. Technical errors in implantation will be more frequent with limited exposure and lead to a higher incidence of early and late failures. Intuitively, these errors will occur more frequently in inexperienced hands. I personally prefer a "moderately invasive" technique for unicompartmental arthroplasty, as discussed in Chapter 18.

METALLIC UNICOMPARTMENTAL HEMIARTHROPLASTY

Metallic hemiarthroplasty of the knee has been available for more than 50 years in the form of the McKeever or McIntosh prosthesis (Fig. 17–9). I have 30 years of experience with selective use of the McKeever technique.[17–19] This method is being revisited by a technique called the UniSpacer.[20] In my experience, metallic hemiarthroplasty is indicated in approximately 1% of my patients. The indications would be a patient in whom an osteotomy would normally be considered, but there is early disease in the opposite compartment or poor range of motion that would not be improved by osteotomy. In addition, the patient would be considered too young, too heavy, or too active for metal-to-plastic knee arthroplasty.[19] Advantages of the metallic arthroplasty are its conservative technique, allowing easy conversion to any other type of arthroplasty. In addition, activity tolerance is permitted. In a review of 24 of my patients under the age of 60 years at the time of arthroplasty with minimum 12-year follow-up, half the knees are still functioning well at average 17-year follow-up. Both Knee Society knee scores and function scores[21] are in the 90s. One patient at 10 years after bilateral McKeever surgery played ice hockey twice a week (Fig. 17–10). A second patient skied daily for 10 years on a resort ski rescue team and was easily converted after 10 years to a metal-to-plastic UKA. Ten years after revision, she still was an active skier.

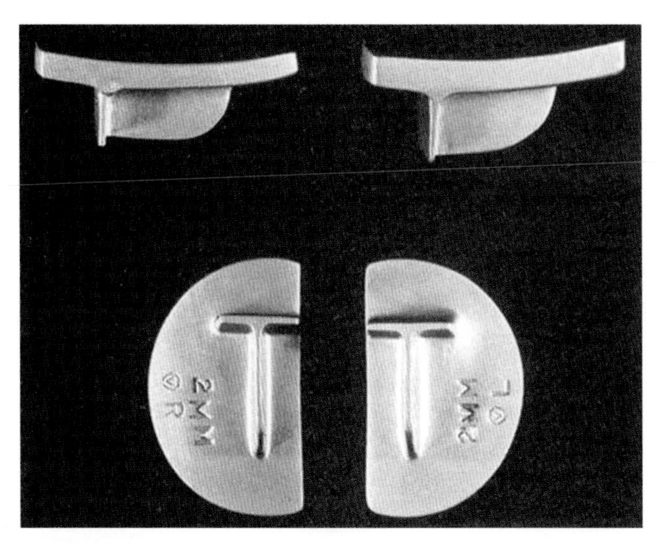

FIGURE 17–9. McKeever metallic hemiarthroplasty components.

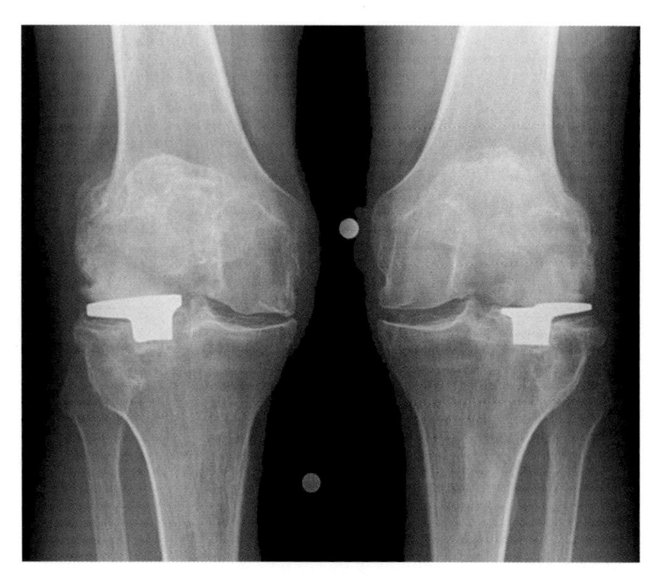

FIGURE 17–10. Ten years after bilateral McKeever arthroplasty, this patient was still playing ice hockey.

SUMMARY

UKA is an attractive alternative to osteotomy or TKA in selected osteoarthritic patients. I would estimate that between 10% and 15% of patients are excellent candidates for this procedure. The operation is being performed in increasing frequency in all age groups, fueled by minimally invasive techniques. To date, there is no peer-reviewed published literature that supports the use of minimally invasive UKA in the young patient.[22,23] The future will bring better surgical techniques and prosthetic designs to minimize the late complication of wear. Mobile-bearing articulations show promise in improving longevity by decreasing wear complications, but the composite thickness of the tibial component required by current FDA regulations eliminates its conservative nature on the tibial side.

References

1. Barrett WP, Scott RD: Revision of failed unicondylar unicompartmental knee arthroplasty. J Bone Joint Surg Am 1987;69:1328–1335.

2. Levine WN, Ozuna RM, Scott RD, Thornhill TS: Conversion of failed modern unicompartmental arthroplasty to total knee arthroplasty. J Arthroplasty 1996;11:797–801.
3. Insall J, Walker P: Unicondylar knee replacement. Clin Orthop 1976;120:83–85.
4. Laskin RS: Unicompartmental tibiofemoral resurfacing arthroplasty. J Bone Joint Surg Am 1978;60:182–185.
5. Scott RD, Santore RF: Unicondylar unicompartmental knee replacement in osteoarthritis. J Bone Joint Surg Am 1981;63:536–544.
6. Scott RD, Cobb AG, McQueary FG, Thornhill TS: Unicompartmental knee arthroplasty eight to twelve year follow-up evaluation with survivorship analysis. Clin Orthop 1991;271:96–100.
7. Insall JN, Hood RW, Flawn LB, Sullivan DJ: The total condylar knee prosthesis in gonarthrosis: a five- to nine-year follow-up of the first one hundred consecutive replacements. J Bone Joint Surg Am 1983;65:619–628.
8. Scott RD: Robert Brigham unicondylar knee surgical technique. Techniques Orthop 1990;5:15–23.
9. Kozinn S, Marx C, Scott RD: Unicompartmental knee arthroplasty: a 4.5 to 6 year follow-up study with a metal-backed tibial component. J Arthroplasty 1989;4 Suppl:S1–S10.
10. White SH, Ludkowski PF, Goodfellow JW: Anteromedial osteoarthritis of the knee. J Bone Joint Surg Br 1991;73:582–586.
11. McCallum JD, Scott RD: Duplication of medial erosion in unicompartmental knee arthroplasties. J Bone Joint Surg Br 1995;77:726–728.
12. Schai PA, Suh JT, Thornhill TS, Scott RD: Unicompartmental knee arthroplasty in middle-aged patients. J Arthroplasty 1998;13:365–372.
13. Goodfellow J, O'Connor J, Murray DW: The Oxford meniscal unicompartmental knee. J Knee Surg 2002;15(4):240–246.
14. Kozinn SC, Scott RD: Unicondylar knee arthroplasty: current concepts review. J Bone Joint Surg Am 1989;71:145–150.
15. Stern SH, Becker MW, Insall JN: Unicondylar knee arthroplasty: an evaluation of selection criteria. Clin Orthop 1993;286:143–148.
16. Repicci JA, Hartman JF: Minimally invasive unicondylar knee arthroplasty for the treatment of unicompartmental osteoarthritis: an outpatient arthritic bypass procedure. Orthop Clin North Am 2004;35:201–216.
17. Scott RD: The mini incision uni: more for less? Orthopedics 2004;27:483.
18. Scott RD, Joyce MJ, Ewald FC, Thomas WH: McKeever metallic hemiarthroplasty of the knee in unicompartmental degenerative arthritis. J Bone Joint Surg Am 1985;57:203–207.
19. Scott RD: The UniSpacer. Clin Orthop 2003;416:164–166.
20. Hallock RH, Fell BM: Unicompartmental tibial hemiarthroplasty: early results of the UniSpacer knee. Clin Orthop 2003;416:154–163.
21. Insall JN, Dorr LD, Scott RD, Scott WN: Rationale of the Knee Society rating system. Clin Orthop 1989;248:13–14.
22. Deshmukh RV, Scott RD: Unicompartmental knee arthroplasty: long term results. Clin Orthop 2001;392:272–278.
23. Deshmukh RV, Scott RD: Unicompartmental knee arthroplasty for young patients. Clin Orthop 2002;404:108–112.

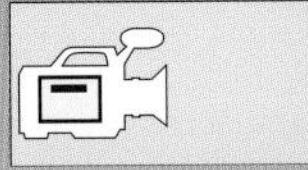

C H A P T E R 18

Unicompartmental Knee Arthroplasty Technique

Before proceeding with unicompartmental knee arthroplasty (UKA), the surgeon must decide at arthrotomy whether the patient is an appropriate candidate. Both cruciate ligaments should be intact, although a deficient anterior cruciate ligament (ACL) occasionally is acceptable if certain criteria are fulfilled. These criteria include a tibial wear pattern that remains in the anterior two thirds of the tibial plateau. A posterior wear pattern represents unacceptable ACL deficiency. There should be no evidence of significant mediolateral tibiofemoral subluxation. Finally, if UKA is performed in an ACL-deficient knee, little or no posterior slope should be applied to the tibial resection during surgery to discourage a posterior wear pattern from evolving.

Changes no greater than grade I[1] should be present in the opposite compartment. The patellofemoral compartment can have up to grade III changes, but the presence of eburnated bone is probably a contraindication to the procedure. Significant inflammatory synovitis is a contraindication as is the presence of crystalline disease in the form of gout or pseudogout.

The technique that follows is as generic as possible regarding UKA. Each prosthetic design will have individualized features regarding alignment and cutting jigs and modes of prosthetic fixation such as lugs or fins.

BASIC PRINCIPLES

A significant advantage of UKA is its potentially conservative nature. It preserves both cruciate ligaments, the opposite compartment, and the patellofemoral articulation. If the prosthetic design and surgical technique remain conservative, bone also is preserved in the compartment being resurfaced. My goal is to prepare a unicompartmental replacement in such a way that no augmentation methods will be necessary at the time of any future revision. The only possible deficiency would occur in a medial compartment replacement on the tibial side due to subsidence of the tibial component. Fortunately, osteolysis compromising bone stock is extremely rare in UKA. The following are my basic principles for unicompartmental arthroplasty:

- Conservative tibia-first resection
- Assessment of the resultant extension and flexion gaps
- Equalization of the gaps
- Distal femoral resection in the proper alignment and amount
- Sizing the femur and aligning it relative to the tibia in 90 degrees of flexion
- Completion of the femoral preparation
- Sizing, orienting, and completing tibial preparation
- Confirmation of limb alignment and component orientation with trial implantation of the real components
- Implantation of real components

PREOPERATIVE PLANNING

To accomplish a conservative tibia-first preparation, the preoperative anteroposterior (AP) radiographs should be utilized to plan the level of the resection. A conservative resection line is drawn on the radiograph at 90 degrees to the long axis of the tibia (Fig. 18–1). The level of this resection is determined on the lateral side 8 to10 mm below the joint line. The level of the initial tibial resection should be no lower than this line whether it is for a medial or a lateral compartment arthroplasty. For medial compartment replacement, the resection begins where this line intersects with the most peripheral aspect of the plateau. For most knees, this will be somewhere between 0 and 2 mm of resection. This amount of resection makes sense, since for every millimeter of elevation of the joint line from the periphery of the

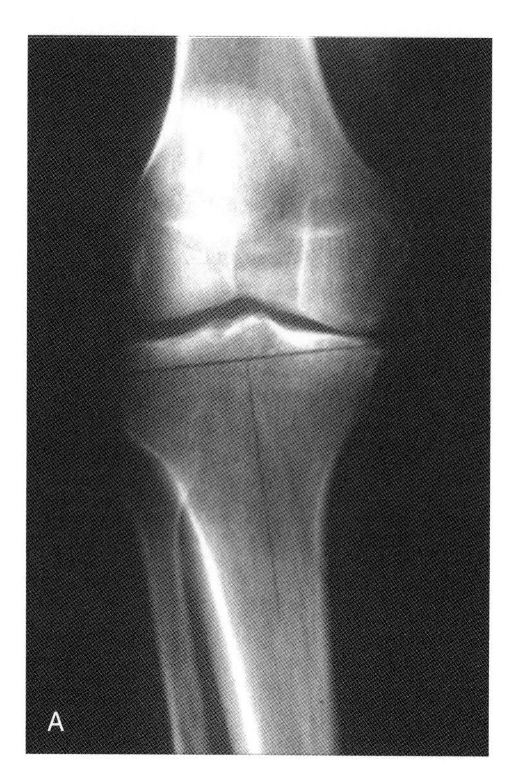

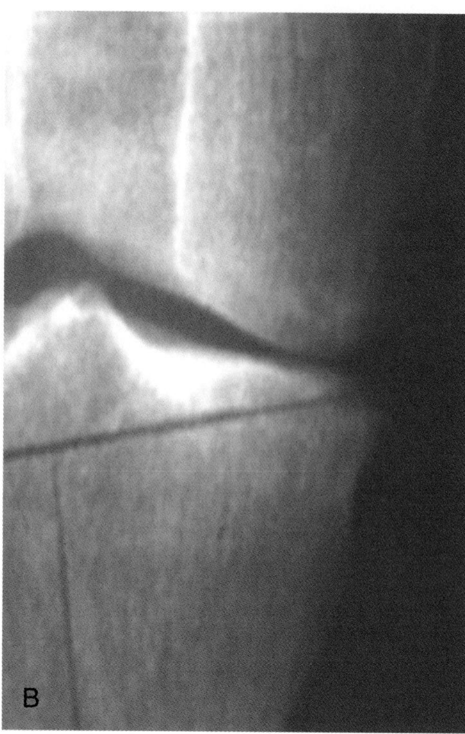

FIGURE 18–1. *A,* Preoperative planning involves drawing a conservative resection for total knee arthroplasty. *B,* An initial conservative medial resection.

plateau, 1 degree of correction is obtained. Therefore, if the peripheral resection is 0 and a 7-mm tibial component is utilized, approximately 7 degrees of correction will be achieved. This would take a typical UKA candidate in 3 degrees of anatomic varus back to 4 degrees of anatomic valgus (Fig. 18–2).

OPERATIVE EXPOSURE

Traditionally, UKA of the medial side was carried out by a standard total knee exposure using a median parapatellar arthrotomy with complete eversion of the patella. Care would be taken not to derange the anterior horn of the lateral meniscus. This exposure gave the surgeon the opportunity to completely explore the knee and make an intraoperative decision about whether the patient was a candidate for UKA.

Minimally invasive unicompartmental surgery and exposure are now popular.[2] The shorter incisions permit a shorter hospital stay and faster recovery. They have several disadvantages, however.[3] The limited exposure does not allow as complete an assessment of the opposite compartment. It also does not allow as thorough an assessment of component orientation. The result could be malpositioning of components and an increased incidence of both early and late failure of the procedure. There is also concern that the amount of stretching of the skin needed for adequate visualization could lead to an increased incidence of wound healing difficulties and subsequent infection. It is my opinion that a more rapid recovery associated with minimally invasive UKA is not so much due to a short incision but rather to the treatment of the quadriceps mechanism. If the patella is subluxated laterally, rather than everted, rapid recovery is possible.

I use a shorter than normal skin incision approximately 10 to 12 cm in length and begin the arthrotomy approximately 1 cm above the superior pole of the patella. The incision into the joint ends distally at the mid portion of the tibial tubercle. Adequate inspection of the joint can usually

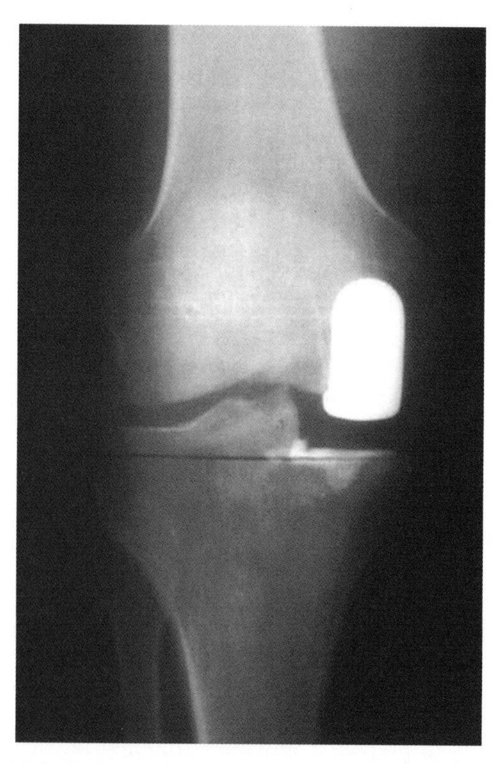

FIGURE 18–2. Postoperative correction can be estimated in degrees by the number of millimeters of polyethylene added to the tibial resection.

be accomplished by flexing the knee 30 to 40 degrees and manually subluxating the patella. Digital palpation of the patella will allow for the detection of eburnated bone on its surface. A retractor such as a bent Hohman is anchored in the intercondylar notch and allows maintenance of the lateral subluxation of the patella during the procedure (Fig. 18–3).

For lateral compartment replacement, many surgeons use a short lateral arthrotomy. My concern with this approach is the fact that a formal lateral parapatellar exposure to the knee would be necessary if the UKA is abandoned for a total knee arthroplasty (TKA). My preference is to use a standard median parapatellar approach for a valgus knee requiring lateral compartment replacement. As the arthrotomy approaches the anterior horn of the medial meniscus, the dissection is taken laterally anterior to the coronary ligament to avoid derangement of the medial meniscus (Fig. 18–4). The patella is everted and the knee flexed. Enough of the fat pad is removed from the anterior aspect of the tibia to expose it for the tibial resection. An incision is made at the mid-coronal plane of the lateral plateau just outside the lateral meniscus for placement of a bent Hohman retractor. Moist wound towels protect the subcutaneous tissue and the medial compartment throughout the remainder of the procedure.

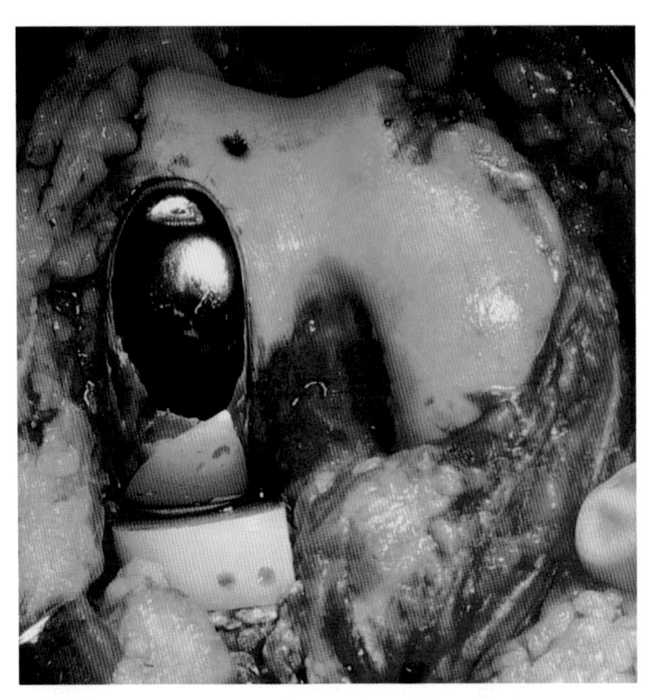

FIGURE 18–4. A medial arthrotomy with preservation of the anterior horn of the medial meniscus provides excellent exposure for a lateral arthroplasty.

Other Elements of the Exposure

Prior to execution of the bony resections, the anatomy should be defined and measures taken to protect the MCL from injury. First, the anterior third of the medial meniscus is removed. This defines an entry point between the deep MCL and the proximal tibial plateau. At this level, a curved 1-cm osteotome is inserted tangential to the plateau with half its surface above and the other half below the level of the plateau. It is then tapped with a mallet along the border of the plateau until it reaches the level of the semimembranosus bursa. This creates a pathway for insertion of a retractor that will protect the MCL during tibial preparation.

As noted above, a bent Hohman-type retractor is placed with its tongue in the intercondylar notch and its blade against the medial border of the patella, subluxating it laterally for adequate exposure of the entire medial femoral condyle. If this exposure is compromised, the arthrotomy can be extended proximally for about a centimeter. Medial and lateral osteophytes are removed to define the true mediolateral dimension of the condyle. Removal of intercondylar osteophytes relieves any potential impingement between them and the tibial spine and provides a pathway for the resection that will take place along the spine. Removal of medial osteophytes releases the MCL and allows passive correction of the deformity.[4]

The chondro-osseous wear pattern on both femur and tibia is defined with a marking pen or electrocautery. This gives an initial guide to the proper rotatory alignment of the femoral and tibial components (Fig. 18–5). Final rotational alignment of each is confirmed as the bone preparation proceeds.

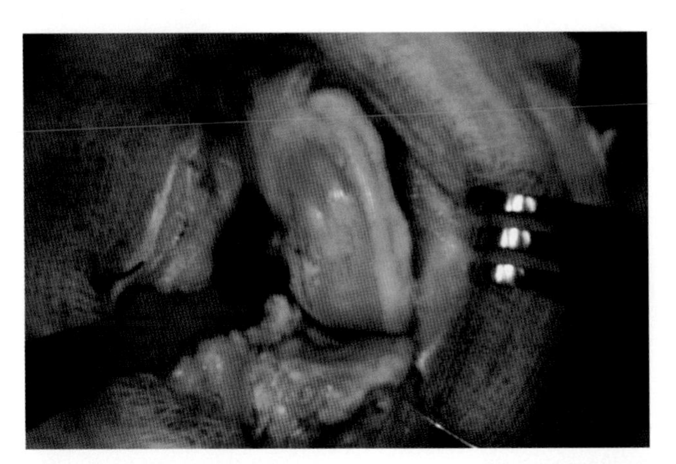

FIGURE 18–3. Excellent exposure is obtained with a short arthrotomy and lateral subluxation of the patella.

PREPARATION OF THE TIBIA

I describe here the technique for an “onlay” type of tibial component. The same general principles of preparation apply for an “inlay” technique.

An external tibial alignment jig is applied, with the level of resection based on the preoperative templating for a conservative cut (see Fig. 18–1). The varus/valgus alignment should be more or less perpendicular to the long axis of the tibia and the amount of initial posterior slope applied between 3 and 5 degrees. The exception to this amount of slope is the rare ACL-deficient knee in which posterior slope is limited to between 0 and 3 degrees.

If the alignment jig is to be stabilized by a fixation pin, I recommend that only one inboard pin be utilized. Outboard pins that come close to the medial cortex are associated with

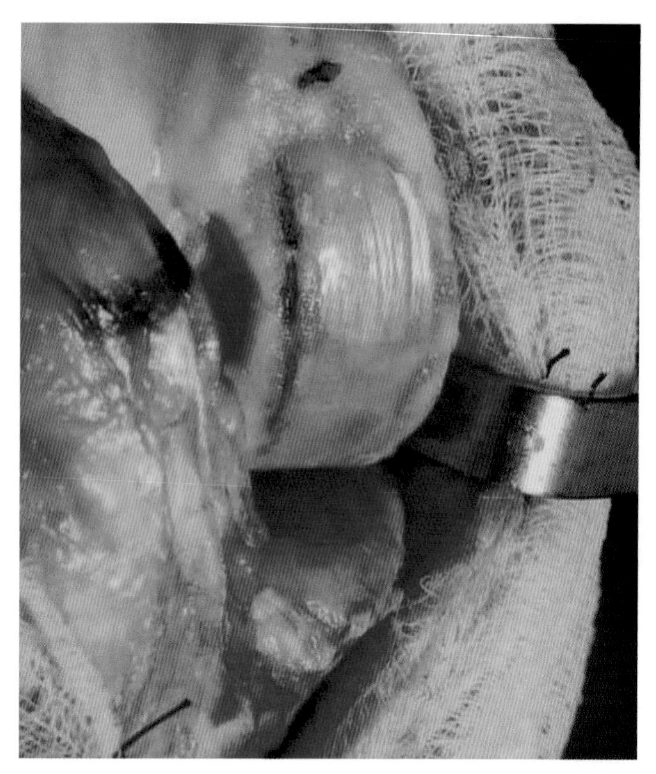

FIGURE 18–5. The chondro-osseous wear pattern provides a good start for determining the rotational alignment of the components.

postoperative stress fractures as are techniques that call for the application of multiple stabilizing pins (Fig. 18–6).[5] It is important to use a narrow oscillating saw blade for this cut to avoid undercutting the tibial spine or injuring medial soft tissues.

Further protection of the medial tissues is afforded by the placement of a 1.5-cm wide retractor into the tissue plane created by the curved 1-cm osteotome in the initial exposure (Fig. 18–7). After completion of the horizontal bone cut, a vertical cut is made along the tibial spine with a reciprocating saw that is parallel to the tibial chondro-osseous wear pattern. Removal of the medial femoral osteophyte creates a pathway for the saw (Fig. 18–8). The lateral placement of this cut is, in general, halfway up the slope of the medial tibial spine. The resected tibial bone is easier to remove with the knee in extension than in flexion because there is usually cartilage remaining posteriorly on both femur and tibia. The resected bone can be grasped with a Kocher clamp while the knee is in flexion and then pulled free when the knee is extended. The resected piece will usually show a wear pattern that is anterior and medial (Fig. 18–9).With the knee now in extension, the thinnest tibial trial is slid into the space created by the tibial resection (Fig. 18–10). If this tibial thickness is correct, the knee should come to full extension and the anatomic alignment should lie between 2 and 5 degrees of valgus. The knee should be stable to valgus stress. It is permissible for the medial side to spring open a millimeter or two with the valgus stress but not remain open by this amount when the stress is released. If the alignment is undercorrected or the medial side is lax, a thicker trial insert is necessary. Alternatively, the distal femoral resection can be less than anatomic to allow tightening of the extension gap. Deciding between these two alternatives depends on the corresponding flexion gap. For example, if both extension gap and flexion gap are loose, a thicker tibial insert is appropriate. If the extension gap is loose but the flexion gap is appropriate, diminished distal femoral resection is recommended.

Once the extension gap has been established, the same thickness of tibial component is given a trial in flexion. The

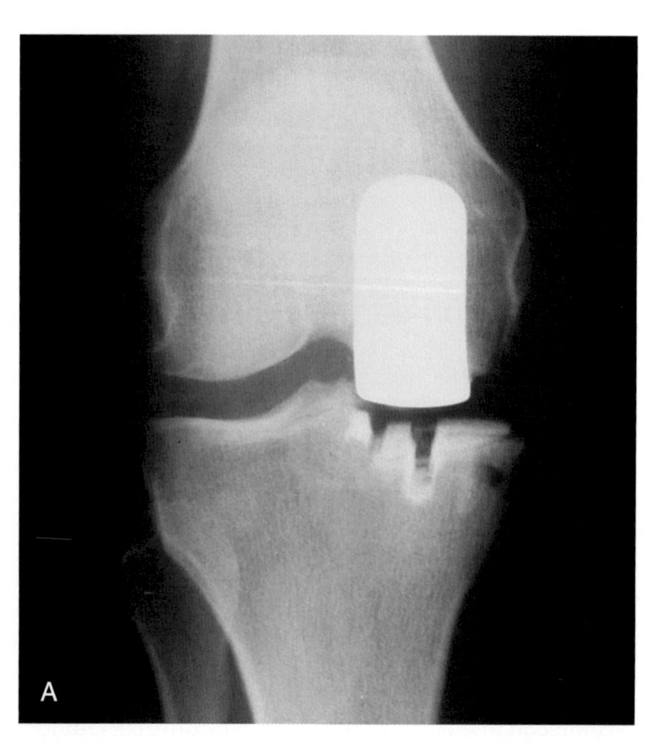

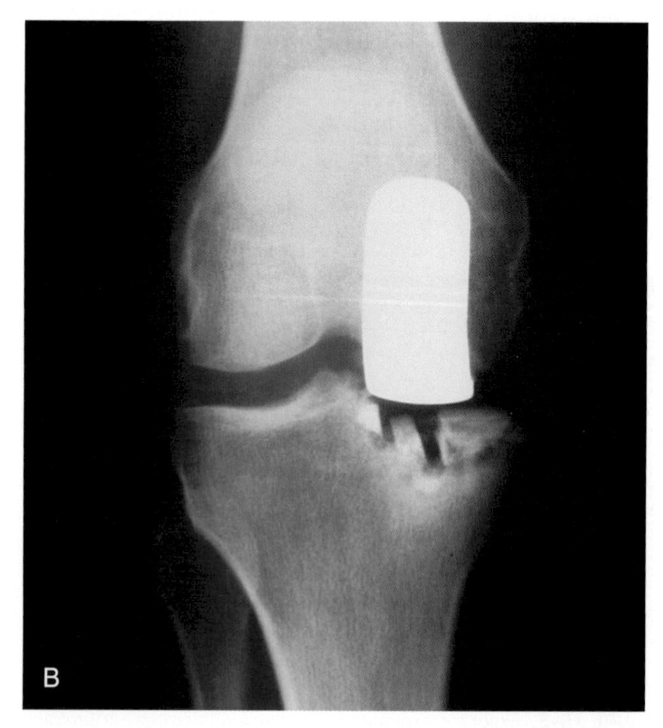

FIGURE 18–6. *A*, A peripheral pinhole for an alignment jig creates a stress riser. *B*, The result can be a stress fracture through the pinhole.

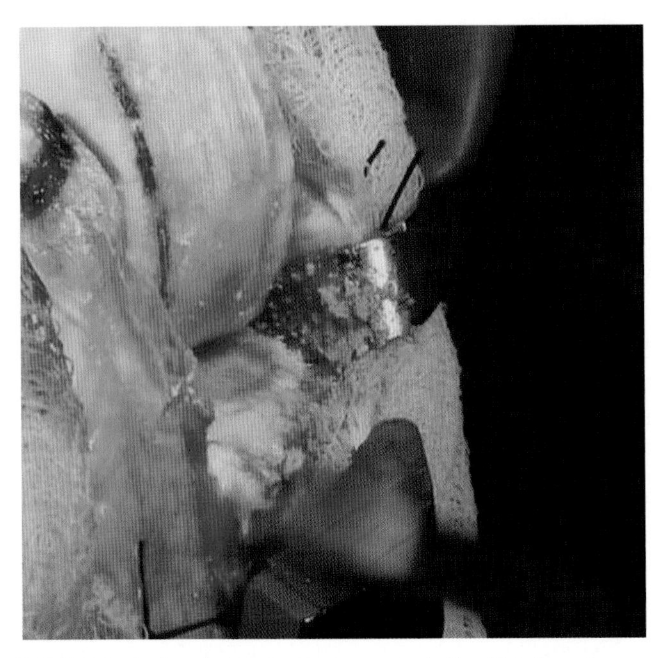

FIGURE 18–7. A well-placed retractor protects the MCL from the saw resecting the proximal tibia.

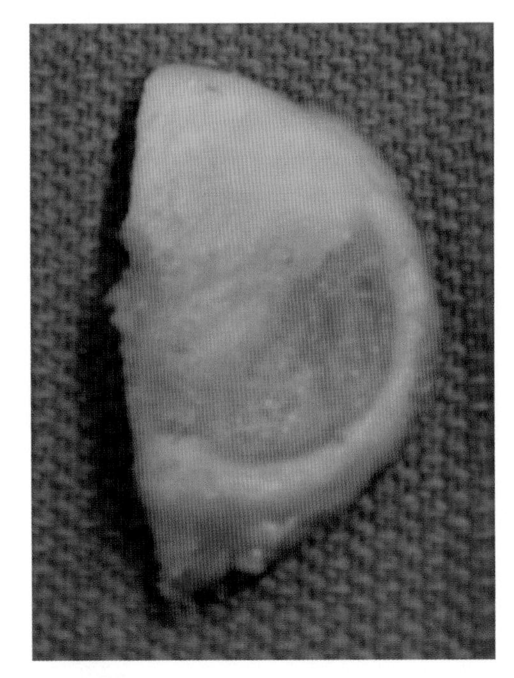

FIGURE 18–9. The typical wear pattern in a varus knee with unicompartmental disease is anterior and medial.

medial retractor should be relaxed during this test or it might create a false sense of tightness. Under ideal circumstances, the appropriate trial for extension stability slides in easily under the posterior condyle with the knee flexed 90 degrees (Fig. 18–11). Erring toward the slightly lax side in flexion is better than erring toward the slightly tight side. To relieve flexion tightness for any given tibial thickness, the trial insert is pushed into the flexion space until it engages the posterior condyle (Fig. 18–12). A line is then drawn parallel to the top side of the insert to show the angle and amount of resection necessary to increase the flexion space. This resection can be performed with the narrow oscillating saw. It usually amounts to 1 or 2 mm and mainly involves removal of residual posterior condylar cartilage.

If both the flexion and extension spaces are too tight, a little more of the tibia may be resected but the surgeon must remain as conservative as possible on the tibial side.

If the spacing is fine in flexion but tight in extension, the surgeon can resect a little more than the anatomic amount of distal femur that corresponds with the thickness of the femoral component. If the gap is fine in flexion but loose in extension, a smaller amount than the thickness of femoral component is resected.

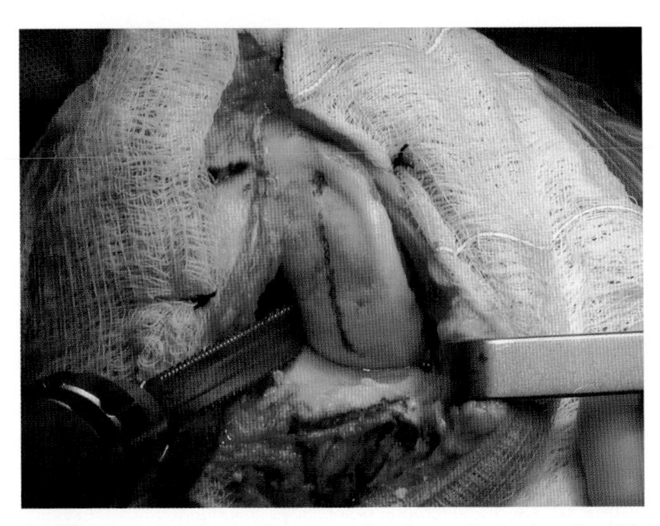

FIGURE 18–8. A reciprocating saw makes the vertical cut on the tibial plateau.

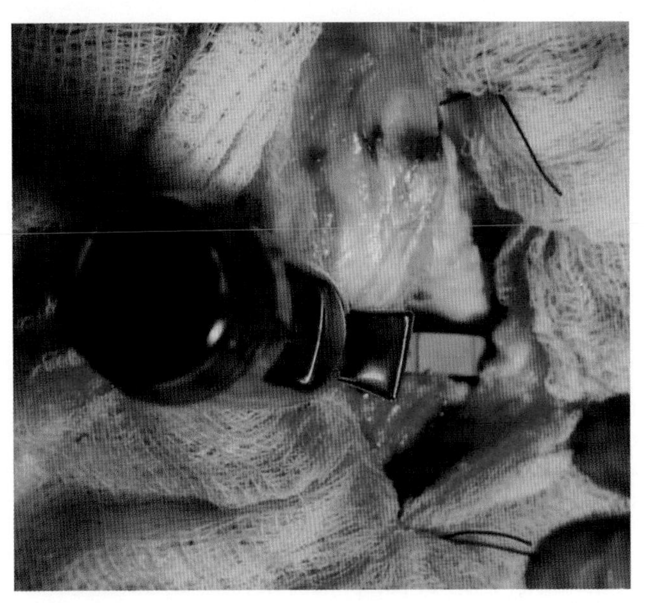

FIGURE 18–10. A trial tibial component is assessed in extension for alignment and stability.

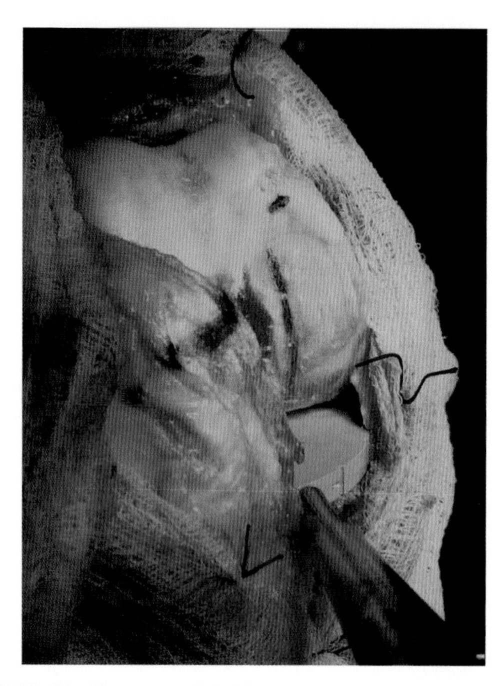

FIGURE 18–11. The same trial tibial component is assessed in flexion.

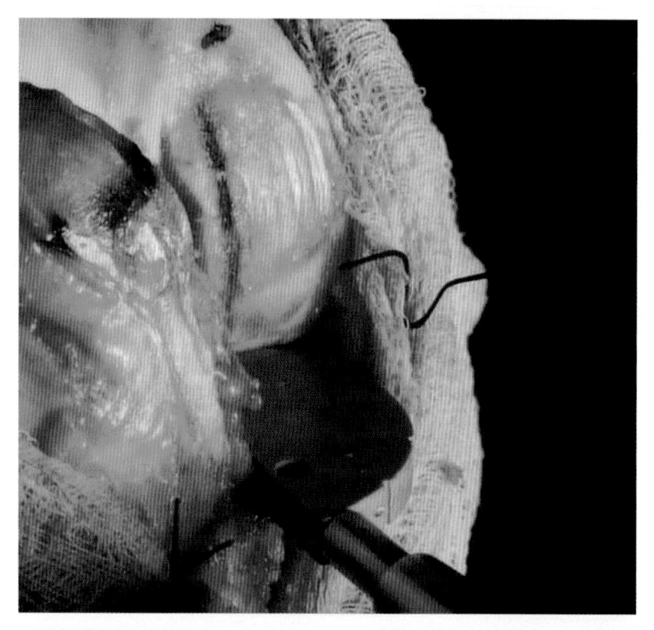

FIGURE 18–12. If the flexion gap is too tight, the trial tibial component is pushed up against the posterior condyle to determine the amount of residual cartilage to be removed to equalize the gaps.

DISTAL FEMORAL RESECTION

Distal femoral resection can be guided by intramedullary or extramedullary alignment. The advantage of intramedullary alignment is its accuracy; its disadvantage is its invasiveness. At the present time, I prefer an extramedullary technique, as described below. Regardless of the technique, the goal is to remove an amount of bone equivalent to the thickness of the metal femoral component in order to attempt to restore the femoral joint line. The ideal angle of resection is probably about 5 degrees of valgus. The forgiveness of varying from this angle depends on the congruency of the femorotibial articulation in the coronal plane. For example, a round-on-round articulation forgives any variation. A flat-on-flat articulation demands complete accuracy in the coronal alignment to avoid any edge-loading of the articulation. Most articulations are a variation of round-on-flat with the amount of forgiveness and the amount of contact area dependent on the difference of the radius of curvature between one articulation and the other.

Intramedullary Femoral Alignment Technique

The medullary canal is entered in a similar way to the technique for TKA. The entry hole is approximately 1 cm above the origin of the posterior cruciate ligament (PCL) in the intercondylar notch. It is often prejudiced several millimeters to the medial side. In minimally invasive techniques, the intramedullary rod can serve to retract the patella.

Extramedullary Femoral Alignment Technique

The varus/valgus alignment of the femoral component is keyed off its relationship with the previously performed tibial resection. The guide has a rectangular spacer block attached to it that is equivalent to the thickness of the tibial component selected to stabilize the knee in extension. The guide is inserted with the knee somewhere between 5 and 15 degrees of flexion, depending on the amount of posterior slope applied to the tibial resection. Hyperextension of the knee while pinning the guide should be avoided because this will impart an extension angle to the resection with resultant extension of the femoral component (Fig. 18–13). Slight flexion can be seen as an advantage because it will enhance metal-to-plastic contact in maximal knee flexion. The guide is pinned to the femur with two fixation pins to

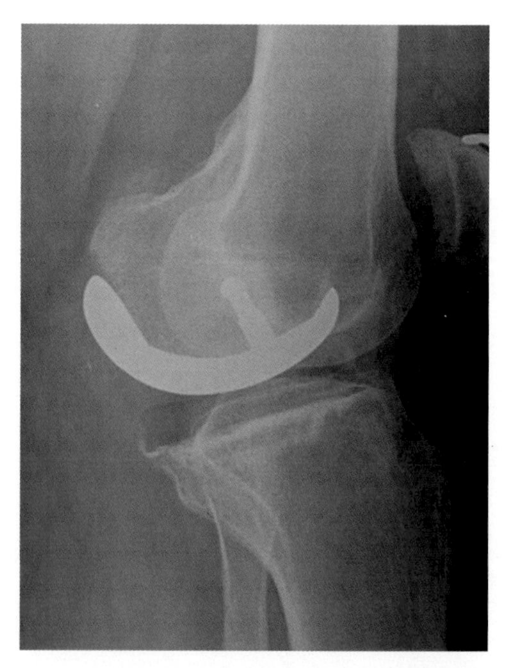

FIGURE 18–13. If the femoral resection is linked to the tibial resection, excessive posterior tibial slope will lead to a hyperextended femoral resection.

create stability. Some surgeons prefer to perform the resection with the knee in extension. A cutting slot in the guide will resect the proper amount of distal condyle to restore the femoral joint line with the femoral component.

An adaptor block can be slid onto the femoral pins to adjust the amount of resection 2 mm proximally or distally depending on the need to either increase or decrease the extension gap.

I prefer to cut the distal femur in flexion to better visualize the progression of the cut. If this technique is chosen in the system I use, the cutting guide that was initially placed in extension must be slid off the pins before the knee is flexed and then slid back into place. Failure to do this may allow the spacer block component of the guide to pry open the knee and possibly avulse the attachment of the ACL.

SIZING OF THE FEMUR

In most UKA systems, any size of femur can be articulated with any size of tibia. For this reason they are sized independently. The size is determined by the AP femoral dimension. For medial replacements, I prefer to use the largest possible size that does not protrude anteriorly and permit patellar impingement during flexion. My rationale is that the larger size will better cap the femoral bone, providing more surface area for fixation and minimizing the chance for femoral component subsidence or loosening. The anatomic landmark for the leading edge of the femoral component is sometimes obvious as the junction between intact trochlear cartilage and eburnated bone on the distal femoral condyle (Fig. 18–14).

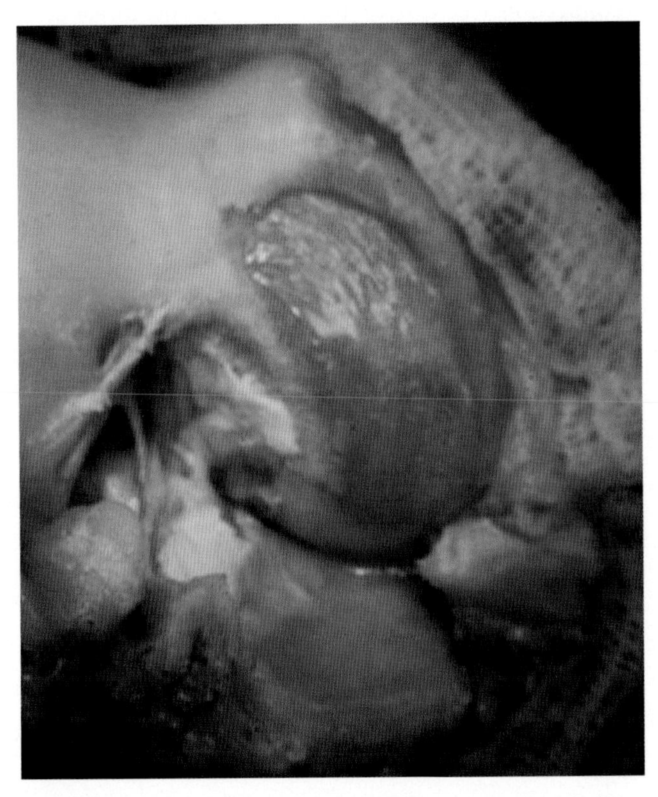

FIGURE 18–14. The leading edge of the femoral component usually extends to the junction between eburnated bone and trochlear cartilage.

If unclear, this landmark can be determined by placing a mark at the estimated spot and then bringing the knee to full extension to confirm that there will be adequate metal-to-plastic contact between the femoral and tibial component with the leg in this position. Virtually all sizing jigs will key off the posterior condyle, with the anterior aspect of the guide mimicking the leading edge of actual femoral component.

ROTATIONAL ALIGNMENT OF THE FEMORAL COMPONENT

The patient's chondro-osseous wear pattern usually suggests the appropriate rotational alignment of the femoral component. Another guide to rotation is to choose an alignment that is perpendicular to the varus/valgus alignment of the tibial component when the knee is flexed to 90 degrees. Choosing this alignment gives maximum congruency between the articulating surfaces in flexion. As in extension, the forgiveness depends on the congruency of the articulating surfaces. Similarly to distal alignment, a flat-on-flat articulation is very unforgiving while a round-on-round articulation is completely forgiving. Most systems are a variation of round-on-flat with the forgiveness again dependent on the difference in radius of curvature between one articulation and the other.

Another critical aspect of femoral component rotation is its effect on the tracking of the components in full extension. The tibial wear pattern of most varus knees undergoing unicompartmental replacement is anterior and peripheral (see Fig. 18–9). If the femoral component is placed in internal rotation, its leading edge will ride on the peripheral aspect of the tibial component in extension, possibly promoting premature wear and loosening (Fig. 18–15). For this reason, the surgeon should usually err toward slight external rotation of the femoral component and bring the leading edge of the femur more laterally in extension.

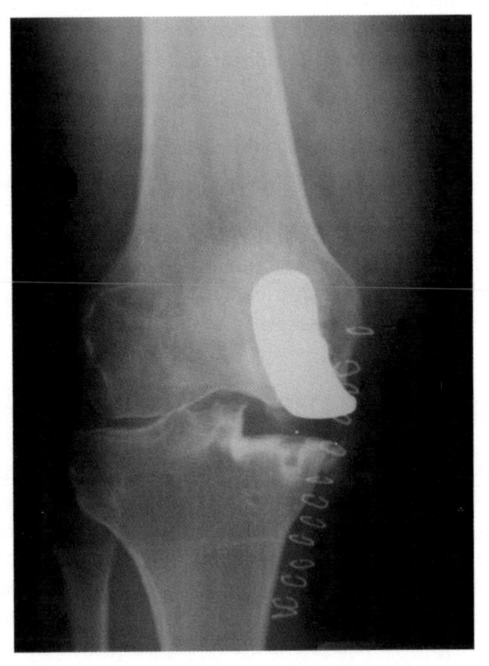

FIGURE 18–15. Internal rotation of the femoral component causes its leading edge to track peripherally.

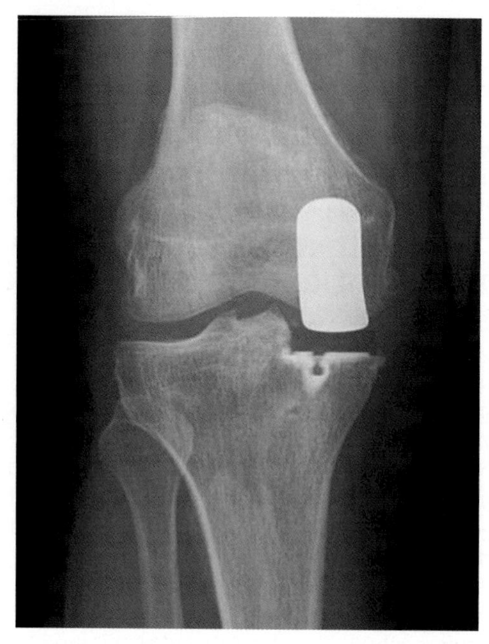

FIGURE 18–16. Erring toward lateral placement of the femoral component improves mediolateral component congruency.

MEDIOLATERAL POSITIONING OF THE FEMORAL COMPONENT

As mentioned above, the usual wear pattern in early osteoarthritis in the varus knee is anterior and peripheral. To avoid adverse effects on the polyethylene due to a return to this wear pattern, the femoral component should be shifted laterally on the condyle (Fig. 18–16). The appropriate amount of shift is determined by checking mediolateral congruency between the femoral and tibial components in full extension before making any fixation holes or slots.

In lateral compartment arthroplasty, the femoral component should also be shifted laterally for a slightly different reason. The periphery of the lateral plateau extends several millimeters beyond the border of the periphery of the lateral femoral condyle. Most surgeons have a tendency to align the tibial component flush with the peripheral cortex. If this is done in a lateral compartment arthroplasty, there will be mediolateral incongruency between the components in extension unless the femoral component is shifted laterally (Fig. 18–17). Alternatively, a larger tibial component in the mediolateral dimension can be utilized, but in most knees the shorter AP dimension of the plateau will not accommodate a larger size.

FINAL PREPARATION OF THE FEMUR

Now that the proper size, rotation, and mediolateral positioning of the femoral component have been determined, the femoral resection can be completed. In most systems, this involves a posterior condylar resection, a posterior chamfer resection, and a partial anterior chamfer resection. In other techniques, a burr is used to prepare a bed for the component, and angle-guided resections are not appropriate. In all cases, a recess must be created for the leading edge of the femoral component to prevent patellar impingement (Fig. 18–18).

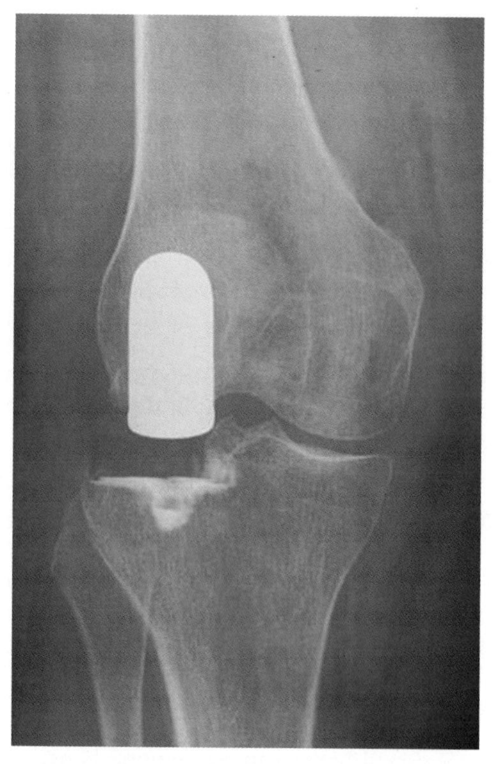

FIGURE 18–17. In a lateral arthroplasty, the femoral component should also be placed laterally for better component congruency.

This recess is more critical in a lateral arthroplasty than in a medial arthroplasty because of the tendency of the patella to track more on the lateral facet during deep flexion. To maximize this recession on the lateral side, the initial distal femoral resection must be adequate (Fig. 18–19). Underresection is most likely to occur when there is residual distal femoral cartilage due to a markedly posterior lateral

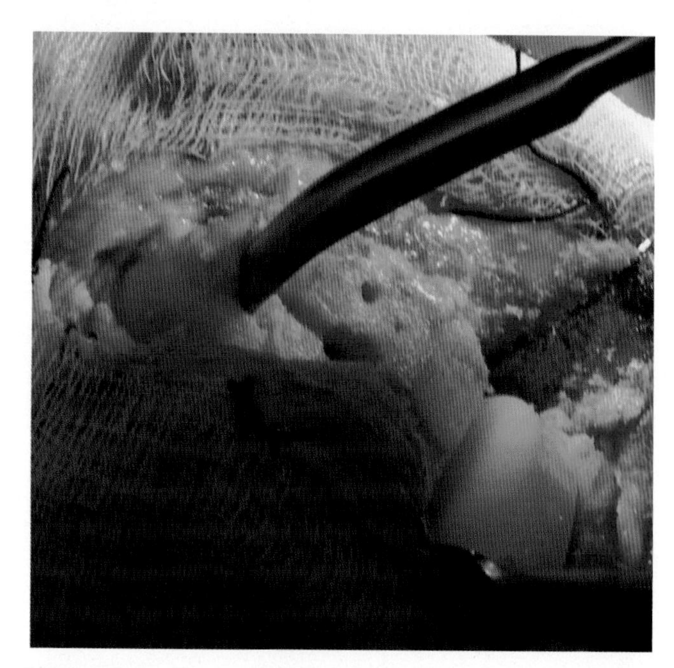

FIGURE 18–18. A recess should be made to countersink the leading edge of the femoral component.

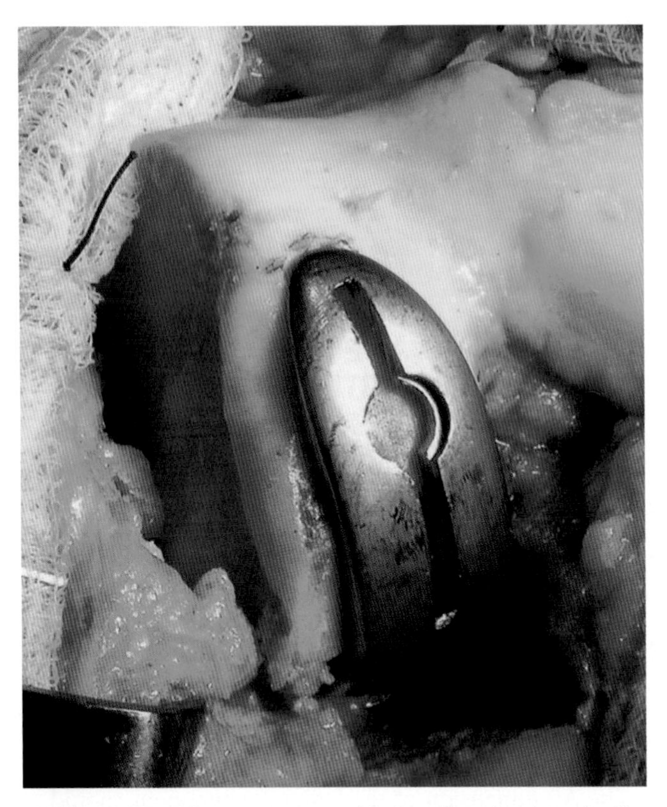

FIGURE 18–19. Failure to remove residual cartilage in a lateral arthroplasty will prevent countersinking the leading edge.

wear pattern or in an arthroplasty necessitated by a lateral tibial plateau fracture. It also is important to err toward undersizing the AP dimension of the femoral component in a lateral arthroplasty to avoid patellar impingement (Fig. 18–20). When undersizing, always check the articulation in full extension to be sure there is adequate metal-to-plastic contact (Fig. 18–21). The final preparation of the femur involves the creation of either lug holes or slots for fixation lugs and fins. These are made through instrument templates provided or possibly through holes or slots on a trial component.

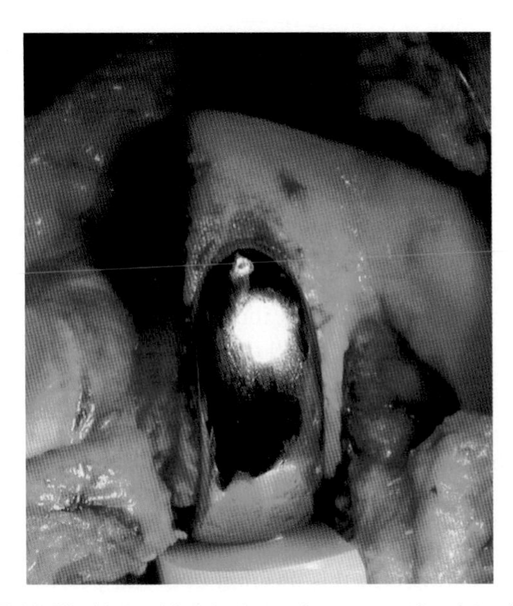

FIGURE 18–20. Undersizing the femoral component in a lateral arthroplasty helps prevent patellar impingement.

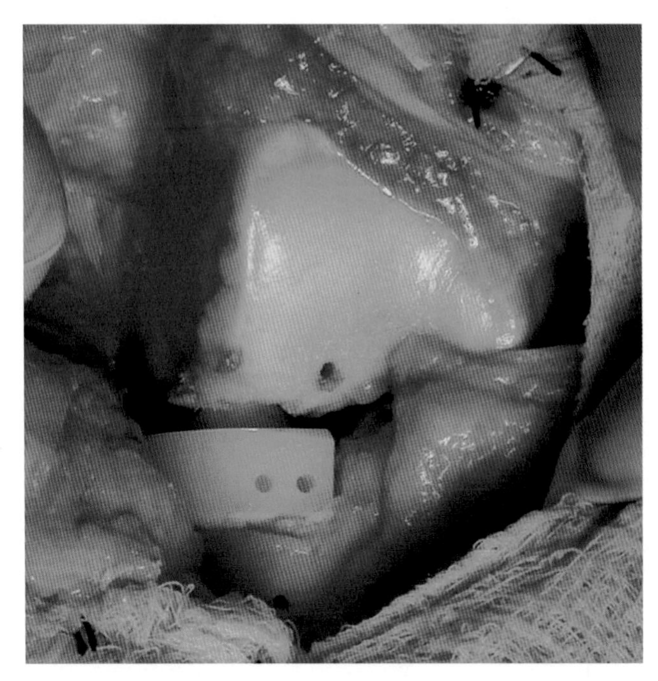

FIGURE 18–21. When undersizing the femur, be certain that there is still adequate metal-to-plastic contact in full extension.

The trial femur is now slid into place on top of the prepared femoral bed. Some systems provide a shim to pressurize the posterior condyle up against the posterior condylar resection. It is important for a good fit be obtained in this section of the prosthesis to resist forces that may promote femoral component loosening. In some systems, the lug fixation is parallel to the posterior condylar resection so that the component is slid into place without the potential to pressurize the cement. In other systems, femoral lugs are angled in such a way that the posterior condyle is compressed as the component is fully seated. In systems in which the fixation lug is parallel to the posterior condyle, it may be helpful to angle the drill for the lug hole in a slightly anterior direction (Fig. 18–22).

This angling will promote slight flexion of the femoral component and compress the posterior condyle. The drill should never be angled posteriorly because this would drive the femoral component into extension and lift the metallic femoral condyle away from the bone.

Once the femur is fully prepared and the trial fully seated, it is helpful to take a curved $\frac{1}{4}$-inch osteotome and outline the back edge of the metallic condyle to define and eventually remove any retained osteophytes or uncapped posterior condylar bone that could cause impingement on the tibial polyethylene during maximum flexion.

FINAL PREPARATION OF THE TIBIAL COMPONENT

Final sizing of the tibial component can now take place. In most systems, the tibia can be sized independently of the femur. I prefer to use the largest size that does not overhang posteriorly or medially in order to maximally cap the cut

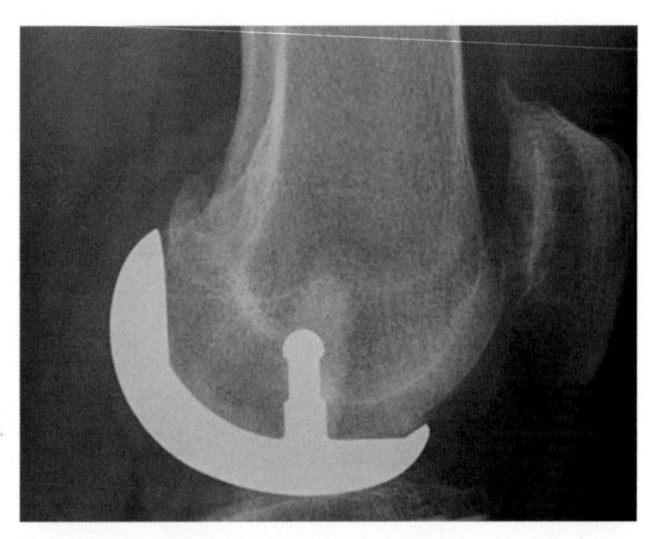

FIGURE 18–22. Angling the drill hole for the fixation lug anteriorly will help pressurize the posterior condyle.

surface of the tibia and decrease focal forces that could promote loosening.

Earlier designs were symmetric so that they could be used on either the medial or lateral compartment in both right and left knees. Asymmetric components are now the rule to allow maximal capping of the cut surface of the tibia. An asymmetric component also provides more polyethylene anteriorly and peripherally to accommodate the common wear pattern in varus osteoarthritic knees. Final mediolateral and rotational positioning of the tibial component is determined by a trial reduction. Congruency should be assessed with the knee in full extension (Fig. 18–23). As noted above, mediolateral congruency is altered by mediolateral placement of the femoral component. Rotational alignment is altered on the tibial side by changing the orientation of the resection along the tibial spine.

If the flexion space is too tight, the tibial component will lift-off anteriorly or the femoral component will lift-off from the distal femoral condylar resection. This can usually be resolved by applying a little more posterior tibial slope to the tibial resection as long as a total posterior slope of approximately 10 degrees is not exceeded. Alternatively, tightness in flexion can be resolved by downsizing the femoral component, which will require a slightly more posterior condylar resection, thereby loosening the flexion gap. When doing so, the surgeon must be sure that the smaller component still provides adequate metal-to-plastic contact in full extension. If not, the same size femoral component is shifted anteriorly on the distal femur by resecting more posterior condyle and reorienting the fixation lugs to a more anterior location.

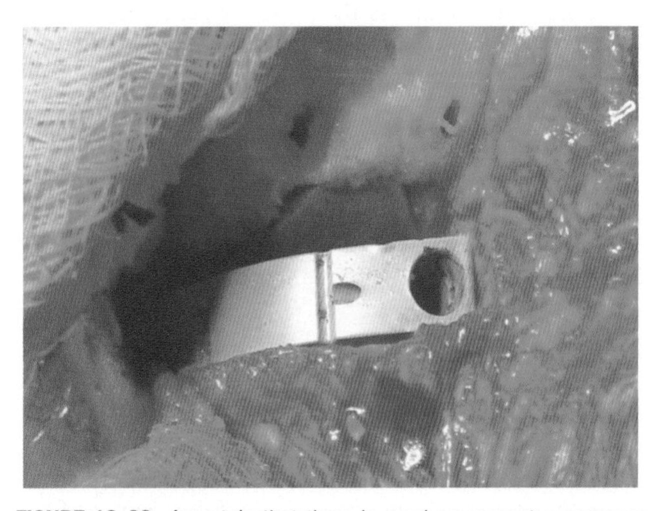

FIGURE 18–23. Ascertain that there is good component congruency with the trial components before making the fixation holes or slots.

TECHNICAL NUANCES IN LATERAL COMPARTMENT ARTHROPLASTY

In my practice, lateral compartment arthroplasties make up only 10% of the UKAs I perform each year. They are technically more difficult and sensitive. It is worth repeating here some technical features of lateral procedures. I believe that lateral compartment arthroplasties are best exposed through a medial arthrotomy that spares the medial meniscus.

The distal femur often has residual cartilage that should be removed prior to the distal femoral resection to avoid under-resection that hinders recession of the leading edge of the femoral component. This increased distal femoral resection calls for a very conservative initial tibial resection to avoid the need for very thick tibial components.

The AP dimension of the femoral component should be undersized to also help avoid patellar impingement. The surgeon should err toward placing the femoral component laterally and the tibial component medially to maximize congruency between the articulating surfaces.

CEMENTING COMPONENTS

Before the real components are cemented, they should be tested in the knee as if they were trials. I do this because the lugs or fins of the real component may make insertion more difficult than that experienced with the lug-free trials. It is better to appreciate and resolve this difficulty before committing to the cementing process.

The tibial component is cemented first. Any lug holes or slots are packed under pressure with cement, and little or no cement is placed on the plateau itself (Fig. 18–24). The remaining cement is placed on the undersurface of the real tibial component (Fig. 18–25), which is inserted so that it makes contact posteriorly first. This prevents pushing any cement to the back of the knee and allows any extruded cement to come forward as the knee is extended and the anterior aspect of the tibial component seats itself (Fig. 18–26). The femoral component is then cemented with a similar technique. Cement is placed on the distal femoral condyle and pressurized into any lug holes or slots. A thin film of cement is smeared onto the posterior condylar bone for cement intrusion there, and the remainder of the cement is placed on the inside of the femoral component (Fig. 18–27). The knee is slowly extended to pressurize the bone-cement interface (Fig. 18–28). Any extruded cement is brought forward and removed. After terminal extension is achieved, the knee is rested in this position until full polymerization takes place. Flexing and extending the knee during the polymerization process may disrupt the prosthesis-cement or

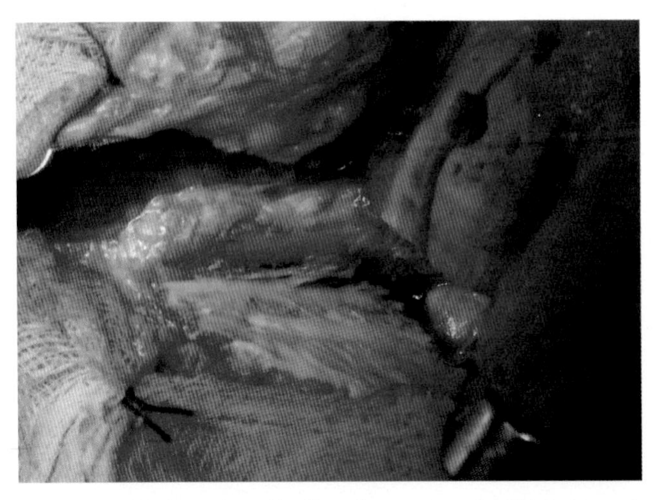

FIGURE 18–24. Put only a thin film of cement on the tibial plateau to prevent posterior cement extrusion.

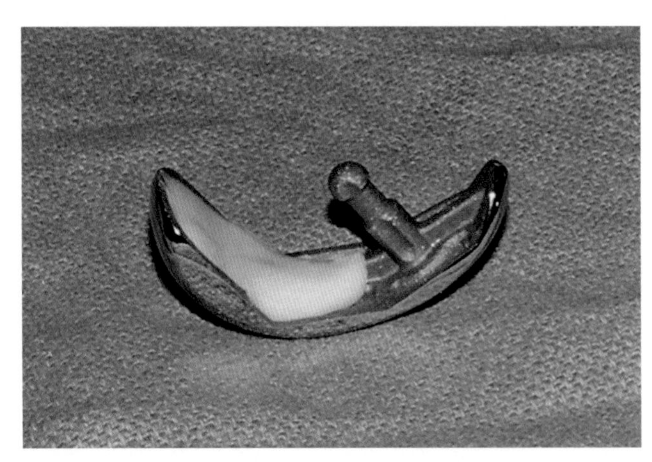

FIGURE 18–27. As is recommended on the tibial side, cement is placed on the back of the femoral component to prevent posterior extrusion.

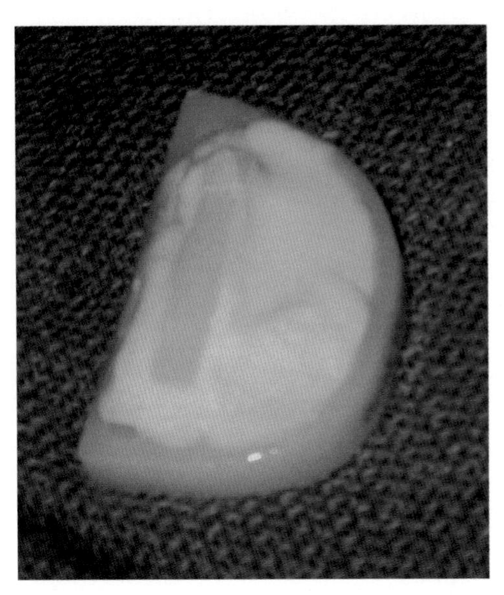

FIGURE 18–25. The remainder of the cement should go on the back of the prosthesis.

bone-cement interface and should be avoided. I leave a little extruded cement anteriorly on either the femur or the tibia so that it can be tested until it is fully polymerized (the cement will usually harden at a faster rate outside the knee).

After full polymerization, the knee is flexed and the tourniquet deflated. Any further extruded cement is removed. I pass an instrument such as a straight pituitary rongeur along the tibial spine to be certain there is no potential impingement between any retained bone or osteophyte. The knee should also be inspected peripherally for any extruded cement that could possibly break off at a later time.

CLOSURE

Two small-caliber drains are inserted and brought out laterally through separate exit points. The wound is closed in layers with monofilament No. 1 PDS (polydioxanone) sutures for the capsule, resorbable No. 3-0 sutures for the subcutaneous layer, and interrupted No. 3-0 nylon for the skin

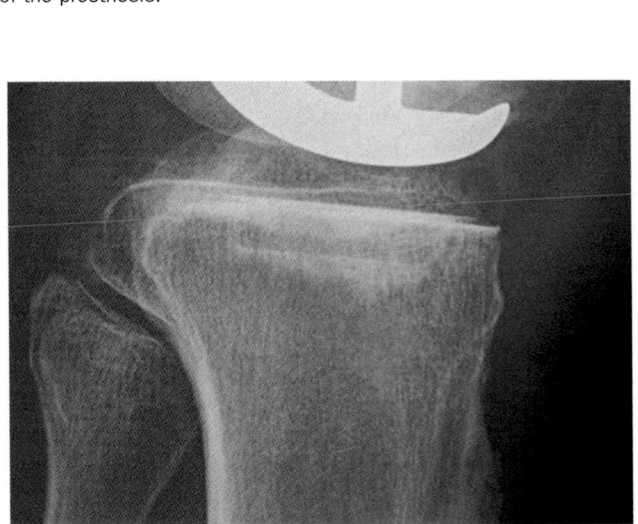

FIGURE 18–26. This radiograph shows good cement penetration into the bone without posterior extrusion.

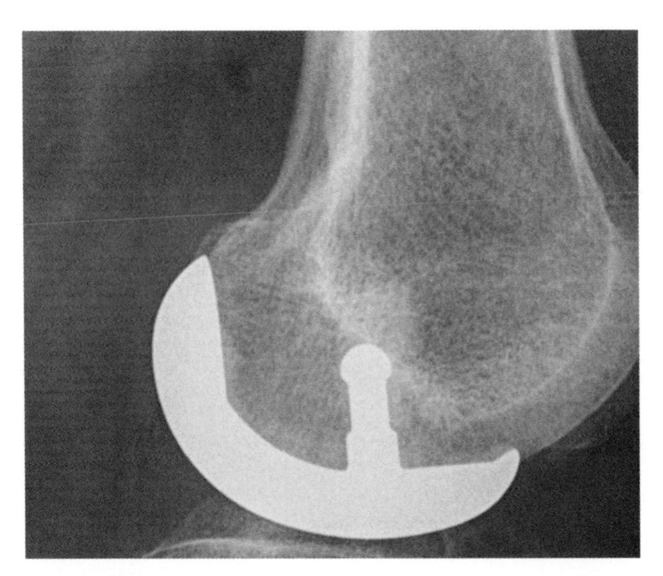

FIGURE 18–28. This femoral component is well seated distally and posteriorly.

sutures. Knee flexion against gravity is measured and recorded. The immediate postoperative treatment is the same as described in Chapter 4 for TKA except that recovery often is accelerated.

References

1. Outerbridge RE: The aetiology of chondromalacia patellae. J Bone Joint Surg 1961;43B:752–757.
2. Repicci JA, Hartman JF: Minimally invasive unicondylar knee arthroplasty for the treatment of unicompartmental osteoarthritis: an outpatient arthritic bypass procedure. Orthop Clin North Am 2004;35:201–216.
3. Scott RD: The mini incision uni: more for less? Orthopedics 2004;27:483.
4. Scott RD, Santore RF: Unicondylar unicompartmental knee replacement in osteoarthritis. J Bone Joint Surg Am 1981;63:536–544.
5. Brumby SA, Carrington R, Zayontz S, et al: Tibial plateau stress fracture: a complication of unicompartmental knee arthroplasty using 4 guide pins. J Arthroplasty 2003;18:809–812.

CHAPTER 19

Frequently Asked Questions Concerning Total Knee Arthroplasty

RATIONALE

Patients are rightfully trying to become more educated about their surgery and recovery. They often obtain (mis)information on the Internet or from friends. They need to be informed about their surgeon's individual postoperative protocol, and they need to have their anxieties relieved when "things happen" during their recovery.

For years, measures were already in place at our hospitals to try to address this. These measures included a preoperative dialogue with the surgeon, and a preoperative teaching class was available that could be attended at the time of the preadmission screening tests.

What was missing was a document that the patient could refer to regarding events that might arise before, during, and after their hospitalization. To address this need, G. Erens and I created a brochure to be given to each patient when surgery was scheduled. Initially, the answers given to each question were our own responses. Since the concept became attractive to all members of the arthroplasty staffs, the brochure was modified for everyone's use.[1] A disclaimer was attached to remind patients that they were being given general information and they should always contact their personal physician with any questions or concerns.

CATEGORIES OF QUESTIONS

Questions from patients were collected in three categories: preoperative, perioperative, and postoperative. Perioperative questions were divided into those that might arise in the hospital and those more likely to be asked soon after discharge.

In addition, three very frequent concerns of patients—depression, insomnia, and constipation—were specifically addressed.

Some things that normally occur following total knee arthroplasty might be alarming to patients unless they are aware that their symptoms are within normal limits. These events include the following: an intermittent clicking sensation inside the knee, an area of skin numbness on the outside part of the knee, swelling after exercise and at the end of the day, warmth around the knee, and palpable sutures under the skin that are not apparent until the swelling begins to resolve.

Worrisome things also can occur during recovery that are definitely abnormal and require an immediate call to the physician. These include increasing redness about the wound, increasing pain and swelling, fever over 101° F, any drainage whatsoever from the wound, calf swelling or pain, ankle swelling that does not decrease or resolve overnight, and bleeding gums or blood in the stool or urine.

THE ANSWERS

Given below are possible answers to frequently asked questions. These are not meant to be definitive answers but rather guidelines that different surgeons might modify to fit their own practice routines.

Preoperative Questions

Q: What is the chance for success?

A: "Success" should not be measured as a quantitative knee score but rather by the ability to answer "yes" to the following three questions:

Are you glad you had the operation?
Did it fulfill your expectations?
Would you do it again?

Approximately 98% of patients at 1 year will answer "yes" to all three questions.

Q: What is the recovery time?

A: Everyone heals from surgery at a different pace. In most cases, however, you will be restricted to the use of a walker or crutches for distances for 1 month after your operation. You will then be allowed to advance to a cane outdoors and no support around the house for several weeks. You will gradually return to normal function without any assistive devices. This usually takes about 3 months but may take longer.

Q: Will I go to a rehabilitation facility or home?

A: It depends. Many people are able to go home after their operation. However, you may go to a rehabilitation facility in order to gain the skills you need to safely return home. Many factors will be considered in this decision. These factors include availability of family or friends to assist with daily activities, home environment and safety considerations, postoperative functional status as evaluated by a physical therapist in the hospital, and overall evaluation by your hospital team.

Q: When can I drive?

A: If you had surgery on your right knee, you should not drive for at least a month. After 1 month, you may return to driving as soon as you feel comfortable. If you had surgery on your left knee, you may return to driving as soon as you feel comfortable if you have an automatic transmission. Do not drive if you are taking narcotics. Some surgeons do not allow their patients to drive until after they have been seen in the office at 4 to 6 weeks after surgery. Check with your surgeon.

Q: When can I travel?

A: You may travel as soon as you feel comfortable. It is recommended that you get up to stretch or walk at least once an hour when taking long trips. This is important to help prevent blood clots.

Q: When can I return to work?

A: It depends on your profession. Typically if your work is primarily sedentary, you may return after approximately 1 month. If your work is more rigorous, you may require up to 3 months before you can return to full duty. In some cases, more or less time is necessary.

Q: What activities are permitted following surgery?

A: You may return to most activities as tolerated including walking, gardening, and golf. Some of the best activities to help with motion and strengthening are swimming and using a stationary bicycle. You should avoid high-impact stresses such as running and jumping, and vigorous sports such as singles tennis or squash.

Q: How long will my knee surgery last?

A: This varies from patient to patient. For each year following your knee replacement, you have a 1% chance of requiring additional surgery. For example, at 10 years postoperatively, there is a 90% success rate without further surgery.

Perioperative Questions (in Hospital)

Q: When can I shower or get the incision wet?

A: You may shower 3 days after your operation, if no drainage is present at the incision. Initially, try to keep the incision dry with a plastic wrap. If it gets wet, pat it dry.

Q: When can I immerse my knee totally such as in a bathtub or swimming pool?

A: Your knee can be totally immersed 2 weeks after surgery as long as the wound is completely healed and the sutures have been removed for 3 or 4 days.

Q: When should I wear the knee immobilizer? When can I discontinue it?

A: The knee immobilizer is generally worn at night for the first few days after surgery or when walking until you are able to independently perform a straight leg raise. Most patients discontinue its use about a week after surgery, but you may continue to wear the knee immobilizer at night for comfort if you wish.

Q: How often should I use the CPM (continuous passive motion) machine?

A: If you are given a CPM machine, you will probably start soon after surgery and use it a total of about 8 hours per day. The amount of bend will be gradually increased. Schedules vary widely from patient to patient.

Q: How long do I need a bandage on my incision?

A: A bandage is applied for approximately 1 week and changed daily to new, dry, sterile gauze. Sometimes its use is continued to protect the incision from irritation due to clothing or the knee immobilizer.

Q: When will my sutures (or staples) be removed?

A: Sutures are removed approximately 10 days after surgery. This may be done by a visiting nurse if you are at home or by the rehabilitation staff if you are in a rehabilitation facility. Sometimes sutures dissolve on their own and do not have to be removed.

Perioperative Questions (Out of the Hospital)

Q: How long will I be on pain medication?

A: It is not unusual to require some form of pain medication for about 3 months. Initially, the medication will be strong (such as a narcotic). Most people are able to discontinue their strong pain medication after about a month and switch to an over-the-counter medication such as acetaminophen or ibuprofen.

Q: How long will I be on a blood thinner?

A: Various options including pills and injections are available to thin your blood and help prevent phlebitis and blood clots. Your surgeon will choose a therapy based on your medical history and possibly on tests done before you leave the hospital.

Q: Can I drink alcohol during my recovery?

A: If you are taking warfarin (Coumadin) as a blood thinner, you should avoid alcohol intake because alcohol modifies the effect of this medication. You should also avoid alcohol if you are taking narcotics. Beyond this, you can use alcohol in moderation at your own discretion.

Q: How long should I take iron supplements?

A: Four weeks of iron after surgery is usually sufficient. These supplements help your body replenish its iron supply and build up your blood count.

Q: What are good and bad positions for my knee during recovery?

A: You should spend some time each day working on both flexion and extension of your knee. It is a good idea to change positions every 15 to 30 minutes. Avoid a pillow or roll under your knee. A roll under the ankle helps improve extension and prevent a contracture.

Q: Should I apply ice or heat?

A: Initially, ice is most helpful to keep down swelling. After several weeks, you may also try using heat and choose what works best for you.

Q: How long should I wear compression stockings?

A: After you are home, you may try going without the stockings and see whether or not your ankles tend to swell. If they do, wear the stockings during the day until the swelling returns to what was normal for you before surgery. Also wear the stockings for several months when you travel in a car or plane.

Q: Can I go up and down stairs?

A: Yes. Initially, you will lead with your unoperated leg when going up stairs and with your operated leg when coming down. As your muscles get stronger and your motion improves, you will be able to perform stairs in a more normal fashion—usually in about a month.

Q: Will I need physical therapy?

A: Yes. The physical therapist plays a very important role in your recovery. You will be seen by a physical therapist soon after your operation and throughout your hospital stay. Once you are home, a therapist will probably visit you two to three times a week to assist with your exercise program. You will also be taught a series of exercises that you can perform on your own without supervision. A written list will be provided by your physical therapist. In addition, swimming and using a stationary bicycle are good exercise options. These exercises can be continued indefinitely even after your recovery is complete.

Q: When can I resume sexual intercourse?

A: As soon as you are comfortable.

Postoperative Concerns

Q: I feel depressed. Is this normal?

A: It is not uncommon to have feelings of depression after knee replacement surgery. This may be due to a variety of factors, such as limited mobility, discomfort, increased dependency on others, and medication side effects. Feelings of depression will typically fade as you begin to return to regular activities. If your feelings of depression persist, consult your internist.

Q: I have insomnia. Is this normal? What can I do about it?

A: Insomnia is a very common complaint following knee replacement surgery. Over-the-counter remedies such as Benadryl or melatonin may be effective. If this continues to be a problem, prescription medication may be necessary.

Q: I am constipated. What should I do?

A: It is very common to have constipation after surgery. This is due to a number of factors and is aggravated by the need to take narcotic pain medication. A simple over-the-counter stool softener (such as Colace) is the best prevention for this problem. In rare cases, you may require a suppository or enema.

Postoperative Concerns (Long Term)

Q: How much range of motion do I need?

A: Most people require 70 degrees of flexion to walk normally on level ground, 90 degrees to ascend stairs, 100 degrees to descend stairs, and 105 degrees to get out of a low chair. To walk and stand efficiently, your knee should come to within 10 degrees of being fully straight.

Q: What range of motion should I expect from my knee after 6 weeks? After 1 year?

A: Everyone's range of motion varies and depends on many individual factors. Your potential will be determined at the time of your surgery. The average patient achieves approximately 115 degrees of flexion by 1 year after surgery. Some patients achieve less and others much more.

Q: I think my leg feels longer now. Is this possible?

A: In the majority of cases, your leg length will essentially be unchanged. In some cases, however, the leg is lengthened.

This is usually the result of straightening out a knee that preoperatively had a significant bow. At first, the increased length may feel awkward. Most people become accustomed to the difference, but occasionally a shoe lift may be necessary in the opposite extremity.

Q: Can I use weights when I exercise?

A: Generally weights are not used for the first 2 months after surgery. As you progress with your physical therapy program, your physical therapist may recommend the use of weights. These should be limited to light weights progressing from one pound to a maximum of five pounds.

Q: Will I set off the security monitors at the airport? Do I need a doctor's letter?

A: You probably will set off the alarm as you progress through the security checkpoint. Be proactive and inform the security personnel that you have had a knee replacement and will most likely set off the alarm. Wear clothing that will allow you to show them your knee incision without difficulty. A letter from your physician or a wallet card is no longer of any help when passing through security checkpoints.

Q: Do I need antibiotics before having dental work or an invasive medical procedure?

A: Yes. You will be given a letter explaining this in detail at your first follow-up visit. Avoid any dental cleaning and other nonurgent procedures for 6 weeks following knee replacement surgery.

Q: Can I kneel?

A: After several months, you may try to kneel. It may be painful at first but will not harm or damage your knee replacement. Much of the discomfort comes from kneeling on your recent incision and the healing local tissues. Kneeling generally becomes more comfortable as times passes. Always use a pad under your knee.

Q: Can I return to downhill skiing?

A: Downhill skiing poses a risk. The risk comes not from the act of skiing but rather from potential injury due to a serious fall or collision with another skier. You should definitely avoid skiing black diamond slopes. If you ski, be aware of the risks, and ski only under good conditions.

Q: When do I need to follow up with my surgeon?

A: Follow-up appointments are usually made postoperatively at 4 to 6 weeks after surgery, followed by 1 year, 2 years, 5 years, 7 years, and 10 years. These follow-up appointments are necessary to monitor the fixation of the prosthesis and the potential wearing out of the plastic articulation.

SUMMARY

Our frequently asked questions brochure has been well received by patients and their families. Important questions are answered, and anxieties are relieved. With continual patient feedback, the content of the brochure will continue to evolve.

Reference

1. Scott RD, Erens GA: Frequently asked questions regarding total knee arthroplasty. Orthopedics 2004;27:1–3.

Index

Note: Page numbers followed by "f" indicate illustrations; page numbers followed by "t" indicate tables.